国家出版基金项目
NATIONAL PUBLICATION FOUNDATION

An Intensively Compiled Practical English-Chinese Library of Traditional Chinese Medicine

（英汉对照）精编实用中医文库

Chief General Compilers　CHEN Kaixian　LI Qizhong（Executive）　HE Xinghai

总主编　陈凯先　李其忠（执行）　何星海

Chief General Translators　SHI Jianrong　HU Hongyi　XU Yao（Executive）

总主译　施建蓉　胡鸿毅　徐　瑶（执行）

Basic Theory of
Traditional Chinese Medicine
中医基础理论

Chief Compiler　　　LI Qizhong

Chief Translator　　　XU Yao

主编　李其忠

主译　徐　瑶

U0312476

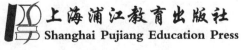
上海浦江教育出版社
Shanghai Pujiang Education Press

(Former Shanghai University of TCM Press)

An Intensively Compiled Practical English-Chinese Library of Traditional Chinese Medicine

Compilation Board of the Library

Chief General Compilers   CHEN Kaixian   LI Qizhong(Executive)   HE Xinghai
Members(Listed in the order of the number of strokes in the Chinese names)

MA Lieguang	He Jiancheng	YU Xiaoping	SHEN Xueyong
ZHANG Tingting	CHEN Hongfeng	CHEN Dexing	ZHAO Yi
GUO Xin	HUANG Ping	YU Jian'er	ZHAN Hongsheng
MIAO Wanhong			

Compilation and Translation Committee of the Library

Chief General Translators   SHI Jianrong   HU Hongyi   XU Yao(Executive)
Translations(Listed in the order of the number of strokes in the Chinese names)

ZHU Aixiu	YANG Yu	XIAO Yuanchun	ZHANG Yiping
ZHU Jianmin	HUANG Guoqi	DONG Jing	HAN Chouping

Basic Theory of Traditional Chinese Medicine

Chief Compiler   LI Qizhong
Chief Translator   XU Yao

《（英汉对照）精编实用中医文库》

编纂委员会

总　主　编　陈凯先　李其忠（执行）　何星海

编　　　委（按姓氏笔画为序）

马烈光　何建成　余小萍　沈雪勇
张婷婷　陈红风　陈德兴　赵　毅
郭　忻　黄　平　虞坚尔　詹红生
缪晚虹

编译委员会

总　主　译　施建蓉　胡鸿毅　徐　瑶（执行）

编　译　者（按姓氏笔画为序）

朱爱秀　杨　渝　肖元春　张亿萍
诸建民　黄国琪　董　晶　韩丑萍

《中医基础理论》

主　　编　李其忠
主　　译　徐　瑶

Foreword
前 言

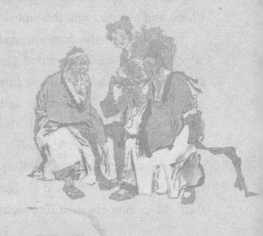

With the traditional medical philosophy and clinical experience as the principal body, the science of Traditional Chinese Medicine (TCM) is a comprehensive subject to study the rules of life activities and the disease prevention, diagnosis, treatment, rehabilitation as well as healthcare. The science of TCM has a long history of development and belongs to a summary of experiences that Chinese nation has fought against diseases for over several thousand years, is also an important component part of Chinese outstanding traditional culture and has contributed greatly to the healthcare undertaking and development of Chinese nation.

By increasing enhancement of modern living standard, change of living modes and acceleration of ageing process, the chronic diseases represented by tumors, cardiovascular diseases and diabetes become gradually the important factors in impacting the health of mankind, but TCM presents the better therapeutic effects. Nowadays, the modern medical mode of "society-psychology-biology" has been advocated in medical science, changing from the medical idea of "disease treatment" to "health promotion". The more and more patients in China and abroad have chosen natural and low side-effect Chinese herbal medicine for their problems. With the changes in medicine modes and in spectrum of diseases in the recent several dozens of years, TCM has increasingly been concerned by the medical experts and ordinary people in China and abroad, and the global "TCM upsurge" keeps rising. In order to meet the growing needs of the domestic and international professionals in learning the knowledge of TCM, we have edited particularly the series books of *An Intensively Compiled Practical English-Chinese Library of Traditional Chinese Medicine*.

The scientific, systematic and practical features have been emphasized in the series books. Based upon the full absorption of new progress in teaching and research achievements of TCM , the series books highlight the academic essentials of TCM, with precise exposition of medical philosophy and down-to-earth clinical practice, to introduce the "original and authentic" TCM to the readers. The series books introduce the commonly used therapeutic methods and clinical skills in Chinese medicine, by the clinically encountered and frequently seen diseases and the relevant ailments predominantly effective by Chinese medical therapies. By studying the series books, the readers can learn the knowledge and techniques of TCM on gradual progress and become proficient gradually in TCM.

The series books highlight"the precise features in three aspects"—capable in authors, refined in contents and accurate in translation. The majority of the authors of the series books are senior experts from the related faculties of Shanghai University of Traditional Chinese Medicine. The translator team is composed of the senior teachers with plentiful expertise in translation of TCM from international education college and foreign language center of Shanghai University of Traditional Chinese Medicine. In order to meet the needs of the readers in China and abroad, the basic and clinical core contents are selected and the latest research achievements are consulted based upon the principle "to seek its essentials but its completion" in the series books.

The series books can satisfy the beginners with certain knowledge of English language in studying TCM systematically and can also be used as the textbooks for education of TCM and pharmacy for foreign students. We sincerely hope the publication of the series books plays its promoting role for TCM going to the world.

Editors
June, 2017

中医学是以传统医学理论与实践经验为主体,研究人体生命活动规律和疾病预防、诊断、治疗、康复以及保健的一门综合性学科。中医学历史悠久,源远流长,是中华民族几千年来同疾病作斗争的经验总结,也是中国传统文化的重要组成部分,长期以来为中国人民的健康保健事业和民族繁衍作出了巨大的贡献。

随着现代生活水平的不断提高、生活方式的改变以及老龄化进程的加剧,以肿瘤、心血管疾病和糖尿病等为代表的慢性病日渐成为影响人类健康的重要因素,而中医药显示了良好的治疗效果。当今的医学倡导"社会—心理—生物"的现代医学模式,医学理念从"疾病治疗"向"健康促进"转变,国内外越来越多的患者选择天然、毒副作用低的中医药治疗疾病。近几十年来,随着医学模式的转变和疾病谱的改变,中医学日益引起越来越多的海内外医学专家和普通民众的关注,全球性的"中医热"正在持续升温。为了满足海内外人士日益高涨的学习中医学知识的需求,我们特地编撰了《(英汉对照)精编实用中医文库》丛书。

本丛书注重"三性"——科学性、系统性、实用性。丛书在充分吸取近年中医教学、科研进展的基础上,突出中医学术精华,理论阐述准确、临床切合实际,向读者介绍"原汁原味"的中医学;丛书介绍中医学常用的治疗方法和临床技能,所涉及的病证均为临床常见病、多发病和中医优势病种。丛书的13个分册涵盖了中医基础与临床的主干课程,通过阅读本丛书,读者可以由浅入深、循序渐进地学习中医药知识和技能。

本丛书突出"三精"——作者精干、内容精炼、翻译精准。丛书的中文作者绝大部分为上海中医药大学各相关教研室的资深专家,翻译团队由上海中医药大学国际教育学院和外语中心具有丰富的中医药学翻译经验的骨干教师组成。为了适合海内外读者的需求,丛书本着"求其精而不求其全"的原则,选取了基础和临床的核心内容,翻译上考了最新的研究成果。

本丛书既可满足具有一定英语水平的初学中医者系统学习中医所用,也可供中医药留学生教育作为教材使用,衷心希望本丛书的出版在中医药走向海外进程中发挥应有的推动作用。

编者

2017 年 6 月

Note for Compilation

编写说明

The basic theory of traditional Chinese medicine (TCM), a science to study and elaborate the basic concept, basic theory, basic regulation and basic knowledge of traditional Chinese medicine, is a theoretical basis to guide the preventive medicine, clinic medicine and rehabilitation of traditional Chinese medicine. The basic theory of TCM is abundant in content of rational knowledge, including theory of yin and yang, theory of five elements, theory of qi, blood and body fluid, theory of zang-fu organs, theory of meridians and collaterals, etiology and pathogenesis and principles of prevention. It has been applied to influence and guide the various doctrines, various schools, various clinic departments of traditional Chinese medicine and various diagnostic methods in the development history of traditional Chinese medicine. It can be seen that the basic theory of traditional Chinese medicine is a gateway course and a required course as well in studying traditional Chinese medicine. During the compilation of the book, we try to retain the inherent terms of traditional Chinese medicine and maintain the conventional characteristics of traditional Chinese medicine in modern vernacular Chinese, for the purpose to make the readers to read more smoothly with easier understanding.

In order to prevent crossing or overlapping in content with other fascicule books of *An Intensively Compiled Practical English-Chinese Library of Traditional Chinese Medicine*, we have made a proper modification in details and omissions of some contents, for examples, locations and running courses of meridians and collaterals, pattern identification according to zang-fu organs, life preservation and disease prevention, referring to *Chinese Acupuncture and Moxibustion*, *Diagnostics of Traditional Chinese Medicine*, *Health Preservation and Rehabilitation of Traditional Chinese Medicine* respectively, no more details hereon.

Traditional Chinese medicine is a unique medicine system, different from modern medicine. Some terms and phrases involved in the books similar to those in modern medicine, as heart, liver, spleen, lung, kidney, etc., have great differences in conceptions, in hope that the readers should pay attention to in studying.

中医基础理论,是研究和阐述中医学的基本概念、基本理论、基本规律及基本知识等的一门学科,是指导中医预防医学、临床医学和康复医学的理论基础,其内容十分丰富,涉及阴阳五行、气血津液、脏腑经络、病因病机、防治原则等理性认识。中医学术发展史上的各家学说、各种流派,中医临床医学中的各个科别、各种诊法,无不受其影响和指导。可见,中医基础理论是学习中医学的入门课、必修课。在本书编写过程中,我们尽量保留中医学的固有术语,保持中医学的传统特色,并采用白话文形式,以使行文流畅,易读易懂。

　　为了防止与《精编实用中医文库》其他分册在内容上的交错重叠,在本书编写过程中,我们对内容的详略作了适当调整,如经络循行部位、脏腑辨证、养生防病等内容,可参阅《中国针灸》《中医诊断学》《中医养生康复学》等分册,在此不作详细介绍。

　　中医学是不同于现代医学的独特的医学体系,书中所涉及的一些与现代医学类同的名词术语,如心、肝、脾、肺、肾等,其在概念上有很大差别,还望读者在学习时加以注意。

Contents
目录

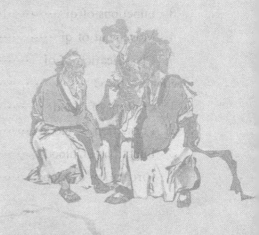

Introduction

绪　论

Traditional Chinese medicine (TCM), one of the component parts of traditional Chinese culture of great splendor, is the summary of the experience in the struggle with the diseases over millennia by Chinese nation, with a rich theoretical speculation and creativity, and a highly clinical practicability as well. Nowadays, when the modern medicine is so highly developed, TCM is still of very strong vitality. It is because that has its own unique theory system, and remarkable therapeutic effects in clinic as well.

1　Formation and development of theory system of TCM

TCM originated in remote antiquity. As early as in the times of primitive tribes, people started to accumulate preliminarily the medical knowledge. In ancient Chinese classics, there are descriptions that "Fuxi made nine needles" and "Shennong tasted hundreds of herbs". These are the real pictures showing that the Chinese ancestors explored the knowledge of medicine and herbs in ancient times. In the Spring and Autumn Period (770 B. C.-476 B. C.) and the Warring States Period (475 B. C.-221 B. C.), the forefathers had a preliminary understanding of diseases, and their medical practice experiences were getting richer. In this period, due to politics, economy, science and culture had been all developed markedly, and the academic thoughts were unprecedentedly vigorous, people summarized

中医学是灿烂中国传统文化的一部分,是对中华民族数千年来与疾病作斗争的经验总结,其不仅具有极为丰富的理论思辨性和创造性,而且具有极强的临床实用性。在现代医学十分发达的今天,中医学依然具有很强的生命力,其重要原因,就在于中医学既有独特的理论体系,又有卓越的临床疗效。

1　中医学理论体系的形成与发展

中医学起源于远古时代。早在原始部落时代,人类就开始了医药知识的初步积累。如中国古典文献有"伏羲制九针""神农尝百草"等记述,就是对上古时期华夏祖先探索医药知识的真实写照。至春秋战国时期,先人对疾病已有初步的认识,医疗实践经验也渐趋丰富,加上这一时期的政治、经济、科学、文化都有显著发展,学术思想空前活跃,因此将世代相传的医药知识加以总结,创造一个较为完整的医学理论体系,则将成为可能。

the medical and herbal knowledge from generation to generation, making it possible to create a rather complete theory system of medicine. It is the symbol that the earliest extant medical classic *Yellow Emperor's Inner Canon* (Huang Di Nei Jing) was published. Huang Di Nei Jing already in circulation in the Warring States Period (475 B. C.-221 B. C.), the Qin Dynasty (221 B. C.-207 B. C.) and the Han Dynasty (206 B. C.-A. D. 220), had collected the massive achievements of medical practice by ancestors. By applying the prevalent theory of yin-yang, five elements, and the knowledge of natural sciences, such as astronomy, geography, biology and meteorology, it illustrated systematically the physiology and pathology of human body, and prevention, diagnosis and treatment of diseases, forming a unique theory system of TCM, and laid a solid foundation for the development of TCM theortically and dinically.

After publication of Huang Di Nei Jing, the physicians in successive dynasties enriched and enhanced the theory of TCM ceaselessly, promoting the further development and completion of the theory system of TCM.

Canon of Perplexities (Nan Jing), another important ancient medical classic slightly later than Huang Di Nei Jing, was further to elaborate and expound some contents of Huang Di Nei Jing, and to make an important supplementary explanation to some deficit contents in the way of questions and answers, regarded as an absolutely necessary medical classic in the study of classic theory of TCM. The theory of "taking Cun Kou pulse" in pulse diagnosis, the theory of triple energizer and the theory of Ming Men (Vital Gate) raised in Nan Jing hare

中国现存最早的医学经典《黄帝内经》的问世，就是其重要标志。《黄帝内经》成书于战国至秦汉时期，其集合了前人大量的医疗实践成果，运用当时盛行的阴阳、五行等学说，参合天文、地理、生物、气象等各种自然科学知识进行归纳、综合，系统地阐述人体的生理、病理及疾病预防、诊治等内容，形成了中医学独特的理论体系，为中医学理论和临床的发展奠定了坚实的基础。

自《黄帝内经》成书以后，历代医家对中医学理论不断进行充实和提高，推动了中医学理论体系的进一步发展和完善。

《难经》是稍晚于《黄帝内经》问世的另一部重要的古典医籍，其以问答的行文方式，对《黄帝内经》的某些内容作了进一步阐发、论述，对《黄帝内经》的某些不足作了重要补充，是研究中医学经典理论必不可少的一部医学典籍。如《难经》提出的诊脉"独取寸口"及三焦之论、命门之说等，对后世医学理

made great influeuce on the development of medical theory in the later generations.

In the late stage of the East Han Dynasty (25-220), ZHANG Zhongjing wrote *Treatise on Cold-Damage Disease and Miscellaneous Diseases* (Shang Han Za bing Lun), a book that had an epoch-making significance in the formation and development of the clinic system of treatment based on pattern identification in TCM, by inheritance of the theories of Huang Di Nei Jing and Nan Jing. With the six meridians (Taiyang, Shaoyang, Yangming, Taiyin, Shaoyin and Jueyin) and zang-fu organs as the guiding principles of pattern identification, ZHANG Zhongjing created many highly effective therapeutic methods and herbal formulas for the treatment of the diseases due to external invasion and the miscellaneous diseases due to internal injury, which is still praised highly in the modern medicine circles at home and abroad. Due to this, ZHANG Zhongjing got the honorific title of "the Sage of Medicine".

The period of the Jin Dynasty (265-420), the Sui Dynasty (581-618) and the Tang Dynasty (618-907) was very important period when the theory and clinic of TCM were summarized and supplemented on a large scale, and the complete theory system of TCM was formed. *Canon of Pulse* (Mai Jing) written by Wang Shuhe in the Jin Dynasty (265-420) was the first monograph on diagnostics of TCM. *Treatise on Sources and Manifestations of All Kinds of Diseases* (Zhu Bing Yuan Hou Lun) compiled by Chao Yuanfang, *et al* in the Sui Dynasty (581-618) was the first monograph on pathogenesis and symptomatology in the history of TCM. *Secret Necessities of A Frontier Official* (Wai Tai Mi Yao) written by

论的发展具有重要影响。

东汉末年,张仲景在继承《黄帝内经》《难经》等理论的基础之上,结合临床实际,撰著了中国医学发展史上具有划时代意义的《伤寒杂病论》一书,为中医临床医学辨证论治体系的形成和发展作出了杰出贡献。张仲景以六经(太阳、少阳、阳明、太阴、少阴、厥阴)和脏腑等为辨证纲领,对外感疾病和内伤杂病的诊治创制了许多卓有疗效的治法和方剂,至今仍为国内外医学界所推崇。张仲景由此而被后人尊称为"医圣"。

两晋隋唐时期,是对中医学理论和临床进行大规模总结、充实,并形成完整理论体系的重要时期。晋代王叔和所著《脉经》,是第一部关于中医诊断学的专门著作;隋代巢元方等人编撰的《诸病源候论》,是中国医学史上第一部病机证候学专著;唐代王焘著《外台秘要》、孙思邈著《备急千金要方》等医籍,是对唐以前医学理论和实践经验进行全面总结的集大成之作。

Wang Tao and *Thousand Ducat Prescriptions for E-mergencies* (Bei Ji Qian Jin Yao Fang) written by SUN Simiao in the Tang Dynasty (618-907) were the epitomized works on the comprehensive summarization of the medical theory and practical experience before the Tang Dynasty (618-907).

In the period of the Song Dynasty (960-1279), the Jin Dynasty (1115-1234) and the Yuan Dynasty (1271-1368), medical schools with various characteristics emerged in large number to develop theory of TCM from different angles, with the representatives of LIU Wansu, ZHANG Congzheng, LI Gao and ZHU Zhenheng. LIU Wansu thought that the nature of a disease often pertained to fire and heat, and it should be treated with the cold and cool herbs. He was addressed "School of Cold and Cool". ZHANG Congzheng thought that a disease was mainly caused by the invasion of the Xie (Pathogenic) Qi. Zheng (Anti-Pathogenic) Qi would be recovered if the Xie (Pathogenic) Qi was eliminated, so the three therapeutic methods of diaphoresis, emesis and purgation could be used to treat the disease. He was addressed "School of Purgation". LI Gao thought that the spleen and stomach were the basis of the Yuan (Primary) Qi. If the spleen and stomach were damaged, the Yuan Qi was deficient, failing to resist the attack of the Xie (Pathogenic) Qi, so as to cause occurrence of various diseases. Therefore, the treatment should be given by regulating and reinforcing the spleen and stomach. He was addressed "School of Reinforcing Earth". ZHU Zhenheng thought that the human body was often in a state of yin qi insufficiency and yang qi excess, so that yin deficiency leading to fire hyperactivity was the major pathogenesis. Therefore, the

宋金元时期，涌现了各具特色的医学流派，从不同的角度发展了中医学理论，其中代表性的医家当推刘完素、张从正、李杲、朱震亨。刘完素提出疾病的性质多偏于火热，用药多以寒凉为主，后人称其为"寒凉派"；张从正认为疾病的发生主要是由邪气入侵人体所致，若邪气去则正气自复，主张用发汗、涌吐、泻下三法治疗，后人称其为"攻下派"；李杲指出脾胃为元气之本，脾胃一伤，元气即虚，抗邪无力，各种疾病随之而生，故治疗重在调补脾胃，后人称其为"补土派"；朱震亨则认为人体常处于阴气不足、阳气有余的状态，阴虚火旺是疾病的主要病机，临床治疗善用滋阴降火的方法，后人称其为"滋阴派"。上述理论都是各自临床实践的总结，各种不同的创见，对丰富中医学理论都起了重要的促进作用，所以受到后人的重视和推崇，被尊称为"金元四大家"。

clinic treatment should be given by the method of nourishing yin and subduing fire. He was addressed "School of Nourishing Yin". All the above theories were the respective summarizations of their clinical practice. Various creative opinions had important promoting function in enriching the theory of TCM, so they were so valued and praised, titled as "Four Eminent Masters in the Jin and Yuan Dynasties".

In the period of the Ming Dynasty (1368-1644) and Qing Dynasty (1644-1911), theory of seasonal febrile disease in TCM was risen. WU Youke in the Ming Dynasty (1368-1644) firstly proposed that the etiology of seasonal febrile disease differed from six pathogenic factors in general. Actually, it was a disease due to invasion of another kind of Xie (Pathogenic) Qi between the heaven and earth, being a new idea on the etiology of seasonal febrile disease. Since then, physicians as YE Tiansi, XUE Shengbai, WU Jutong and WANG Mengying in the Qing Dynasty (1644-1911) had more deeply understanding on the infectious ways, pathogenesis, pattern identification, therapeutic methods, formulas and herbs in the treatment of seasonal febrile diseases, creating the system of pattern identification with Four Phases (Wei-Defensive Phase, Qi-Energy Phase, Ying-Nutrient Phase and Xue-Blood Phase) and triple energizer as the guiding principles.

In modern and contemporary times, the theory of TCM will enter a completely new historic phase on the basis of inheriting and exploring the ancestors' medical theory and practical experience, integrating the modern scientific theory and applying modern techniques and measures to study TCM.

明清时期,中医温病学说兴起。明代吴又可首先提出,瘟疫病的病因不同于一般的六淫,而是天地间另有一种异气侵袭所致,对瘟疫病的病因提出了新的见解。之后,清代的叶天士、薛生白、吴鞠通、王孟英等医家,通过大量的临床实践,对温病的传染途径、发病机理、辨证方法、治法方药等,都有更深刻的认识,创立了以卫气营血和三焦为纲领的温病学辨证体系。

中医学发展至近、现代,在继承、发掘前人医学理论和实践经验的基础上,结合现代科学理论、应用现代技术手段研究中医学,中医学理论的发展将会进入一个崭新的历史阶段。

2 Fundamental characteristics of TCM

In brief, the fundamental characteristics of TCM are holistic concept and treatment based on pattern identification.

(1) Nolistic concept: It is believed in TCM that the human body is an organic holism and that the human body and nature form up a closely related entirety.

It is believed in TCM that all the tissues and zangfu organs, meridians and collaterals, five sense organs, nine orifices, four limbs and skeleton and bones are closely related in their shape, property, structure, physiological function and pathological change, forming up an organic holism. For example, in the structure, the human body, with the heart, liver, spleen, lung and kidney as the center, connects them with the six fu organs, five tissues and sense organs to form up a whole entirety with the upper-lower communication and the exterior-interior link through the network of meridian system and the circulation of qi, blood and body fluid. For example, the heart and small intestine, the liver and gallbladder, the spleen and stomach, the lung and large intestine, the kidney and bladder compose an exterior-interior relationship respectively. A certain zang organ connects with other zang organs in the inter-promoting and inter-acting relations physiologically, so as to establish the conception of human body entirety with the five zang organs as the center. Pathologically, the disease of any zang or fu organ of the human body may influence on other tissues and organs. For example, if the liver is sick and fails to maintain free flow of qi, the transportation and transformation function of the spleen and

2 中医学的基本特点

中医学的基本特点,概括而论,一是整体观念,二是辨证论治。

(1) 整体观念:中医学的整体观念,强调人体是一个有机统一的整体,并认为人与自然界也是一个互相关联的整体。

中医学认为,人体的脏腑经络、五官九窍、四肢百骸等组织器官,在形质结构、生理功能、病理变化等方面都是密切关联的,是一个有机统一的整体。如在结构方面,人体以心、肝、脾、肺、肾为中心,通过经络系统的联系,气血津液的流通,将其与六腑、五体、官窍等形成一个上下沟通、表里相连的统一整体。在生理方面,虽然脏腑各有其不同的生理功能活动,但又互相配合协作。如心与小肠、肝与胆、脾与胃、肺与大肠、肾与膀胱等构成表里关系,而某一脏与他脏之间又存在五行生克制化的生理联系,由此形成以五脏为中心的人体整体观。在病理方面,人体任何脏腑病变都有可能影响到其他组织器官,如肝气失于疏泄,可影响脾的运化、胃的受纳功能;肝的阴血不足,可影响五官之目、五体之筋等的生理活动。

the receiving function of the stomach may be affected. If the liver blood is insufficient, the physiological activities of the eyes and tendons may be affected. Therefore, it is necessary to consider the whole condition in the diagnosis and treatment of diseases in TCM, thus the diagnostic and therapeutic characteristics of TCM can fully be embodied.

The human body exists in the nature, where the necessary conditions for the human beings living exist. For example, the climatic changes of warmth in spring, heat in summer, coolness in autumn and cold in winter of the whole year may produce various influences on human body. It is pointed out in Huang Di Nei Jing that in spring and summer, the yang qi outflows to the exterior and the qi and blood of human body flow to surface, so manifesting looseness of skin, opening of sweating pores, more sweats and less urine, and superficial and large pulse. In autumn and winter, the yang qi inflows to the interior and the qi and blood of human body flow to the internals, so manifesting contraction of skin, closure of sweating pores, less sweats and more urine, and deep and small pulse. This example shows that the physiological functions and pulse changes of human body may be regulated automatically by the influence of the seasons and climates. If the climatic changes are too violent and go beyond the human regulating ability, or if the human body resistance decreases, leading to abnormality of the regulating function, there may be seasonal frequently-occurring diseases and epidemic diseases, as the wind diseases in spring, the summer-heat diseases in summer, the dryness diseases in autumn and the cold diseases in winter. Some old people or patients with chronic diseases, due to their poor adaptability,

因此,中医临床诊治疾病时必须从整体出发,才能充分体现中医学的诊疗特色。

人类生活在自然界之中,自然界存在着人类赖以生存的必要条件。同时,自然界的各种变化,又会直接或间接影响人体的生理病理。如一年之中春温、夏热、秋凉、冬寒的气候变化,会对人体产生不同影响。早在《黄帝内经》中就指出:春夏阳气升发在外,人体气血趋于体表,所以多见皮肤松弛,毛窍开张,汗出较多而排尿减少,脉也相对浮大;秋冬阳气收敛内藏,人体气血趋行于内,所以多见皮肤收缩,毛窍固密,汗出减少而排尿增多,脉也略显沉小。这一例子说明人体的生理功能、脉象变化等均会受到四时气候影响而自动调节。若气候变化过于剧烈,超过了人体的调节能力,或人体本身抵抗力下降,调节功能失常时,就可引起季节性的多发病、流行病,如春多风病、夏多暑病、秋多燥病、冬多寒病等。又如某些老年人或慢性病患者,由于适应能力比较差,往往在季节转换之际感到身体不舒,容易导

may feel unwell when the seasons change, so as to cause the attack or severity of the diseases.

Not only the seasonal and climatic changes, but also the changes of the geographic environment produce a certain influence on the human body physiologically and pathologically. In the northern area where it is cold and dry, the skin of human body is fine and close, the body constitution is strong, so people there are not attacked by the exogenous factors, and their diseases are often caused by internal injury. Therefore, if someone moves to a different area, his original body constitution cannot adapt the new geographic environment, leading to various diseases or discomforts known as "not in getting acclimated".

(2) Treatment based upon pattern identification: Treatment based upon pattern identification refers to the diagnostic process of collecting the symptoms and signs through four diagnostic methods (inspection, auscultation and olfaction, inquiring and palpation) to analyze, induce, synthesize and judge, to summarize as a certain pattern. then, according to the result of the pattern identification, the corresponding therapeutic methods to establish. Treatment based upon pattern identification is the fundamental principle to understand and treat diseases in TCM.

Pattern is the summarization of the pathological change of a certain phase in the process of the occurrence and development of a disease, including the location, cause and nature of the disease and the relation between the Xie (Pathogenic) Qi and Zheng (Anti-Pathogenic) Qi, reflecting the nature of the disease more completely, deeply and correctly than a single symptom. For example, a patient

致疾病发作或加重。

不仅季节气候变化对人体有影响,地理环境的不同对人体的生理、病理也会有一定影响。如我国东南沿海地区,气候温热多雨,人体的肌肤松弛,体质相对较弱,容易感受外邪;而气候寒冷干燥的北方地区,人体肌肤致密,体质相对较强,一般不易受外邪侵犯,其病多为内伤。因此,一旦易地而居,若原来的体质状况不能适应新的地理环境,就会出现"水土不服"的种种病变或不舒。

(2) 辨证论治:所谓辨证论治,是指通过四诊(望、闻、问、切)所收集的症状、体征等临床资料,进行分析、归纳、综合和判断,概括为某种性质的证。然后,再根据辨证的结果,确定相应的治疗方法。辨证论治是中医学认识疾病和治疗疾病的基本原则。

证,即证候,是对疾病发生、发展过程中某一阶段的病理变化的概括,包括了疾病的部位、原因、性质以及邪正关系等内容,它比单一的症状能更全面、更深刻、更正确地反映疾病的本质。例如,患者表现为恶寒轻、发热

has manifestations of mild aversion to cold, heavy fever, sore throat, and superficial and rapid pulse. After analysis and induction, it is confirmed that the cause of disease is windheat, the location of disease is the exterior, the nature of disease is heat, the relation between Xie (Pathogenic) Qi and Zheng (Anti-Pathogenic) Qi is excess. The result of pattern identification is the exterior pattern of wind-heat, treated by eliminating wind and relieving the exterior, clearing heat and benefiting throat. It is clear that pattern identification is the premise and basis for establishing the treatment, while treatment is the purpose of pattern identification, and also the method and measure to examine if the pattern identification is correct or not as well.

Clinically, the disease and pattern are interrelated, but also different as well. Generally speaking, a disease is the whole pathological process due to a certain pathogen, while a pattern is a pathological summarization of a certain phase of the whole process of the disease. Therefore, a disease may pertain to several different patterns, while some different diseases may pertain to a same pattern during the progress. Therefore, in TCM, the understanding and treatment of disease stress on pattern identification and on the general character and individual character during the whole process of pattern identification. As for one kind of disease, due to different body constitutions of the patients, different time and places of occurrence and different phases in the progress, different symptoms and signs may occur, thus the therapeutic methods are different accordingly. Take common cold for example. Because of the different types of Xie (Pathogenic) Qi attacked, there is the wind-cold pattern and

重、咽喉肿痛、脉浮数等症，通过分析归纳，确定其病因为风热，病位在表，疾病性质为热，邪正关系是实，辨证结果为风热表证，治以疏风解表，清热利咽。可见，辨证是确定治疗的前提和依据，论治是辨证的目的，也是检验辨证是否正确的方法和手段。辨证与论治是诊治疾病过程中相互联系而不可分割的两个方面。

临床上疾病与证候之间既有内在联系，又有一定区别。通常认为，疾病是病因作用下整个病理全过程的概念，而证候则是疾病过程中某一阶段的病理概括。因此，同一种疾病可表现出不同的证，而不同的疾病在发展过程中又可出现相同的证。所以，中医认识疾病和治疗疾病，主要是着眼于辨证，着眼于辨证的过程中找出证的共性或个性。如同一种疾病，由于患者的体质不同，或发病的时间、地域不同，或处于不同的发展阶段等，可以表现出不同的证候，其治法也随之而异。再以感冒为例，由于患者感受的邪气不同，临床上有风寒证和

wind-heat pattern. For the former, it is advisable to treat with spicy and warm herbs to relieve the exterior, while for the latter, it is advisable to treat with spicy and cool herbs to relieve the exterior. It is called "different treatments for the same disease" in TCM. For different diseases with same symptoms and signs during their progress, it is advisable to apply the same therapeutic methods. For example, dysentery and jaundice are two different diseases, but both are diagnosed as damp-heat pattern, for that, it is advisable to treat with the method to clear heat and dissolve damp. It is called "same treatment for different diseases" in TCM. In summary, it is stressed on "same treatment for same pattern and different treatments for different patterns" in clinic of TCM, showing the important function of "pattern" in the diagnosis and treatment of diseases.

风热证的区别,前者治以辛温解表,后者治以辛凉解表,中医学把这种情形叫做"同病异治"。又如不同的疾病,在其发展过程中,只要出现相同的证候,便可采用相同的治疗方法,如痢疾和黄疸,是两种不同的疾病,但如果都表现为湿热证,就都可用清热利湿的方法来进行治疗,中医学把这种情形叫做"异病同治"。由此可见,中医临床强调"证同治亦同,证异治亦异",尤其突出"证"在疾病诊治过程中的重要作用。

10 Heavenly Stem (HS)十天干

Jia	甲	The First Heavenly Stem (HS 1)
Yi	乙	The Second Heavenly Stem (HS 2)
Bing	丙	The Third Heavenly Stem (HS 3)
Ding	丁	The Fourth Heavenly Stem (HS 4)
Wu	戊	The Fifth Heavenly Stem (HS 5)
Ji	己	The Sixth Heavenly Stem (HS 6)
Geng	庚	The Seventh Heavenly Stem (HS 7)
Xin	辛	The Eigth Heavenly Stem (HS 8)
Ren	壬	The Ninth Heavenly Stem (HS 9)
Gui	癸	The Tenth Heavenly Stem (HS 10)

Chapter 1 Yin-Yang and Five Elements

第1章
阴阳五行

Theories of yin-yang and five elements are the important propositions in the study of ancient Chinese philosophy, the major thinking way of ancient Chinese people to understand and explain the nature. After permeating into TCM, they promoted the formation and development of the theory system of TCM and became the theoretical fundament and guiding ideology of TCM.

阴阳五行是中国古代哲学研究的重大命题,是中国古人认识自然、解释自然的主要思维方法,其渗透到医学领域后,促进了中医理论体系的形成和发展,并成为中医学的理论基础和指导思想。

Section 1 Yin-Yang

第 1 节　阴阳

The theory of yin-yang, originating in the remote antiquity, is a kind of philosophical theory about the origin of the universe and the motion and mutation of all things. It is believed in the theory of yin-yang that all natural events and states of being are rooted in yin and yang. The material world originates, develops, moves and mutates constantly by the mutual influence of yin and yang. The ancient Chinese physicians applied the theory of yin-yang to explain the phenomena and essences of the whole universe and life, and called the motion and mutation principles of the opposition and consuming-supporting of yin-yang "the way of the heaven and earth".

阴阳学说产生于中国远古时代,是一种关于宇宙起源及万物运动变化的哲学理论。阴阳学说认为,世界是由物质构成的,物质世界是在阴阳二气的相互作用下滋生、发展和不断运动变化着的。中国古代医家即用阴阳学说来解释整个宇宙和生命的一切现象和本质,并将阴阳对立与消长的运动变化规律,称之为"天地之道"。

1　Implication of yin-yang and attributive division of yin-yang in things

1.1　Implication of yin-yang

The initial implication of yin-yang was rather intuitive and concrete, referring to that the side of a mountain facing the sun was yang, while the side opposite to the sun was yin. Then the implication was extended and developed gradually to the sense that two separate phenomena with opposing natures or different and opposite aspects within the same phenomenon were summarized by yin and yang. The side facing the sun was extended to the things and phenomena with the characteristics and attribution of brightness, warmth and heat, upward direction and motion pertaining to yang. The side opposite to the sun was extended to the things and phenomena with the characteristics and attribution of darkness, cold and coolness, downward direction and quietness pertaining to yin. Therefore, "yin-yang" ascended from the specific directivity concept to the theory of universal law.

Since the attribution of yin-yang is rather abstract, it takes the water and fire as the representatives of yin and yang in Huang Di Nei Jing, to point out that they are "the symbols of yin and yang". "Fire" has the properties of warmth and heat, brightness, motion and upward direction, which embody the attribution of yang; while "water" has the properties of cold and coolness, darkness, quietness and downward direction, which embody the attribution of yin.

1　阴阳的含义与事物阴阳属性的划分

1.1　阴阳的含义

阴阳的最初含义是比较直观、具体的，主要指日光的向背，向阳者为阳，背阳者为阴。后来由此而逐渐引申，不断扩展，乃至把一切事物或现象本身所存在的相互对立的两个方面，均用阴阳加以概括。如由向阳而引申至凡是明亮、温热、向上、运动等特性、属性的事物和现象，都归属于阳；由背日而引申至凡具晦暗、寒凉、趋下、静止等特性、属性的事物和现象，都归属于阴。从而使"阴阳"由特定的指代概念上升为能够普遍运用的理论。

由于阴阳所表达的事物属性较为抽象，《黄帝内经》以水火为例，指出其为"阴阳之征兆也"。"征兆"，就是象征的意思。"火"具有温热、明亮、运动、向上的特征，典型地体现了阳的属性；"水"具有寒凉、晦暗、静止、向下等特性，典型地体现了阴的属性。

1.2 Division of yin-yang attributions of things and phenomena

Generally speaking, the things and phenomena with the properties of warmth and heat, brightness, motion, upward direction, excitement, outward movement and dispersing pertain to yang, while those with the properties of cold and coolness, darkness, quietness, downward direction, inhibition, inward movement and restraining pertain to yin.

The yin-yang attribution is relative but not absolute. Therefore, it should be paid attention to in the division of yin and yang as follows.

Firstly, the yin-yang attribution of a thing may vary along with the elapse of time and the different application scope. For example, in the comparison of the warmth in spring and heat in summer, the warmth in spring pertains to yin. In the comparison of the warmth in spring and cold in winter, the warmth in spring pertains to yang.

Secondly, any thing or phenomenon may be infinitely divided into its yin and yang aspects, thus the phenomenon of yang within yin and yin within yang occurs. For example, day is yang, while night is yin. During the day, morning with yang qi ascending pertains to yang (yang within yang), while afternoon with yang qi descending pertains to yin (yin within yang). During the night, the first half of night with yin qi ascending pertains to yin (yin within yin), while the second half of night with yin qi descending pertains to yang (yang within yin).

1.2 事物阴阳属性的划分

一般地说,凡是具有温热、明亮、运动、上升、兴奋、外向、发散等特征的事物和现象,都属于阳;凡是具有寒凉、晦暗、静止、下降、抑制、内守、收敛等特性的事物和现象,都属于阴。

由于事物的阴阳属性是相对的,而不是绝对的,所以在事物划分阴阳属相时,须注意以下两点。

一是事物的阴阳属性,随着时间的推移和适用范围的不同,可以发生相应的变化。如春温与夏热相比较,春温(温为次热)属阴;春温与冬寒相比较,春温属阳。

二是事物阴阳属性的每个方面还可以再分阴阳,并且可以无限地分下去,这就形成了阴中有阳、阳中有阴的现象。如以昼夜分阴阳,则白天为阳而晚上为阴。但白天还可以分为上午和下午,则上午阳气上升故属阳(阳中之阳),下午阳气下降故属阴(阳中之阴)。同理,晚上可以分为前半夜和后半夜,则前半夜阴气增长故属阴(阴中之阴),后半夜阴气消退故属阳(阴中之阳)。

2　Mutual actions between yin and yang

The two aspects of yin and yang in a thing or phenomenon are not the simple division, but a kind of complicated mutual action state, leading to the occurrence, development and mutation of a thing. The mutual actions between yin and yang are as follows.

2.1　Opposition and restraint of yin and yang

The opposition and restraint of yin and yang means that due to their opposite properties, yin and yang are always in a condition of mutual repellency and restraint. If both sides of yin and yang are proportionate in force, this kind of mutual repellency and restraint may lead to a whole harmony and equilibrium of the thing. If each of the both sides of yin and yang is stronger or weaker in force, the weak may be restrained by the strong, causing the destruction of the whole equilibrium of the thing. According to the action principle of yin-yang opposition, one of the therapeutic principles in TCM is "to treat by counteracting the nature of the disease". For example, it is to apply the warm and hot formulas and herbs to treat the cold-natured diseases, while to apply the cold and cool formulas and herbs to treat the hot-natured diseases.

2.2　Mutual depending and mutual functioning of yin and yang

It means that yin and yang in the whole entirety, based upon each other and using each other. That is to say yin and yang cannot exist singly without the opposite. There is no yin without yang,

2　阴阳之间的相互作用

事物或现象之间的阴阳两个方面,不是一种简单的划分,而是处于一种极为复杂的相互作用之中,由此而导致了事物的发生、发展和变化。阴阳之间相互作用有多种形式,主要表现在以下几个方面。

2.1　阴阳对立制约

阴阳对立制约,是说阴阳双方由于其性质相反,总是处于相互排斥、相互制约之中。如果阴阳双方力量相当,那么这种相互排斥和相互制约就会导致事物整体平和协调状态。若阴阳双方力量有强弱盛衰的变化,那么弱者将受强者制约,事物整体的平衡就会被破坏。根据阴阳对立的作用原理,中医治疗疾病的基本原则之一是"逆其疾病性质而治"。如寒凉性质的疾病用温热方药治疗;温热性质的疾病用寒凉方药治疗。

2.2　阴阳互根互用

阴阳互根互用,是说阴阳双方存在于一个统一体中,二者互为根基,相互为用。从概念上说,阴和阳的

while there is no yang without yin. Actually, the yin-yang aspects of a thing may be transformed each other, so either side cannot exist singly by separating itself from the other. Therefore, it is said in TCM that "there is no production of yang without yin" and that "there is no production of yin without yang". According to the mutual depending and functioning principles of yin and yang, it is stressed in TCM on the mutual transformation and production of qi and blood and the mutual depending and mutual functioning of yin and yang in the treatment of insufficiency qi, blood, yin or yang. For example, in the treatment of blood deficiency, it is advisable to add the qi-reinforcing herbs at the same time to reinforce the blood, because qi functions to produce the blood. In the treatment of qi deficiency, it is advisable to add the blood-reinforcing herbs at the same time to reinforce qi, because the blood functions to produce qi. With the same reason, it is advisable to add yang-reinforcing herbs at the same time to reinforce yin for yin deficiency, because yang helps to produce yin (so-called "searching for yin in yang"). It is advisable to add yin-reinforcing herbs at the same time to reinforce yang for yang deficiency, because yin helps to produce yang (so-called "searching for yang in yin").

2.3 Inter-waning-waxing relation of yin and yang

Inter-waning-waxing relation refers to that as one wanes, another waxes, or as one waxes, another wanes in the process of yin-yang inter-action. The concrete forms of expression are as follows: As yin wanes, yang waxes. As yang wanes, yin waxes. As yin waxes, yang wanes. As yang wa-

任何一方都不能孤立存在。没有阳无所谓阴,没有阴无所谓阳。事实上,事物内部的阴阳之间可以相互化生,任何一方都不能脱离另一方而单独存在。因此,中医理论中有"独阳不生""孤阴不长"的说法。根据阴阳互根互用的原理,中医在治疗气血阴阳不足时,特别重视气血的相互化生及阴阳的互根互化。如治疗血虚时,在补血的同时,往往配以补气之药,因补气有助于生血。治疗气虚时,在补气的基础上,往往伍以补血之品,因补血有利于生气。同样,阴虚者在补阴之时,适当配以补阳药,补阳有助于以生阴(称为"阳中求阴")。阳虚者在补阳之时,适当伍以补阴药,补阴有助于生阳(称为"阴中求阳")。

2.3 阴阳消长和调

阴阳消长和调,是指在阴阳的相互作用过程中,双方总是表现出此消则彼长,此长则彼消的运动变化形式。其具体表现形式如:阴消则阳长,阳消则阴长;阴长

xes, yin wanes.

In general condition, the inter-waning-waxing of yin and yang is always kept in a certain scope. "Waning" to a certain degree changes into "waxing", while "waxing" to a certain degree changes into "waning". Therefore, both "waning" and "waxing" do not go too far. "Waning" and "waxing" alternate mutually, and go round and begin again, forming a kind of dynamic harmony state of yin and yang, i.e. the healthy state of the human body.

If waning or waxing of yin and yang surpasses the normal scope, the preponderance or weakness of yin or yang occurs. In this situation, the yin-yang harmony is destroyed, leading to disharmony of yin and yang, i.e. the sick state of the human body.

2.4 Inter-transformation of yin and yang

The inter-transformation of yin and yang refers to that on the premise of yin-yang waning and waxing, either of the two may transform into its opposite if "waning" or "waxing" reaches its extreme point, i.e. yin may transform into yang, while yang may transform into yin. It is necessary to point out that the transformation of yin and yang often occurs in the phase when the thing develops to its extreme point. It is said in Huang Di Nei Jing that "extreme cold gives birth to heat", "extreme heat gives birth to cold", "extreme yin turns into yang", and "extreme yang turns into yin". All these quotations pertain to the scope of yin-yang transformation.

The yin-yang mutation of the climates in four seasons is the typical progress of yin-yang transformation. From spring to summer, it turns from

则阳消,阳长则阴消。

在通常情况下,阴阳双方的互为消长总是保持在一定的范围之内。"消"至一定程度会转为"长","长"至一定程度则转为"消",因此"消"与"长"都不会太过。"消"与"长"相互交替,周而复始,形成一种动态的阴阳和调状态,在人体即是健康状态。

如果阴阳消长超出了正常范围,就会出现阴阳偏盛或偏衰的变化,于是动态的阴阳和调就会被打破,从而导致阴阳失调,在人体即是疾病状态。

2.4 阴阳互相转化

阴阳互相转化,是指在阴阳消长的前提下,如果"消"或"长"至极点,可以向相反的方向转化,即阴可以转变为阳,阳可以转变为阴。需要指出的是,引起阴阳转化常常出现在事物发展至极点的阶段。《黄帝内经》所指出的"寒极生热""热极生寒""重阴必阳""重阳必阴"等理论,都属于阴阳转化的范畴。

一年四季气候的阴阳变化,即是阴阳转化的典型过程。从春至夏,气候由温至

warm into hot, pertaining to the process of yang waxing and yin waning. When it reaches the Summer Solstice, the certain turning point, yin-yang waning and waxing will reverse. Then it turns from hot to cool, pertaining to the process of yin waxing and yang waning. From autumn to winter, it turns from cool to cold, pertaining to the process of yin waxing and yang waning. When it reaches the Winter Solstice, another certain turning point, it reverses to yang waxing and yin waning again. It can be seen that the yin-yang mutation of the climates in four seasons centrally embodies the progress that "extreme yin turns into yang, and extreme yang turns into yin".

3　Application of yin-yang theory in TCM

3.1　Illustrate the organic structure of human body

It is believed in TCM that the human body, an organic entirety, has all the tissues and structure with the yin-yang opposition and restraint relations. Therefore, yin-yang theory is applied to illustrate the attributions of these tissues and structure. It is said in Huang Di Nei Jing that "man has a physical shape which is inseparable from yin and yang". In terms of anatomical location, the upper part of human body pertains to yang, while the lower part to yin. The body surface pertains to yang, while the internals to yin. The back pertains to yang, while the chest-abdomen to yin. The lateral aspects of four limbs pertain to yang, while the medial aspects to yin. In terms of zang-fu organs, the five zang organs, storing the essence and qi without draining,

热,属于阳长而阴消的过程,但到达特定的时间转折点——夏至,阴阳消长出现逆转,气候由热转凉,进入阴长而阳消的过程;从秋至冬,气候由凉至寒,属于阴长而阳消的过程,而到达另一个特定的时间转折点——冬至,又逆转为阳长而阴消。可见四季气候的阴阳变化,集中体现了"重阴必阳、重阳必阴"的过程。

3　阴阳学说在中医学中的应用

3.1　用于说明人体的组织结构

中医学认为,人体是一个有机的整体,其体内一切相关的组织结构之间,都存在着阴阳对立依存的关系,因此也都可用阴阳来说明这些组织结构的属性,故《黄帝内经》有"人生有形,不离阴阳"的说法。从人体部位来说,人体上部属阳,下部属阴;体表属阳,体内属阴;背部属阳,胸腹部属阴;四肢外侧属阳,四肢内侧属阴。若以脏腑来分,五脏藏精气而不泻,属阴;六腑传化物而不藏,属阳。五脏之中,心肺居

pertain to yin, while the six fu organs, transporting and transforming materials without storing, to yang. Among the five zang organs, the heart and lung, locating in the chest, pertain to yang, while the liver, spleen and kidney, locating in the abdomen, to yin. Furthermore, within each of the zang-fu organs, there are yin and yang aspects according to the different functional states, as the heart yin and heart yang, the kidney yin and kidney yang.

3.2 Explain the physiological functions of human body

It is believed in TCM that the normal vital activities of human body are based upon the coordination of yin and yang in a unity of opposites, and that there is a close relation between the organic structure and physiological functions. The organic structures, including all the material basis of zang-fu organs, meridians and collaterals, qi, blood and body fluid, pertain to yin, while their functional activities pertain to yang. There exist the opposition, dependence, waning-waxing and transformation relationships of yin and yang between the yin-attributed materials and the yang-attributed functions. In terms of mutual depending and functioning relations of yin and yang, the production and maintenance of human body's physiological functions are based upon the materials of zang-fu organs, meridians and collaterals, qi, blood and body fluid. Simultaneously, the metabolic process of qi, blood and body fluid is also based upon the functional activities of the related zang-fu organs. In the process of metabolic movement and mutation, there exists the yin-yang transformation relation between the materials and functions as well. Only when the series of physio-

胸中,属阳;肝脾肾居腹中,属阴。而每一脏腑又依据其功能状态的不同而各有阴阳之分,如心阴与心阳、肾阴与肾阳等。

3.2 用于解释人体的生理功能

中医学认为,人体的正常生命活动,是阴阳两个方面保持着协调平衡的结果,而组织结构与生理功能之间有着密切联系。人体的组织结构,包括脏腑经络和气血津液等物质基础均属于阴,其功能活动则属于阳。属阴的物质与属阳的功能之间,存在着阴阳的对立、依存、消长以及转化的关系。就阴阳互根互用的关系而言,人体生理功能的产生和维持,要以脏腑经络、气血津液等作为物质基础,而气血津液的新陈代谢过程,也要依赖相关脏腑的功能活动。新陈代谢的运动变化过程中,还存在着物质与功能之间阴阳转化的关系。只有这一系列的生理过程保持着阴阳平和的状态,人体才能维持正常生命活动。

logical process keeps a yin-yang harmony state, can the human body maintain the normal vital activities.

3.3　Analyze the pathological changes of human body

When the harmonious relation between yin and yang in the human body is destroyed, there can be a series of pathological changes, called "yin-yang disharmony" in TCM. The pathological changes of human body are complicated, but they are nothing but preponderance and weakness of yin and yang by application of yin-yang theory to analyze their basic pathogenesis.

3.3.1　Preponderance of yin or yang

Preponderance of yin or yang refers to a kind of pathological change due to yin or yang waxing beyond the normal scope, including preponderance of yang and preponderance of yin.

Preponderance of yang is often caused by the invasion of the yang pathogens into the human body or by the heat transformed from the yin pathogens, leading to the preponderance of the yang heat in the body with the manifestations of the heat pattern of excess type, as it is said in Huang Di Nei Jing that "preponderance of yang leads to heat". The Xie (Pathogenic) Qi of different properties may damage the Zheng (Anti-Pathogenic) Qi opposite to it inside the human body, so the yang pathogens may damage the yin fluid inside the body during the progress. For example, the pathogenic heat invades the human body, causing preponderance of yang inside the body with the manifestations of high fever, sweating, red complexion and rapid pulse, pertaining to the heat pattern of excess. Along with the further

3.3　用于分析人体的病机变化

当人体阴阳之间的平和协调关系遭到破坏时,便会出现一系列病理变化,中医学统称其为"阴阳失调"。人体的病机变化虽然复杂,但用阴阳学说来分析其基本的病机,不外乎阴阳偏盛和阴阳偏衰两个方面。

3.3.1　阴阳偏盛

阴阳偏盛,是由于阴阳亢盛超过了正常的范围而出现的一种病理变化,包括阳偏盛和阴偏盛两个方面。

阳偏盛,多由阳邪侵犯人体,或感受阴邪从阳化热,以致体内阳热之气亢盛,而表现出实热性质的病证表现,即《黄帝内经》所说的"阳胜则热"。由于不同性质的邪气能够损伤人体与之相对的正气,所以在病变过程中,阳邪还容易损伤人体的阴液。例如热邪侵入人体,使体内阳气偏盛,出现高热、汗出、面红、脉数等实热证候,随着病情进一步发展,阳邪耗伤了机体的阴液,可出现口渴、尿少、便秘等阴液受损的症状。

development of the disease, yang pathogens consume the yin fluid inside the body, leading to yin deficiency pattern with the manifestations of thirst, scanty urine and constipation.

Preponderance of yin is often caused by the invasion of the yin pathogens into the human body, leading to the preponderance of yin qi inside the body with the manifestations of the cold pattern of excess type, as it is said in Huang Di Nei Jing that "preponderance of yin leads to cold". The yin pathogens may further damage the yang qi of the human body. For example, the pathogenic cold invades the human body, causing the cold pattern of excess with the manifestations of aversion to cold, cold limbs and cold pain in abdomen, and causing the yang deficiency pattern with the manifestations of bright white complexion, tiredness, sleepiness, and slow and weak pulse as well.

According to the principle of yin-yang transformation, when the disease of yin or yang preponderance develops to the extreme point, it may transform to its opposite under certain conditions. For example, the yin cold pattern may transform into the yang heat pattern, and vice versa.

3.3.2 Weakness of yin or yang

Weakness of yin or yang refers to a kind of pathological change due to yin or yang waning beyond the normal scope, including weakness of yin and weakness of yang. Weakness of yin or yang pertains to the scope of Zheng (Anti-Pathogenic) Qi insufficiency of human body. Weakness of yin refers to the yin fluid insufficiency inside the human body, while weakness of yang to the yang qi insufficiency inside the human body.

阴偏盛,多由阴邪侵犯人体,导致体内阴寒之气亢盛,从而引起实寒性质的病证表现,即《黄帝内经》所说的"阴胜则寒"。阴邪还可以进一步损伤人体的阳气。例如寒邪侵入人体,患者一方面可出现恶寒肢冷、腹部冷痛等实寒症状,另一方面也可表现出面色㿠白、倦怠喜卧、脉迟无力等阳虚之象。

此外,根据阴阳转化的原理,阴阳偏盛的病变发展到极点,还可在一定的条件下发生相互转化,如阴寒证可转化为阳热证,阳热证可转化为阴寒证。

3.3.2 阴阳偏衰

阴阳偏衰,是由于阴阳消减超过了正常范围而出现的病理变化,包括阴偏衰和阳偏衰两个方面。阴阳偏衰属于人体正气不足的范畴,其中阴偏衰指人体的阴液不足,阳偏衰指人体的阳气不足。

Weakness of yang refers to the insufficiency of yang qi, which fails to restrain the yin qi and to warm and nourish the zang-fu organs, leading to the cold pattern of deficiency with the manifestations of pale-white complexion, fear of cold, spontaneous sweating and slow and weak pulse, as it is said in Huang Di Nei Jing that "yang deficiency leads to cold".

Weakness of yin refers to the insufficiency of yin fluid, which fails to restrain the yang qi and to moisturize and nourish the zang-fu organs, leading to the heat pattern of deficiency with the manifestations of red cheeks, tidal fever, nocturnal sweats and thready and rapid pulse, as it is said in Huang Di Nei Jing that "yin deficiency leads to heat".

Since yin and yang are mutually depended and transformed, either of the two cannot exist singly without the opposite. Therefore, the further development of weakness of yin or yang may affect the opposite, i. e. prolonged yin deficiency may cause the depletion of yang qi, while prolonged yang deficiency may lead to the insufficiency of yin fluid. As a result, the deficiency pattern of both yin and yang occurs.

Preponderance of yin or yang and weakness of yin or yang may develop to a very severe degree, leading to exhaustion of the Zheng (Anti-Pathogenic) Qi of the human body, thus the specific pathological changes of "collapse of yin" and "collapse of yang" occur. The final result of collapse of yin or collapse of yang is separation of yin and yang, causing death.

3.3.4　Guide the diagnosis of the diseases

It is believed in the yin-yang theory that the

阳偏衰,指人体阳气不足,不能制约阴寒之气,脏腑失于温养,出现虚寒性质的病证表现,临床可见面白、畏寒、自汗、脉迟弱等症状,即《黄帝内经》所谓"阳虚则寒"。

阴偏衰,指人体阴液不足,不能制约阳热之气,脏腑失于滋养,出现虚热性质的病证表现,临床可见面红、潮热、盗汗、脉细数等症状,即《黄帝内经》所谓"阴虚则热"。

由于阴阳双方互相依赖,互相化生,任何一方都不能脱离对方而单独存在,因此阴阳偏衰的病变进一步发展,还可以互相影响,即阴虚日久会引起阳气虚损,阳虚日久也会引起阴液不足,从而出现阴阳两虚证。

阴阳偏盛和阴阳偏衰发展到极其严重的程度,还可能导致人体正气衰竭,出现所谓"亡阴"和"亡阳"的特殊病机变化。亡阴、亡阳的最终结果是导致阴阳离决而死亡。

3.3.4　用于指导疾病的诊断

阴阳学说认为,由于疾

fundamental cause of the occurrence, development and mutation of a disease is disharmony of yin and yang, so the manifestations of various diseases, such as color, voice and pulse, can be summarized and explained by the yin-yang theory in the clinic.

In the diagnosis, it is advisable to analyze the information collected from the four diagnostic methods, so as to judge the yin-yang property of the disease, as it is said in Huang Di Nei Jing that "it is advisable to observe the patient's complexion and feel his pulse, thus take the first step in determination if it is a yin or yang disease". In terms of color, the fresh and bright color pertains to yang, while the dim and dark color to yin. In terms of speaking voice, the loud and heavy voice pertains to yang, while the light and weak voice to yin. In terms of preference and aversion, the preference for cold and aversion to heat pertain to yang, while the preference for heat and aversion to cold to yin. In terms of pulse, the superficial, slippery, rapid and surging pulses pertain to yang, while the deep, choppy, slow and thready pulses to yin.

In the pattern identification, it is advisable to determine the property of the disease from the aspects of yin-yang, exterior-interior, deficiency-excess and cold-heat, which are believed as the guiding principles to identify all types of diseases, the so-called "pattern identification according to eight principles". Among the eight principles, "yin and yang" are regarded as the leading principles in pattern identification according to eight principles. Generally speaking, the exterior pattern, excess pattern and heat pattern pertain to the yang pat-

病的发生、发展和变化的根本原因均在阴阳失调，所以临床上各种疾病，包括其色泽、声音、脉象等症状表现，都可以用阴阳来加以概括和说明。

诊断方面，对四诊所收集的资料来进行具体地分析，首先要判明疾病的阴阳性质，正如《黄帝内经》所说"察色按脉，先别阴阳"。如从色泽的明暗来看，色泽鲜明者为阳，色泽晦暗者为阴；从语声的高低来看，声音高亢洪亮者为阳，声音低微无力者为阴；从性情的喜恶来看，喜寒恶热者为阳，喜热恶寒者为阴；从脉象形态来看，凡浮、滑、数、洪等脉象皆属阳，凡沉、涩、迟、细等脉象属阴。

辨证方面，临床上往往首先从疾病性质的阴阳、表里、虚实、寒热等方面来进行，认为这是辨别一切病证的纲领，所以称之为"八纲辨证"。但其中的"阴阳"两纲，又可看作是八纲辨证的总纲。也就是说，表证、实证、热证皆属阳证，里证、虚证、寒证皆属阴证。又如在脏腑辨证中，也常结合阴阳来进

tern, while the interior pattern, deficiency pattern and cold pattern to the yin pattern. In pattern identification according to zang-fu organs, it is advisable to combine the yin-yang theory to analyze the diseases, such as the heart yin deficiency, heart yang deficiency, kidney yin deficiency, kidney yang deficiency, spleen yang deficiency and liver yin deficiency in the category of the deficiency patterns of zang-fu organs. Therefore, the identification of yin pattern and yang pattern of the diseases is the fundamental principle in pattern identification, possessing the important guiding significance in the clinic.

3.3.5 Guide the treatment of the diseases

In terms of preponderance of yin or yang, it is advisable to apply "the heating method for cold disease" in the treatment of the cold pattern of excess due to yin preponderance, while to apply "the cooling method for heat disease" in the treatment of the heat pattern of excess due to yang preponderance.

In terms of weakness of yin or yang, it is advisable to apply the method "to search for yin in yang" in the treatment of the heat pattern of deficiency due to yin weakness, by adding yang-reinforcing herbs when reinforcing yin, while to apply the method "to search for yang in yin" in the treatment of cold pattern of deficiency due to yang weakness, by adding yin-reinforcing herbs when reinforcing yang. These are the therapeutic principles based upon the mutual depending and functioning relation of yin and yang.

Furthermore, the functional performance of the herbs, as the four properties, five flavors, ascending-descending, floating-sinking, etc. can also be concluded with the yin-yang theory.

行分析,如脏腑虚证分类中有心阴虚、心阳虚、肾阴虚、肾阳虚、脾阳虚、肝阴虚等证候。所以辨别疾病的阴证、阳证,是辨证的基本原则,在临床上具有重要的指导意义。

3.3.5 用于指导疾病的治疗

针对阴阳偏胜,阴偏胜而出现寒实证,应用"寒者热之"来治疗,阳偏胜而出现实热证,应用"热者寒之"来治疗,这便是依据阴阳对立制约所确定的治疗原则。

针对阴阳偏衰,阴偏衰而出现虚热证,应用"阳中求阴"来治疗,即补阴之时适当加入补阳之品,阳偏衰而出现虚寒证时,应用"阴中求阳"来治疗,即补阳之时适当加入补阴之药,这便是依据阴阳互根互用确立的治疗原则。

此外,药物的四气、五味、升降浮沉等性能,也都可以阴阳理论加以归纳。

The four properties refer to cold, hot, warm and cool properties. The hot and warm herbs pertain to yang, while the cold and cool herbs to yin. The warm and hot natured herbs are used to treat the cold pattern, while the cold and cool natured herbs are used to treat the heat pattern.

The five flavors refer to the pungent, sweet, sour, bitter and salty flavors. Besides, another flavor, called bland flavor, is a kind flavor in which all the above five flavors are light. Different flavors function differently, with different yin-yang attributions. For example, the pungent flavor functions to disperse, the sweet flavor to reinforce, and the bland flavor to permeate and discharge, therefore the sweet, pungent and bland flavors pertain to yang. The sour flavor functions to restrain, the bitter flavor to reduce and descend, and the salt flavor to moisturize and purge, therefore, the sour, bitter and salty flavors pertain to yin.

Ascending-descending and floating-sinking are the summarization of the action tendency of the herbs. The herbs with the ascending and floating actions pertain to yang, while the herbs with the descending and sinking actions pertain to yin.

It is to serve the clinic treatment based upon pattern identification by applying the yin-yang theory to summarize the functional performance of herbs. In the treatment of a disease clinically, it is advisable to determine the preponderance or weakness of yin and yang, establish the correct therapeutic principles and choose the proper herbs according to the properties, flavors and functional performance of the herbs, then a good effect will be received.

四气,也称四性,有寒、热、温、凉之别。其中热药、温药属阳,寒药、凉药属阴。温热性质的药物一般用来治疗寒证,寒凉性质的药物一般用来治疗热证。

五味,包括辛、甘、酸、苦、咸五种。另有一种五味皆轻薄的成为淡味。不同的药味具有不同的作用,阴阳属性也不相同。如辛味能发散,甘味能补益,淡味能渗泄,故甘、辛、淡属阳;而酸味可收敛,苦味可泻降,咸味可润下,故酸、苦、咸属阴。

升降浮沉,是对药物作用趋向的一种概括。凡是具有升浮(上升、发散)作用的药物均属阳,凡是具有降沉(下降、重镇)作用的药物均属阴。

用阴阳理论归纳药物性能,是为临床辨证论治服务的。临床治疗疾病,只有在辨清阴阳偏盛或偏衰并制定正确治疗原则基础之上,再结合药物的性味功能,选用适宜的药物,才能收到良好的疗效。

Section 2 Five Elements

The theory of five elements also originated in remote antiquity, a kind of understanding to the material world in the ancients' prolonged life and production practice. It became a thinking way to explain and analyze all the things and phenomena in the natural world and their mutations in the ancient times. With the theory of yin-yang, it became a unique world outlook in ancient China. After it was applied in the fields of TCM, the theory of five elements became an important component part of the theory system of TCM.

1 Implication of five elements

The ancients believed that the five materials of wood, fire, earth, metal and water were necessary in their daily life and productive labor, and the fundamental elements to form up the normal mutation of the nature. For example, water and fire are the necessities of the people's food, metal and wood are the necessities in manufacturing various tools, while earth functions to transform all things to cultivate the human beings. All these materials are mutually related and functioned. This is the theory of five elements.

In the theory of five elements, "five" refers to the five materials of wood, fire, earth, metal and water in the natural world, while "elements" have two meanings as: one is order, referring to the certain sequential order, motion and mutation among the five materials, another is movement, referring to the regulations of motion and mutation of the

第 2 节 五行

五行学说同样产生于中国的远古时代,是古人在长期的生活和生产实践中所形成的对物质世界的一种认识,并成为古代用来解释和分析自然界中的所有事物及其变化的思维方法,其与阴阳学说一起构成了中国古代一种独特的宇宙观。五行学说被运用于中医学领域后,便成为中医学理论体系的重要组成部分。

1 五行的含义

远古之人认为,木、火、土、金、水五种物质是日常生活及生产劳动中不可缺少的,是构成自然界正常变化的五种重要的基本元素,如水、火是人们饮食所必需的,金、木可制成各种用具所必备的,土则能化生万物以养人类,这些物质之间又是相互联系、相互作用的,由此而逐渐形成了五行理论。

五行之"五",是指自然界中的木、火、土、金、水五种物质;五行之"行",其义有二:一是指行列,指五行之间的相生相克均有一定的排列次序运动和变化。二是指运动,强调五行阐述其所指代

five categories of things. Therefore, the theory of five elements refers to the five categories of things of wood, fire, earth, metal and water and their motion and mutation and mutual relations among the five categories of things.

2 Attributive division of five elements in things

Wood, fire, earth, metal and water are the five elements that constitute the whole world. They each have their own characteristics, and yet are mutually interdependant. Therefore, their characteristics are used to classify and illustrate the attribution of everything.

As for the characteristics of the five elements, the ancients recognized the intuitive attributions of the five materials of wood, fire, earth, metal and water in the nature. It is said in *A Collection of Ancient Works* (Shang Shu) that the wood is featured by bent branches and straight trunk, the fire by hotness and flaring up, the earth by sowing and harvesting, the metal by clearance and variation, and the water by moisture and downward flowing.

In order to illustrate and explain the attributions of more things and phenomena, the features of five elements were further abstractly extended and applied, to possess a more extensive implication. For example, those with the features of bending and straightness, growing, ascending and dispersing, free flowing, etc. pertain to the category of wood, those with warmth and heat, upward movement, rising, luxuriance, etc. pertain to the category of fire, those with receiving, carrying, growing and transforming, nourishing, etc. pertain to the category of earth, those with desolating, restraining,

的五类事物间运动变化规律。由此而言,所谓五行,是指木、火、土、金、水这五类物质及其所指代的五类事物的运动变化及其相互关系。

2 事物五行属性的划分

由于木、火、土、金、水是构成世界的五种基本物质,彼此之间既各有特性,又相互依存,因此人们就利用五行的特性来划分和说明一切事物的属性。

关于五行特性,人们最早认识到的是自然界木、火、土、金、水五种物质的直观属性,如早在《尚书·洪范》对五行特性就有明确记载:木性枝曲、干直,火性炎热、向上,土可播种、收获,金可销铄、变革,水性滋润、向下。

为了说明和解释更多的事物属性,人们又将五行特性进一步抽象地加以引申运用,使其具有了更广泛的涵义,如:凡具有曲直、生长、升发、舒畅等特性的事物,均属于木的一行;凡具有温热、向上、升腾、繁茂等特性的事物,均归于火的一行;凡具有受纳、承载、生化、长养等特性的事物,均属于土的一行;凡具有肃杀、收敛、潜降、洁

subsurface and descending, clearance, etc. pertain to the category of metal, and those with moisturizing, downward flowing, cold and cool, closing and storing, etc. pertain to the category of water.

On the basis of mastering the basic features of five elements, we can apply the inductive method and deductive method to classify all the things to determine their attributions of five elements.

First, it is advisable to compare the image, property and action of a thing with the abstract features of five elements. If it is similar to one of the elements, it pertains to the category of this element.

In terms of the geographic environment of China, the sun rises from the east, similar to the ascending and dispersing features of the wood, so the east pertains to wood. It is hot and warm in the south, similar to the warming and heating features of the fire, so the south pertains to fire. There are many high mountains which are high and steep, similar to the desolating and restraining features of the metal, so the west pertains to metal. It is very cold in the north, similar to the cold and cool features of the water, so the north pertains to water. It is properly cool and warm in the central part of China with rich products, similar to the growing and transforming features of the earth, so the center pertains to earth.

In terms of the seasons, meteorological phenomena and phonological conditions, the yang qi starts to rise and all things on earth germinates in spring, similar to the free flowing, growing and dispersing features of the wood, so the spring pertains

净等特性的事物,均属于金的一行;凡具有滋润、向下、寒凉、闭藏等特性的事物,均属于水的一行。

在把握五行基本特性的基础上,就可以运用归类法和推演法,对所有事物进行分类,以确定不同事物的五行属性。

首先,将事物的形象、性质、作用等分别与五行的抽象特性进行比较,如果与某一行的特性相类似,就归属于某一行之中。

如就中国的地理环境而言,太阳从东方升起,与木的升发特性相类似,故东方属木;南方气候炎热,与火的炎热特性相类似,故南方属火;西方多崇山峻岭,地势高峭,与金的肃杀特性相类似,故西方属金;北方气候寒冷,地气潜藏,与水的寒凉特性相类似,故北方属水;中国中原地区气候寒温适宜,物产丰富,与土的生化特性相类似,故中央之地属土。

又如就季节气象物候特点而言,春天阳气渐升,万物萌生,与木的舒展生发特性相类似,故春季属木;夏天气候炎热,万物盛长,与火的炎

to wood. It is warm and hot in summer when all things on earth grow luxuriantly, similar to the warming and rising features of the fire, so the summer pertains to fire. It is humid in the "late summer" after summer and before autumn when all things on earth are ripe, similar to the growing, transforming and nourishing features of the earth, so the "late summer" pertains to earth. The yang qi starts to descend and all things on earth are withered in autumn, similar to the features of restraining and descending features of the metal, so the autumn pertains to metal. It is very cold in winter when all things on earth are stored, similar to the cooling and storing features of the water, so the winter pertains to water.

Secondly, for those things that cannot be compared directly with the abstract features of five elements, it is advisable to apply the deductive method. According to the known five-element attribution of some thing, we can deduce the other things that are related to it, so as to reach a conclusion of its five-element attribution. For example, the physiological functions of the liver, one of the five zang organs of the human body, are to maintain dredging and draining and to prefer to free growing, similar to the features of the wood, so the liver pertains to wood. The gallbladder, one of the fu organs, the tendons, one of the five body constituents, and the eyes, one of the five sense organs cannot be compared with the features of any of the five elements directly, but these organs and tissues have an inner link with the liver, thus they pertain to wood as well.

Therefore, the inductive and deductive methods are applied in TCM to classify all things on earth and

热升腾特性相类似,故夏季属火;夏秋之交的"长夏"湿气偏重,万物成熟,与土的生化长养特性相类似,故"长夏"属土;秋天阳气下降,万物凋落,与金的收敛肃杀特性相类似,故秋季属金;冬天气候寒冷,万物潜藏,与水的寒凉闭藏特性相类似,故冬季属水。

其次,对于一些与五行的抽象特征无法进行直接比较的事物,可以采用推演的方法,即根据已知的某些事物的五行属性,再推演至与其相关的其他事物,从而得知这些事物的五行属性。如人体五脏之肝的生理功能是主疏泄、喜条达,其与木的特性相类似,故肝的五行属性为木,而六腑之胆、五体之筋、五官之目等因无法与五行的特性直接类比,而这些器官组织与肝有着内在的密切联系,于是都随肝而归属于木。

因此,中医学理论用归类和推演的方法,将自然界

the zang-fu organs, organs and tissues of the human body in the five categories of the wood, fire, earth, metal and water according to their attributions, so as to form up a structure system of five elements with the mutual relations between the internal and external environments of the human body. The structure system of five elements include the five flavors, five colors, five climatic phenomena, five directions and five seasons in the nature, and the five zang organs, five fu organs, five sense organs, five body constituents, five emotions and five fluids of the human body as well.

的各种事物和人体的脏腑、器官、组织,按其不同的属性均可分别归类于木、火、土、金、水五行之中,从而形成人体内外环境相互联系的五行结构系统。五行结构系统的主要内容包括自然界中五味、五色、五气、五方、五季及人体中五脏、五腑、五官、五体、五志、五液等。

Structure System of Five Elements

Nature					FIVE ELEMENTS	Human Body					
Five Flavors	Five Colors	Five Climatic Phenomena	Five Directions	Five Seasons		Five Zang Organs	Five Fu Organs	Five Sense Organs	Five Body Constituents	Five Emotions	Five Fluids
Sour	Green	Wind	East	Spring	WOOD	Liver	Gallbladder	Eyes	Tendons	Anger	Tear
Bitter	Red	Heat	South	Summer	FIRE	Heart	Small Intestine	Tongue	Vessels	Joy	Sweat
Sweet	Yellow	Dampness	Central	Late Summer	EARTH	Spleen	Stomach	Mouth	Muscles	Worry	Xian (Thin) Saliva
Pungent	White	Dryness	West	Autumn	METAL	Lung	Large Intestine	Nose	Skin	Grief	Snivel
Salty	Black	Cold	North	Winter	WATER	Kidney	Bladder	Ears	Bones	Fear	Tuo (Thick) Saliva

五行结构系统表

自 然 界					五行	人 体					
五味	五色	五气	五方	五季		五脏	五腑	五官	五体	五志	五液
酸	青	风	东	春	木	肝	胆	目	筋	怒	泪
苦	赤	暑	南	夏	火	心	小肠	舌	脉	喜	汗
甘	黄	湿	中	长夏	土	脾	胃	口	肉	思	涎
辛	白	燥	西	秋	金	肺	大肠	鼻	皮	悲	涕
咸	黑	寒	北	冬	水	肾	膀胱	耳	骨	恐	唾

3　Mutual actions among five elements

Each of the five elements possesses its own features, while the five elements are mutually acted and related. The relations among the five categories of things classified according to the features of the elements are complicated and varied, but they can be explained with the theory of five elements. There are normal relations and abnormal relations among the five elements.

3.1　Normal mutual relations among five elements

The normal mutual relations among the five elements refer to the inter-promoting relation and interacting relation.

(1) Inter-promoting relation implies that one element has the promoting and generating function on the other. The inter-promoting order of five elements is regular, forming up an inter-promoting cycle as, wood promotes fire, fire promotes earth, earth promotes metal, metal promotes water, and water, in turn, promotes wood. The element "to promote" is regarded as "the mother", while the element "to be promoted" as "the son". Therefore, the inter-promoting relation of five elements is also called the mother-son relation. Take the fire as the example. The element to promote the fire is the wood, while the element to be promoted by the fire is the earth. The wood is the mother of fire, while the earth is the son of fire.

(2) Interacting relation implies that one element has the restraining and controlling function on the other. The interacting order of five elements is regular, forming up an interacting cycle as, wood

3　五行之间的相互作用

五行各有其特性，而五行之间又相互作用，相互联系，故根据五行特性而划分的五类事物，虽然彼此之间关系复杂多变，但仍可用五行理论进行说明。五行之间相互作用有正常和异常两种情形。

3.1　五行之间正常的相互关系

五行之间正常的相互关系，主要是相生与相克关系。

（1）相生，是指五行之中的某一行对另一行具有促进和资生作用。五行相生的次序是有规律排列的，并构成一个循环相生环，即木生火，火生土，土生金，金生水，水又复生木。由于"生我"者为"母"，"我生"者为"子"，所以五行相生关系又叫做母子关系。如以火行为例，生我者为木，我生者为土，故称木为火之母，土为火之子。

（2）相克，是指五行之中的某一行对另一行具有克制、制约作用。其相克次序也是有一定规律的，并构成

acts on earth, earth acts on water, water acts on fire, fire acts on metal, and metal, in turn, acts on wood.

The inter-promoting and interacting relations of five elements are the two aspects that cannot be separated. Without promoting, it is impossible to possess the growth and generation of things. Without acting, it is impossible to prevent the over-development of things that leads to damage. Therefore, only when there is acting in promoting and promoting in acting, can the things maintain their normal development and mutation, and keep a harmonious and balanced state.

3.2 Abnormal mutual relations among five elements

The abnormal mutual relations among the five elements refer to the overacting relation, counteracting relation and mutual mother-son involvement.

3.2.1 Overacting relation and counteracting relation

Overacting relation implies the abnormal state in which one element restrains another too excessively. The order of overacting relation is same as that of interacting relation as, wood overacts on earth, earth overacts on water, water overacts on fire, fire overacts on metal, and metal, in turn, overacts on wood. The causes of overacting relation are as follows:

Firstly, if one of the elements is too strong, it may restrain and control the other too much, so as to destroy the normal interacting relation between the two. For example, the wood that is too strong may overact on the earth, the water that is excessive may overact on the fire, etc.

一个循环相克环,即木克土,土克水,水克火,火克金,金又复克木。

五行的相生与相克,是不可分割的两个方面。没有生,就没有事物的发生和成长;没有克,就不能防止事物因过于发展而造成的危害,所以只有生中有克,克中有生,才能维持事物的正常发展变化及其平和协调状态。

3.2 五行之间异常的相互关系

五行之间异常的相互关系主要表现在相乘、相侮及母子相及两个方面。

3.2.1 相乘与相侮

相乘,是指五行之中的某一行对另一行制约过度的异常状态。相乘的次序与相克的次序是一致的,即木乘土,土乘水,水乘火,火乘金,金又复乘木。引起相乘的原因有两方面:

一是五行中的某一行力量太强,导致对其所克的一行克制太过,从而破坏了两者之间正常相克的关系。如木旺则乘土,水盛则乘火等。

Secondly, if one of the elements is too weak, it may be restrained and controlled by the other too much, so as to destroy the normal interacting relation between the two. For example, the earth that is deficient may be overacted by the wood, the water that is deficiency may be overacted by the earth, etc.

Counteracting relation implies the abnormal state in which the originally acted element acts on the other, preying upon the other. The order of counteracting relation is just opposite to that of interacting relation as, wood counteracts on metal, metal counteracts on fire, fire counteracts on water, water counteracts on earth, and earth, in turn, counteracts on wood. The causes of counteracting relation are as follows:

Firstly, if one of the elements is too strong, it cannot be acted, but acts on the counterpart, leading to the abnormality of the interacting relation. For example, the wood that is excessive may counteracts on the metal, the fire that is hyperactive may counteracts on water, etc.

Secondly, if one of the elements is too weak to act on the other, but acted by the counterpart, leading to the abnormality of the interacting relation. For example, the metal that is too weak may be counteracted by the wood, the earth that is deficiency may be counteracted by the water, etc.

3.2.2　Mutual mother-son involvement

The interacting relation of the five elements is called the mother-son relation, while the abnormal mother-son relation is called the mutual mother-son involvement. "The mother disease involving the son" refers to that the mother abnormality may af-

二是五行中的某一行力量太弱,导致克其的一行克制太过,从而破坏了两者之间正常相克的关系。如土虚则木乘,水虚则土乘等。

相侮,是指五行之中的某一行对另一行反向克制的异常状态,故又叫"反侮"。相侮的次序与相克的次序是相反的,即木侮金,金侮火,火侮水,水侮土,土侮木。引起相侮的原因也有两方面:

一是五行中的某一行出现太过,便反向制约克其的一行,导致两者之间的相克关系出现异常。如木旺则侮金,火旺则侮水等。

二是五行中的某一行出现不及,无力制约其应克的一行,而导致反向克制,导致两者之间的相克关系异常。如金虚则木侮,土虚则水侮等。

3.2.2　母子相及

五行相生关系称为母子关系,五行母子关系异常称为母子相及。其中母病及子,是指母行异常可影响及子行,其次序与相生次序一

fect the son, with the same order as that of the interacting relation. "The son disease involving the mother" refers to that the son abnormality may affect the mother, with the opposite order as that of the interacting relation. For example, the water (kidney) failing to moisturize the wood (liver) pertains to the mother disease involving the son, while the wood (liver) disease affecting the water (kidney) pertains to the son disease involving the mother.

4   Application of the theory of five elements in TCM

4.1   Illustrate the physiological features and mutual relations of five zang organs

The theory of five elements is applied to illustrate the physiological features of the five zang organs, so as to classify the five zang organs into five elements. For example, the wood is featured of free growing, ascending and dispersing, illustrating that the liver prefers to unblocked and is averse to inhibition. The fire is featured of warming, heating and up-flaring, illustrating that the heart yang functions to warm the whole body. The earth is featured of receiving, producing and transforming, illustrating that the spleen dominates the transportation and transformation of food essence, as the source to produce qi and blood. The metal is featured of clearance, descending and restraining, illustrating that the lung qi is stored internally, with preference for descending. The water is featured of moisturizing and storing, illustrating that the kidney dominates the storage of essence and the water metabolism.

The inter-promoting and interacting relations of five-element theory are applied to explain the

致;而子病犯母,是指子行异常可影响及母行,其次序与相生次序相反。如水(肾)不涵木(肝),为母病及子;木(肝)病及水(肾),为子病犯母。

4   五行学说在中医学中的应用

4.1   用于说明五脏生理特性及其相互关系

运用五行特性来说明五脏的生理特性,从而将五脏分别归属于五行。如以木性舒展升发,表述肝喜调畅而恶抑郁;以火性温热炎上,表述心阳温煦周身;以土性受纳生化,表述脾主运化饮食精微,为气血生化之源;以金性肃杀收敛,表述肺气内守,以肃降为顺;以水性滋润闭藏,表述肾主藏精,主宰水液代谢。

运用五行相生相克的理论,以说明五脏生理功能之

mutual generating and mutual restraining relations of the physiological functions of five zang organs. In terms of the inter-promoting relation, wood promotes fire, so correspondingly the liver promotes the heart, displaying that the liver blood nourishes the heart spirit. Fire promotes earth, so correspondingly the heart promotes the spleen, displaying that the heart spirit regulates the transporting and transforming functions of the spleen. Earth promotes metal, so correspondingly the spleen promotes the lung, displaying that the food essence transported and transformed by the spleen nourishes the lung. Metal promotes water, so correspondingly the lung promotes the kidney, displaying that the clearing and descending functions of the lung assist the kidney to accept qi. Water promotes wood, so correspondingly the kidney promotes the liver, displaying that the kidney yin moisturizes and nourished the liver yin.

In terms of the interacting relation, wood acts on earth, so correspondingly the liver acts on the spleen, displaying that the smooth-flowing liver qi disperses and drains the blockage of the spleen-earth, so as to make its transporting and transforming functions to elaborate normally. Earth acts on water, so correspondingly the spleen acts on the kidney, displaying that the spleen's transporting and transforming functions on water prevents the overflow of the kidney water, leading to edema. Water acts on fire, so correspondingly the kidney acts on the heart, displaying that the sufficient kidney yin goes upward to nourish the heart, so as to restrain the hyperactivity of the heart fire. Fire acts on metal, so correspondingly the heart acts on the

间相互资生与相互制约的关系。如五脏的相生方面，木生火，对应于肝生心，表现为肝血可营养心神；火生土，对应于心生脾，表现为心神可调节脾的运化功能；土生金，对应于脾生肺，表现为脾运化水谷精微可濡养于肺；金生水，对应于肺生肾，表现为肺主肃降有助于肾主纳气；水生木，对应于肾生肝，表现为肾阴可滋养肝阴。

又如五脏的相克方面，木克土，对应于肝克脾，表现为肝气调畅能疏泄脾土的壅滞，使其运化功能正常发挥；土克水，对应于脾克肾，表现为脾主运化水液可防止肾水泛滥而生水肿等症；水克火，对应于肾克心，表现为肾阴充足而上济于心，可制约心火亢盛；火克金，对应于心克肺，表现为心阳温煦能抑制肺气肃降太过；金克木，对应于肺克肝，表现为肺气肃降下行能制约肝气，防止肝气过于升发而出现逆乱。

lung, displaying that the warming function of the heart yang inhibits the over-clearing and over-descending activities of the lung qi. Metal acts on wood, so correspondingly, the lung acts on the liver, displaying that the lung's clearing and descending function inhibits the liver, so as to prevent the counter-flow disturbance due to over-ascending activity of the liver qi.

4.2　Illustrate the mutual pathological relations of five zang organs

The five zang organs not only possess the mutual coordination and mutual operation physiologically, but also the mutual affection and mutual transference pathologically, i. e. the disease of one zang organ may transfer to other zang organs. The theory of five elements is applied to illustrate the mutual pathological relations of the five zang organs, including the overacting, counteracting and mother-son relations.

The overacting and counteracting relations are the pathological transferences due to the abnormality of the interacting relations. The overacting relation is a kind of pathological transference due to excessive interaction, with the same order as the interacting relation. For example, in the condition of the liver qi attacking the spleen transversely, the spleen qi is restrained to cause decrease of its function, leading to the spleen failing to transport and transform as the result. The counteracting relation is a kind of pathological transference due to the reverse action, with the opposite order as the interacting relation. For example, the lung acts on the liver in normal condition, but if the liver fire is too hyperactive, it counteracts on the lung instead, leading to the lung failing to clear and descend.

4.2　用于说明五脏病变的相互影响

五脏之间不仅在生理功能上互相协调,互相配合,在病理上也会相互影响,相互传变,即一脏有病可以传及他脏。运用五行学说来说明五脏病变的相互影响,包括相乘、相侮和子母相及两个方面。

相乘、相侮是相克关系异常所导致的病理传变。相乘是相克太过而发生的疾病传变,其次序与相克一致,如肝气横逆犯脾,脾气受制而功能减退,可导致脾失健运。相侮是反向克制而引起的疾病传变,其次序与相克相反,如肺本克肝,若肝火太亢反可侮肺,可导致肺失清肃等。

The mother-son involvement is the pathological transference caused by the abnormality of the inter-promoting relation. The mother disease involving the son refers that the disease is transferred from the mother zang organ to the son zang organ. For example, the hyperactive liver fire may affect the heart to cause the heart fire hyperactivity, leading to the pattern of heart and liver fire hyperactivity. This is the so-called the mother disease involving the son. The son disease involving the mother refers that the disease is transferred from the son zang organ to the mother zang organ. For example, the liver yin deficiency may involve the kidney to cause the kidney yin deficiency, leading to the pattern of liver and kidney yin deficiency as the result. This is the so-called the son disease involving the mother.

4.3 Guide the diagnosis of the diseases

In the theory of five elements, the five colors and five flavors correspond to the five zang organs of the liver, heart, spleen, lung and kidney respectively, and may be applied in the diagnosis of the diseases of the five zang organs. For example, the condition with green complexion, preference for sour-tasted food, or feeling of sour taste in mouth, can be diagnosed as the liver disease. The condition with red complexion and bitter taste in mouth can be diagnosed as the heart disease. The condition with the yellow complexion and sweet taste in mouth can be diagnosed as the spleen disease. The condition with the black complexion and salty taste in mouth can be diagnosed as the kidney disease.

4.4 Guide the treatment of the diseases

The theory of five elements applied in the treatment of the diseases includes the two aspects of

子母相及是相生关系异常导致的病理传变。母病及子是指疾病从母脏传变及子脏,如肝火亢盛,可影响及心,导致心火也亢盛,从而形成心肝火旺的证候,这便是母病及子的传变。子病及母是指疾病从子脏传变及母脏,如肝阴亏虚,日久及肾,引起肾阴也虚,这便是子病及母的传变。

4.3 用于疾病的诊断

在五行学说中,五色、五味,分别对应五脏,可直接用于五脏疾病的诊断。如面色青,喜食酸味,或口味酸,多可诊断为肝病;面色赤,口味苦,多可诊断为心病;面色黄,口味甘,多可诊断为脾病;面色黑,口味咸,多可诊断为肾病等。

4.4 用于疾病的治疗

五行学说在疾病治疗方面的运用,主要体现在控制

controlling the disease transference and of establishing the therapeutic principles.

4.4.1　Control the disease transference

According to the pathological overacting, counteracting and mother-son relations, the five zang organs in the diseased conditions can affect and transfer each other. Therefore, in the treatment of the disease, besides to treat the diseased zang organ directly, it is advisable to consider the possible affected zang organs to apply some preventive treatment, so as to control the disease transference. The application, the points for attention are as follows:

Firstly, it is necessary to choose the most easily-transferred zang organ to treat. For example, the liver disease, according to the theory of five elements, may transfer to the heart, lung, spleen or kidney. But in the actually clinic practice, the most easily affected zang organ is the spleen, so it is necessary to apply the preventive treatment for the spleen.

Secondly, it is necessary apply the treatment according to the functional state of the zang organ. It depends on the functional state of the spleen if the liver disease can transfer to the spleen. If the spleen qi is sufficient and its function is normal, the liver disease is not easy to transfer to the spleen. If the spleen is weak and cannot resist the liver disease transference, the spleen will be sick. Thus it is necessary to apply the treatment to strengthen the spleen, so as to prevent the transference.

4.4.2　Establish the therapeutic principles

It is necessary to consider the two aspects of the inter-promoting and interacting relations in establishing

疾病的传变以及确定治疗原则两个方面。

4.4.1　控制疾病传变

根据五行相乘相侮和子母相及的理论,五脏之间的病变是可以相互影响和传变的,因此在临床治疗时,除了针对有病内脏进行直接治疗外,还要考虑到可能被影响的内脏,及早采取一些预防性的治疗措施,以控制疾病的传变不过,在具体运用时,要注意以下两点:

一是选择容易被传及的内脏进行治疗。如按照五行理论来解释,肝脏有病是可以传及心、肺、脾、肾四脏的,但从临床实际来看,最容易受其影响的则是脾,所以应首先考虑对脾采取预防性的治疗措施。

二是根据内脏的功能状态来进行治疗。肝有病是否传及于脾,取决于脾脏本身的功能状态。若脾气充足,功能健全,则肝病不易传脾,也无需治脾;若脾脏虚弱,不能抵御肝病的传变,就会导致脾病,此时就必须配合健脾法治疗以防止传变。

4.4.2　确定治疗原则

根据五行理论确定治疗原则,可从相生与相克两个

the therapeutic principles according to the theory of five elements. The therapeutic principles established according to the inter-promoting relation are called "to reinforce the mother and to reduce the son".

"To reinforce the mother" is the therapeutic principle applied in the treatment of the deficiency pattern. It is said in Nan Jing that "reinforce the mother for the deficiency". The therapeutic principle to reinforce the mother is applied to treat the deficiency pattern caused by the deficiency of the mother which fails to promote the son. The method to reinforce "the mother" may support the depleted "son" so as to make strong for weak. For example, if the kidney yin is insufficient, the liver-wood loses its moisture and nourishment, leading to both liver and kidney yin deficiency. Therefore, it is advisable to apply the method to reinforce the kidney yin so as to moisturize and nourish the liver yin, called "to moisturize the water so as to support the wood".

"To reduce the son" is the therapeutic principle applied in the treatment of the excess pattern. It is said in Nan Jing that "reduce the son for the excess". The therapeutic principle to reduce the son is applied to treat the excess pattern caused by the mother disease involving the son. The method to reduce "the son" may discharge the preponderant Xie (Pathogenic) Qi. For example, if the liver fire is hyperactive, the heart fire fails to be restrained, leading to both heart and liver fire hyperactivity. Therefore, it is advisable to apply the method to reduce the heart so as to assist to clear and reduce the liver fire.

The therapeutic principles established according to the interacting relation are called "to restrain the

方面进行。根据相生关系确定的治疗原则,称为"补母泻子"。

补母,是应用于虚证时的治疗原则,《难经》称其为"虚则补其母"。补母的治则主要应用于因母虚不能生子而出现的虚证,通过补其"母"的方法使虚损的"子"得到资助而由弱转强。如肾阴不足,肝木失于滋养,而致肝肾之阴俱虚,可用补肾阴的方法以滋养肝阴,此法称为"滋水涵木"。

泻子,是应用于实证时的治疗原则,《难经》称其为"实则泻其子"。泻子的治则主要应用于因母病及子所出现的实证,通过泻子的方法使偏盛的邪气顺势而泄去。如肝火上炎,心火无制,而致心肝之火俱盛,可着重采取泻心之法,以助清泄肝火。

根据相克关系确定的治疗原则,称为"抑强扶弱"。

strong and to foster the weak", which are applied to regulate and adjust the great disparity state of strengthen between the two, so as to guide the recovery of the balanced and harmonious state of the five zang organs.

To restrain the strong and to foster the weak are two different methods, which are mutually related. To restrain the strong may reduce the excessive qi without bullying the weak, while to foster the weak may reinforce the deficient qi without being controlled by the strong. The methods to restrain the strong and to foster the weak can be single-applied, but they are applied together in most conditions. For example, the liver qi tends to attack the spleen-earth transversely, while the depleted spleen qi tends to be attacked by the liver qi. Therefore, for the pattern of liver qi attacking spleen, it is advisable to apply the method to restrain the wood and to foster the earth (i. e. to restrain the liver and to foster the spleen), to reduce the liver qi on one hand, and reinforce the spleen qi on the other hand, for the purpose to cure the disease by regulating both the liver and spleen simultaneously.

抑强扶弱,就是针对强弱不和的力量悬殊状态,引导五脏恢复平和协调状态。

抑强与扶弱虽为两种不同之法,但二者之间是相互关联的。只有通过抑强,才能泻其太过之气而不致对弱者进行欺侮;只有通过扶弱,才能补其不及之气而不受强者的克制。抑强和扶弱可以单独使用,但大多数情形下宜联合使用。如肝气横逆则易乘犯脾土,而脾气虚弱也易受肝气的乘袭,所以对于肝气犯脾的病证,就可采取抑木扶土(即抑肝扶脾)的方法,一方面泻肝气,一方面补脾气,肝脾同调,以利病愈。

Chapter 2 Qi, Blood and Body Fluid

Qi, blood and body fluid are the foundational substances which maintain the normal vital activities of the human body. They are the material products of the transforming functions of the zang-fu organs, and function to warm, moisturize and nourish the zang-fu organs, sense organs and tissues as well.

In terms of the properties of qi, blood and body fluid, qi is intangible and motive and functions to warm and promote, pertaining to yang, while the blood and body fluid are tangible and visible and function to nourish and moisturize, pertaining to yin.

Section 1 Qi

1 Concept of qi

According to ancient Chinese philosophy, qi is the fundamental substance constituting the universe and all things on earth. All things in the nature are constitutes of qi, as well as the life which is produced by the movement and mutation of qi. The survival and perishing of all creatures depend on the aggregation and scatter of qi. They survive if qi aggregates, while they perish if qi scatters.

Qi is featured of the strong mobility, being in the constant movement. In terms of its shape and property, qi is a refined substance, in a dispersing

---

第 2 章
气血津液

气血津液是人体生命活动的基本物质,其既是脏腑气化功能的产物,又对脏腑等器官组织起到温煦濡养作用。

就气血津液的性质而言,气无形而动,具有温养、推动作用,故属阳;血与津液,有形可见,具有濡养、滋润作用,故属阴。

第 1 节 气

1 气的概念

中国古代哲学认为,气是构成宇宙万物的本原性物质,自然界的一切皆由气构成,生命也是在气的运动变化中产生的,一切生命的存亡在于气的聚散,气聚则生,气散则亡。

气的特征是活力很强,并处于不断运动之中。气的形质极其精微,气呈弥散状

state, invisible to the naked eyes, so it is said that "qi is originally intangible". "Qi" in TCM is deeply influenced by ancient Chinese philosophy.

In terms of the concept of qi in the human body, it is believed in TCM that qi is a kind of essential substance to constitute human body and maintain the vital activities of human body.

The reasons why qi is the fundamental substance to constitute the human body are as follows: Firstly, the production of all creatures is from qi, while human being is one of the creatures, which are produced from qi of the heaven and earth. It is said in Huang Di Nei Jing (*Yellow Emperor's Inner Canon*) that "the human being is produced from qi of the heaven and earth, and naturally regulated by the four seasons", and that "the merged qi of the heaven and earth is called the human being". Secondly, all the fundamental substances to form up the human body, as the blood, essence and body fluid, and all the basic structures of the human body, as the zang organs, fu organs, tissues and orifices are produced from qi aggregation.

The reasons why qi is the essential substance to maintain the vital activities of the human body are as follows: Firstly, the human body, produced in the natural world, cannot exist without the necessary nutrient materials supported by qi of the heaven and earth, for example, the Qing (Clear) Qi inhaled by the lung, and the Gu (Grain) Qi taken in by the stomach. Secondly, the up-flowing, down-flowing, out-flowing and inflowing movements of qi in the human body are the fundamental forms and

态,肉眼难以觉察,故有"气本无形"之说。中医学中的"气",深受中国古代哲学的影响。

作为人体之气的基本概念,中医学认为气是构成人体的最基本物质和维持人体生命活动具有很强活力的精微物质。

强调气是构成人体的最基本物质,其立论依据主要有二:一是强调万物化生皆源于气,人为万物之一,也由天地之气所生,即《黄帝内经》所说的"人以天地之气生,四时之法成","天地合气,命之曰人"。二是组成人体的最基本物质,如血、精、津液等,人体的基本组织如脏、腑、体、窍等,也是由气聚合而成的。

强调气是维持人体生命活动的精微物质,其立论依据也主要有二:一是人生成于自然界之中,一刻也离不开天地之气对人体生命活动所提供的必需的营养物质,如肺吸入的清气,胃摄入的谷气等。二是人体之气的升降出入运动是维持其生命活动的基本形式和动力来源,

motive power to maintain the vital activities. Because of its features of strong activity and constant movement, qi stimulates and promotes the vital activities of human body. If the movement of qi ceases, the vital activities stop.

2　Formation of qi

The formation of qi is based upon three sources, i. e. the congenital Jing (Essence) Qi gained from the parents, the Jing (Essence) Qi of water and grain gained from the food intake and the Qing (Clear) Qi in the nature. The synthetically physiological functions of the kidney, spleen-stomach and lung integrate the three into qi.

The congenital Jing (Essence) Qi comes from the reproductive essence of the parents. The reproductive essence of the parents is the primary substance to constitute the embryo of human body and make it grow and develop, so it is called "the congenital essence". It is believed in the theory of TCM that the congenital essence, stored in the kidney, is the major component part of the Jing (Essence) Qi in the kidney and functions to govern the growth, development and reproduction of the human body. Without the congenital Jing (Essence) Qi, there is no possibility to produce the human life and no possibility to constitute qi of the human body.

The Jing (Essence) Qi of water and grain, coming from the food intake, is the nutrient substance in the food. The human body takes in the food, while the spleen and stomach transport and transform the food, to absorb the food's nutrient composition and distribute it all over the body, be-

因为气具有活力很强、不断运动的特性,人体的生命活动实际上都是在气的激发推动下产生的,如果气的运动一旦停息,就意味着生命活动的终止。

2　气的生成

人体之气的生成来源主要有三个方面,即禀受于父母的先天精气、饮食物中的水谷精气和存在于自然界中的清气,通过肾、脾胃和肺等脏腑生理功能的综合作用,将三者结合起来而生成的。

先天精气,源于父母的生殖之精。由于父母的生殖之精是构成人体胚胎发育的原始物质,故称为"先天之精"。中医学理论认为,先天之精藏于肾中,是肾中精气的主要组成部分,人体的生长、发育和繁衍后代均以此为基础。没有先天精气,也就不可能产生人的生命,更无从谈论人体之气的生成。

水谷精气,来源于饮食物,即饮食物中的营养物质。人体摄入饮食后,经脾胃的运化作用,吸收其中的营养成分,输布于全身,成为维持人体生命活动的营养和化生

coming the nutrient to maintain the vital activities of human body and the major substantial source to transform and produce qi and blood. Since it originates from the taken-in food after birth, it is also called "the acquired essence".

The Qing (Clear) Qi in the nature is inhaled by the respiratory function of the lung. After birth, the human starts to respire. The inhaled Qing (Clear) Qi is the important component part of qi of the human body, so the vital activities of human body cannot be conducted without the constant inhalation of the Qing (Clear) Qi in the nature.

The source of human qi is divided into the congenital Jing (Essence) Qi, the Jing (Essence) Qi of water and grain, and the Qing (Clear) Qi in the nature. After the human qi is formed, it is necessary to realize the physiological functions of the kidney, spleen-stomach and lung in a mutual coordination, so as to make the human qi abundant, and bring the qi's physiological efficacy into full play. On the contrary, if the physiological functions of the kidney, spleen-stomach and lung are abnormal, it may influence the formation of qi and the normal implementation of qi's physiological efficacy. For example, if the kidney fails to store essence or the congenital essence is insufficient, if the transporting and transforming function of the spleen and stomach is abnormal, leading to the poor production of the Jing (Essence) Qi of water and grain, or if the respiration of lung is abnormal or the gas exchange *in vivo* and *in vitro* is abnormal, it may influence the formation of qi and its physiological function, leading to the reduction of qi or the decrease of the qi's functions. This is also the theoretical basis why

气血的主要物质来源。由于其来源于出生后摄入的饮食物,故又可称之为"后天之精"。

自然界清气,依靠肺的呼吸功能吸入。人出生后,即开始呼吸。吸入的清气,是人体气的重要组成部分,人体生命活动一刻也离不开自然界清气的不断吸入。

人体之气的来源,虽然可分为先天精气、水谷精气和自然界清气三个方面,但人体之气的生成,必须通过肾、脾胃、肺等生理功能的作用,并相互协调,才能使人体之气充沛,气的生理效应得以充分发挥。反之,肾、脾胃、肺等生理功能失常,均会影响气的生成,或影响气的生理效应的正常发挥。如肾失封藏或先天禀赋不足,脾胃运化功能失调,水谷精气生化匮乏,肺的呼吸功能失常,体内外气体交换受阻等种种因素,都会影响气的生成及其生理作用,从而导致人体之气的衰少或气的功能减退。临床上调治气虚每从肾、脾胃、肺入手,其理论依据即在于此。

it is necessary to stress on the kidney, spleen-stomach and lung in the clinic treatment of the qi deficiency pattern.

Furthermore, we should pay great attention to the transporting and transforming function of the spleen and stomach in the process of qi formation of the human body. The reason is that after birth, the human body relies on the food essence transported and transformed from the spleen and stomach to maintain the vital activities. So it is said that "one will be prosperous when he gains the food, while one will perish when he loses the food". Besides, the congenital Jing (Essence) Qi in the kidney must rely on the constant cultivation and support of the acquired Jing (Essence) Qi of water and grain, so as to give full play to its normal physiological efficacy.

3　Functions of qi

Qi is the fundamental substance to form up the human body and to maintain various physiological activities of human body. Qi has various kinds of physiological functions in different zang-fu organs and other the organs and tissues. Qi has five types of physiological functions as follows:

3.1　Promoting function

The promoting function of qi is the primary motive power of the functional activities of all zang-fu organs and tissues of human body, so called the basis of the human life. Due to various kinds of zang-fu organs and tissues where qi stays, its physiological functions are different. For example, the kidney qi functions to promote the growth, development and reproduction of human body, and to transform the water. The heart qi functions to pro-

此外,在人体之气生成过程中,尤其要重视脾胃运化功能的作用。这是因为,人出生以后,必须依赖于脾胃运化而来的水谷精微才能维持其生命活动,即所谓"得谷者昌,绝谷者亡"。同时,肾中的先天精气,也必须依赖于后天水谷精气的不断培育和补充,才能持满而发挥其正常的生理效应。

3　气的作用

气是构成人体和维持人体各种生理活动的基本物质。气在不同脏腑、器官中发挥着多种多样的生理作用。归纳而言,气主要具有以下五种生理作用。

3.1　推动作用

气的推动作用,是人体所有脏腑器官功能活动的原动力,所以气被称为人体生命之根本。由于气所在脏腑器官的不同,所发挥的生理作用也各不相同。如肾气,能推动人体的生长发育和生殖功能,并能气化水液;心气,能推动血液运行;肺气,

mote the blood circulation. The lung qi functions to govern the respiratory movement, and to regulate and open the water passage. The spleen qi functions to promote the digestion and absorption of food, and to control the blood. The liver qi functions to regulate the qi activities so as to give full play to its regulating and adjusting function. If the promoting function of qi decreases, the various kinds of deficiency patterns of the related zang-fu organs may occur.

3.2 Warming function

The warming function of qi is the source of the thermal energy of human body, possessing the important significance in maintaining the normal body temperature and guaranteeing the physiological functions of all zang-fu organs. The warming function of qi is a kind of yang-attributed functional manifestation, so called "the yang qi". Each of the five zang organs has its yang qi. For example, the heart yang functions to warm and open the blood vessels, so as to promote the blood circulation. The lung yang functions to warm and nourish the skin and hair, so as to defend the body from invasion of the exogenous Xie (Pathogenic) Qi. The spleen yang functions to warm and transform the food, so as to promote the digestion and absorption. The liver yang functions to lift and stimulate the qi activities and to inspire the transforming function of five zang and six fu organs. The kidney yang functions to inspire the reproduction and to transpire and transform water. If the warming function of qi decreases, the patterns of endogenous yin cold, unsmooth circulation of qi and blood, and dysfunction of zang-fu organs may occur.

能主宰呼吸运动、主管通调水道;脾气,能推动对饮食的消化吸收,并能统摄血液;肝气,能疏泄气机而发挥多种调节功能等。气的推动作用减退,便可出现相关脏腑的各种虚损性病证。

3.2 温煦作用

气的温煦作用,是人体热能产生的来源,对于人体维持正常体温,保证各脏腑器官生理功能的发挥,具有十分重要的意义。气的温煦作用是一种属阳的功能表现,所以气被称为"阳气"。五脏各有阳气。如心阳能温通血脉,促进血液运行;肺阳能温养皮毛腠理,防御外邪侵袭;脾阳能温化水谷饮食,促进消化吸收;肝阳能升发气机,鼓舞五脏六腑之气化;肾阳能激发生殖功能,同时对水液有蒸腾气化作用。气的温煦作用减弱,主要表现为阴寒内生,气血运行不畅,相关脏腑功能低下。

3.3　Defending function

The defending function of qi is the essential condition of the human body in resisting various kinds of Xie (Pathogenic) Qi and to prevent the occurrence of diseases. Opposite to the Xie (Pathogenic) Qi, the qi with the defending function is called the Zheng (Anit-Pathogenic) Qi. The defending function of the Zheng (Anti-Pathogenic) Qi includes two aspects: one is to defend the body surface to prevent the invasion of the exogenous pathogens, while another is to fight against the Xie (Pathogenic) Qi and to remove the exogenous pathogens so as to cure the disease that is caused by the invasion of the Xie (Pathogenic) Qi. If the defending function of qi decreases, the anti-disease ability and recovery ability of body will decrease, or the body will be easier to be attacked by the Xie (Pathogenic) Qi, or the body will be difficult to recover after disease.

3.4　Checking function

The checking function of qi refers that qi functions to restrain and accept the liquid-state substances of blood, body fluid and essence and to prevent them from losing. For example, qi functions to check the blood, to make the blood circulate inside the vessels and to prevent it from spilling over the vessels. Qi functions to check the sweat, urine and saliva, to control their secretion and excretion, to make them moderate in discharging and to prevent them from abnormal loss. Qi functions to check the sperms, to make the sexual function harmonious and to prevent the abnormal loss of sperms. Besides, the defecation and the constant positions of internal organs are also influenced by the checking function of

3.3　防御作用

气的防御作用,是人体抵御各种邪气、防止疾病发生的根本条件。针对"邪气"而言,发挥防御作用的气被称为"正气"。正气的防御作用具体表现在两方面:一是能护卫全身肌表,防御外邪入侵;二是一旦邪气入侵而发病后,正气能与邪气抗争,消除外邪,促使病愈。气的防御作用减弱,主要变现为机体抗邪、康复能力低下,或易受邪气侵犯,或病后不易康复。

3.4　固摄作用

气的固摄作用,主要是对血液、津液、精液等液态物质具有收敛、摄纳并防止其流失的功能。如气能固摄血液,使血液循脉而行,防止其逸出脉外;气能固摄汗液、尿液、唾液等,控制其分泌与排泄,使其有节制地排出,防止异常流失;气能固摄精液,使性功能协调,防止精液无故流失。此外,大便的排泄和内脏位置的恒定也受气的固摄作用的影响。若气的固摄作用减弱,主要表现为出血、

qi. If the checking function of qi decreases, there will be the diseases of hemorrhage, spontaneous sweating, excessive urination, salivation, seminal e-mission, chronic diarrhea, incontinence of defecation or urination, prolapse of rectum or uterus.

3.5　Transforming function

The transforming function of qi implies various mutations caused by the activities of qi. The transforming function of qi is the essential cause of the life process of birth, growth, development and ageing. The transforming function of qi involves a broad scope of vital activities as: Firstly, the human body obtains the nutrients from the outside through food intake and respiration, and then transforms them into the vital substances of essence, qi, blood and body fluid for the human body. Secondly, qi regulates and controls the mutual transformation of various essential substances inside the body, so the transforming function of qi is the process of self-regulation, self-perfection and self-balance of the body. Thirdly, qi functions to discharge the waste and the Zhuo (Turbid) Qi produced in the vital process. If the transforming function of qi decreases, the whole vital process will be disturbed or depleted, so as to cause various kinds of diseases.

4　Movement of qi

Qi is a kind of essential substance with strong vitality, with the feature of constant movement. The forms of qi movement different in various zang-fu organs and tissues, but the basic forms are nothing but four types of up-flow, down-flow, outflow and inflow.

The up-flow and down-flow of qi are the

自汗、多尿、流涎、遗精以及久泄、二便失禁，以及脱肛、子宫脱垂等症。

3.5　气化作用

气化，泛指由气的运动而产生的各种变化。气具有气化作用，是生命产生、发育、成长、衰老等一系列过程的根本原因。气化所涉及的生命运动极其广泛，大体可以概括为三个方面：第一，人体通过饮食、呼吸等从外界摄取营养物质，并把它转化成人体自身所需要的精、气、血、津液等生命物质；第二，调控体内各种精微物质的相互转化，是机体自我调整、完善、平衡的内在过程；第三，在生命过程中产生废物、浊气，向体外排出。气的气化作用减弱，整个生命过程就会紊乱或衰退，从而导致各种疾病。

4　气的运动

人体的气，是具有很强活力的精微物质，其主要特征在于不断地运动。气的运动形式，随所在脏腑器官的不同而各异，但其基本形式，不外乎升、降、出、入四种。

升降是上下之间的运

up-down movements. The up-flow and down-flow are the opposite movements, but they may transform mutually. When qi up-flows to the extreme point, it then down-flows, the so-called "extreme up-flow causing down-flow". When qi down-flows to the extreme point, it then up-flows, the so-called "extreme down-flow causing up-flow". It is the up-down circular movement of qi in the normal situation.

The outflow and inflow of qi are the out-in movements. The outflow and inflow are the opposite movements, but they are always in a circular movement. When qi spreads outwards (outflows) to a certain degree, it then converges inwards (inflows). When qi converges inwards (inflows) to a certain degree, then it spreads outwards (outflows). It is the out-in circular movement of qi in the normal situation.

Actually, the up-flow, down-flow, outflow and inflow are two different types of yin-yang movements, which possess a mutually coordinating function. The up-flow and outflow pertain to yang, while the down-flow and inflow to yin. Therefore, there is mutual coordination between the up-flow and outflow as well as between the down-flow and inflow. That is to say, it will influence the outflow and inflow if the up-flow and down-flow are normal or not, while it will influence the up-flow and down-flow if the outflow and inflow are normal or not.

The up-flow, down-flow, outflow and inflow of qi in human body are realized through the zang-fu organ and meridians. Qi of each of the zang-fu organ may possess the different movement forms of

动。升与降虽然相反，但两者之间可以相互转化。当升到极点时，就会转而下降，这叫做"升已而降"；当降到极点时，就会转而上升，这叫做"降已而升"。这是正常情况下气的上下循环运动。

出入是内外之间的运动。出与入虽然相反，但两者之间也是交替进行的。当气向外发散（出）到一定阶段，就会转而向内收敛（入）；当气向内收敛（入）到一定阶段时，就会转而向外发散。这是正常情况下气的内外循环运动。

升降与出入实际上是阴阳运动的两种不同形式，两者具有某种相互协调作用。如升、出皆属阳，降、入皆属阴，所以，升与出、降与入之间也是相互协调的。也就是说，升降正常与否会影响到出入，出入正常与否也会影响到升降。

人体之气的升降出入，是通过脏腑、经络来实现的。每一脏腑之气都可以具有升降出入不同的运动方式，但

up-flow, down-flow, outflow and inflow, but it has its own particular emphasis. For example, the liver qi gives priority to the up-flow, while the lung qi to the down-flow. The spleen qi gives priority to the up-flow, while the stomach qi to down-flow. Such related zang-fu organs are mutually coordinated in the up-flow, down-flow, outflow and inflow movements, so as to form up a unique regulating mode of qi activities in the human body. There is a mutual depending and mutual restraining relation between the up-flow of liver qi and down-flow of lung qi, and between the spleen qi dominating the up-flow of the clear and the stomach qi dominating the down-flow of the turbid. The meridians and collaterals are the important passage of qi activities. Due to different course directions of the meridians and collaterals, the up-flow, down-flow, outflow and inflow of the meridian qi are different. The meridians inside runs from the internal to the surface, qi inside the meridians moves outwards. The meridians on body surface run from the surface to the internal, qi inside the meridians moves inwards. The meridians run from the head to foot, qi inside moves downwards. The meridians run from the foot to head, qi inside moves upwards.

The up-flow, down-flow, outflow and inflow movements of qi are very important to the human life. When the up-flow, down-flow, outflow and inflow movements of qi are normal, the functions of the zang-fu organs and meridians will be normal, and vice versa. When the up-flow, down-flow, outflow and inflow movements of qi stop, the life stops.

各有侧重不同。如肝气以升为主,肺气则以降为主;脾气以升为主,胃气则以降为主,等等。脏腑间有侧重的升降出入相互配合协调,形成了人体独特的气机调节方式。如肝气升发与肺气肃降、脾气主升清与胃气主降浊之间,就存在着互相依赖、互相制约的关系。经络是气机运动的重要通道,由于经络的走向不同,其经络之气的升降出入也有所不同。在内的经络从里出表,气也随之向外运行;体表的经络从外入内,气也随之向内运行。经脉从头下行,气也随之下降;经脉从足上行,气也随之上升。

气的升降出入运动,对于人体生命是极其重要的。升降出入功能正常,脏腑、经络的功能才会正常;反之亦然。升降出入运动停止,生命就会停息。

5　Classification of qi

According to the productive sources, distributive positions and functional characteristics, qi of human body has many different names, but the Yuan (Primary) Qi, Zong (Pectoral) Qi, Ying (Nutrient) Qi and Wei (Defensive) Qi are the four major ones.

5.1　Yuan (Primary) Qi

The Yuan (Primary) Qi is the most essential qi of the human body. Yuan implies source and basis. The primary motive power of human life relies on the Yuan (Primary) Qi.

5.1.1　Production of the Yuan (Primary) Qi

The Yuan (Primary) Qi comes from the congenital essence, transformed from the kidney qi of the parents in the embryonic period. Therefore, this type of Yuan (Primary) Qi in TCM is called "the congenital qi". After birth of a person, the strength and volume of his congenital Yuan (Primary) Qi has been determined, but it needs further support. The human body obtains the nutrient substances from food to support the congenital Yuan (Primary) Qi, to make the Yuan (Primary) Qi more substantial, and to distribute it over the whole body to realize the normal physiological efficacy. Therefore, the sufficiency of the Yuan (Primary) Qi also relies on the supports of the acquired qi.

5.1.2　Distribution of the Yuan (Primary) Qi

The Yuan (Primary) Qi is stored in the kidney and distributes over the whole body through the triple energizer. All the tissues and organs, including the zang-fu organs, meridians and collaterals, tissues and orifices, are the place of the up-flow,

5　气的分类

由于气的生成来源、分布部位、功能特点的不同，人体之气有许多不同名称，主要有元气、宗气、营气、卫气四种。

5.1　元气

元气是人体最根本的气。元，有本源、根本之义。人体生命力的原动力在于元气。

5.1.1　元气的生成

元气来源于先天，是在胚胎时期禀受于父母的肾气。因此，中医学常把这种元气称为"先天之气"。人出生以后，先天元气的强弱多少即已确定。但出生以后，元气还有一个充养的过程。人体通过后天饮食获取营养物质，以充养先天之元气，使元气进一步充实，才能布散全身而发挥正常的生理效应。所以，元气的充盛，同样有赖于后天之气的供养。

5.1.2　元气的分布

元气藏于肾中，通过三焦流布到全身，脏腑经络、形体官窍等组织器官均为元气升降出入之所。总之，肾为元气之根源，三焦为元气运

down-flow, outflow and inflow of the Yuan (Primary) Qi. In brief, the kidney is the source of the Yuan (Primary) Qi, while the triple energizer is the circulatory passage of the Yuan (Primary) Qi, which spreads over the whole body to realize its physiological efficacy.

5.1.3　Functions of the Yuan (Primary) Qi

The Yuan (Primary) Qi has two physiological functions as: Firstly, it functions to promote and inspire the growth, development and reproduction of the human body. The strength and volume of the Jing (Essence) Qi in the kidney are closely related to the birth, growth, development, ageing and death. When the Jing (Essence) Qi in the kidney starts to be sufficient, the human body starts to grow and develop. When the Jing (Essence) Qi in the kidney is the most sufficient, the human life enters a luxuriant stage. When the Jing (Essence) Qi in the kidney is getting deficient, the human body enters an ageing stage. Secondly, it functions to promote and inspire the physiological functions of the zang-fu organs, and the meridians and collaterals. The constant movement and mutation of the Yuan (Primary) Qi promote various physiological activities of the human body. Generally, the Yuan (Primary) Qi is the primary motive power of the human vital activities. If the Yuan (Primary) Qi is sufficient, the growth and development of the human body are normal, the body constitution is strong, and the zang-fu organs, meridians and collaterals are vigorous. If the Jing (Essence) Qi in the kidney is not sufficient due to congenital deficiency, or acquired dystrophy, or exhaustion in chronic diseases, the Yuan (Primary) Qi will be lack of sub-

行之通道,流布周身于发挥其生理效应。

5.1.3　元气的功能

元气的主要生理功能有二:一是推动和激发人体的生长、发育和生殖。肾中精气的盛衰对人体生、长、壮、老、有着密切关系。肾中精气始盛,人体因此而生长、发育;肾中精气充盛,人体生命过程进入旺盛阶段;肾中精气始衰,人体也随之进入衰老过程。二是推动和激发脏腑、经络的生理功能。元气的不断运动和变化,推动着机体的各种生理活动。总之,元气是人体生命活动的原动力。机体的元气充沛,人体的生长、发育就正常,体质就强健,脏腑、经络的活力就旺盛。若因先天禀赋不足,或因后天失养,久病耗损,肾中精气不足,元气生化乏源,即可产生种种病变。若年迈之体,元气渐趋耗竭,生命亦随之终止。

stance to be produced and transformed. As a result, various diseases may occur. In an aged body, the Yuan (Primary) Qi is getting exhausted gradually, and the life will stop in the end.

5.2 Zong (Pectoral) Qi

The Zong (Prctoral) Qi is a type of qi locating in the chest. The place where the Zong (Pectoral) Qi gathers is called "Danzhong", also termed as "the sea of qi", because it is the place where the whole body qi is the most convergent.

5.2.1 Production of the Zong (Pectoral) Qi

The Zong (Pectoral) Qi is composed of the natural Qing (Clear) Qi inhaled by the lung and the food essence absorbed and transported from the spleen. Therefore, it may influence the sufficiency or deficiency of the Zong (Pectoral) Qi if the lung's respiratory function and the spleen's transporting-transforming function are normal or not.

5.2.2 Distribution of the Zong (Pectoral) Qi

The Zong (Pectoral) Qi converges in the chest, where is called "the sea of qi". The heart and lung locate in the chest, so the Zong (Pectoral) Qi infuses in the heart vessels and circulates in the blood vessels and respiratory tract. The sufficiency or deficiency of the Zong (Pectoral) Qi may influence the functions of the heart vessels and lung system.

5.2.3 Functions of the Zong (Pectoral) Qi

The Zong (Pectoral) Qi has two major functions as: Firstly, it functions to warm and nourish the heart vessels, so as to maintain the circulation of qi and blood. Secondly, it functions to warm and nourish the lung system, so as to maintain the respiratory and speaking functions. Therefore, if the Zong (Pectoral) Qi is not sufficient, there may be

5.2 宗气

宗气,是积聚于胸中的气。宗气积聚之处称为"膻中",因其为全身气最集中的地方,故又名"气海"。

5.2.1 宗气的生成

宗气是由肺吸入的自然之清气和由脾吸收转输而来的水谷之精微相结合而生成。肺的呼吸功能和脾的运化功能正常与否,都会影响宗气的盛衰。

5.2.2 宗气的分布

宗气积聚于胸中,故称胸中为"气海"。心肺居于胸中,故宗气能贯注于心脉,并能行于血脉和呼吸道。宗气的盛衰,可以影响心脉、肺系的功能。

5.2.3 宗气的功能

宗气的主要功能有二:一是温养心脉,以维持其运行气血的功能;二是温养肺系,以维持其司呼吸和发声的功能。因此,若宗气不足,可出现心悸、呼吸气短、声音低弱等症。

symptoms of palpitation, shortness of breath, light and weak voice in speaking, etc.

5.3   Ying (Nutrient) Qi and Wei (Defensive) Qi

The Ying (Nutrient) Qi circulates inside the vessels along with the blood, so there is such a saying of "the Ying (Nutrient) Qi and blood". In comparison with the Wei (Defensive) Qi that circulates outside the vessels, the Ying (Nutrient) Qi pertains to yin, so it is also called "the Ying (Nutrient) Yin". The Wei (Defensive) Qi pertains to yang, so it is also called "the Wei (Defensive) Yang".

5.3.1   Production of the Ying (Nutrient) Qi and Wei (Defensive) Qi

The Ying (Nutrient) Qi is produced from the food essence obtained in the transportation and transformation of the spleen and stomach. The refining and nourishing part of the food essence enters the vessels to transform into the Ying (Nutrient) Qi. It is called "the Jing (Essence) Qi of water and grain" in Huang Di Nei Jing (*Yellow Emperor's Inner Canon*). The so-called Jing (Essence) Qi refers to the refining substance with nourishing function.

The Wei (Defensive) Qi is also produced from the food essence. The vigorous part of the food essence which is not restrained by vessels transforms into the Wei (Defensive) Qi. It is called "the Han (Fierce) Qi of water and grain" in Huang Di Nei Jing (*Yellow Emperor's Inner Canon*). The so-called Han (Fierce) Qi refers to the vigorous qi that circulates outside the vessels.

5.3.2   Distribution of the Ying (Nutrient) Qi and Wei (Defensive) Qi

Because of the difference of the Ying (Nutrient) Qi and Wei (Defensive) Qi in yin and yang at-

5.3   营气与卫气

营气行于脉中,与血同行,故多"营血"并称。营气与行于脉外的卫气相对而言,营气属阴,故称"营阴";卫气属阳,故称"卫阳"。

5.3.1   营气与卫气的生成

营气的生成,是以脾胃运化而生成的水谷精微为主要成分,水谷精微中的精专部分得以入于脉中而化为营气,《黄帝内经》称其为"水谷之精气"。所谓精气,是指极具濡养功能的精微物质。

卫气的生成,也是以水谷精微作为其主要成分。水谷精微中活力极强而不受脉道约束的这类物质,化为卫气,《黄帝内经》称其为"水谷之悍气"。所谓悍气,是指其气慓疾滑利而运行脉外。

5.3.2   营气与卫气的分布

由于营气与卫气在性质上有阴、阳之别,所以在运行

tributions, they circulate differently inside and outside the vessels respectively. The Ying (Nutrient)
Qi transformed from the Jing (Essence) Qi of water
and grain, pertaining to yin, so it circulates inside
the vessels. The Wei (Defensive) Qi transformed
from the Han (Fierce) Qi of water and grain, pertaining to yang, so it circulates outside the vessels.
Simultaneously, because the Ying (Nutrient) Qi
pertains to yin, while the Wei (Defensive) Qi to
yang, the Ying (Nutrient) Qi mostly distributes in
the internal organs, while the Wei (Defensive) Qi
mostly in the body surface. Of course, there is also
the Wei (Defensive) Qi in the internal organs,
while there is also the Ying (Nutrient) Qi in the
body surface. The only difference is the particular
emphasis on the distributive areas of the Ying (Nutrient) Qi and Wei (Defensive) Qi.

5.3.3　Functions of the Ying (Nutrient) Qi and Wei (Defensive) Qi

The Ying (Nutrient) Qi and Wei (Defensive)
Qi have different functions.

The major functions of the Ying (Nutrient) Qi
are as: Firstly, it functions to transform and produce the blood. Secondly, it functions to nourish
the whole body. The Ying (Nutrient) Qi circulates
inside the vessels, combining with the body fluid infused into the vessels, so as to produce the blood.
The saying that "qi produces the blood" implies the
blood transformed from the Ying (Nutrient) Qi.
The Ying (Nutrient) is transformed from the
refining part of the food essence, becoming the necessary nutrient substance for the physiological activities of the zang-fu organs, and meridians and collaterals, so it is important to maintain the human vi-

径路上有脉内、脉外之异。
营气得水谷精微之精气,性
质属阴,故运行于脉内;卫气
得水谷精微之悍气,性质属
阳,故运行于脉外。同时,由
于营气属阴,卫气属阳,所以
营气得以分布于内脏,卫气
的分布则偏于体表。当然,
内脏也有卫气,体表也有营
气,只是营气与卫气的主要
分布部分有所侧重而已。

5.3.3　营气与卫气的功能

营气与卫气的功能特点
各不相同。

营气的主要功能,一是
化生血液,二是营养全身。
营气行于脉中,并使津液亦
渗入脉内,两者结合,生成血
液。所谓气能生血,主要是
对营气化生血液而言。营气
由水谷精微中的精专部分所
化生,是脏腑、经络等生理活
动所必需的营养物质,对人
体生命活动的维持起着重要
作用。

tal activities.

The major functions of the Wei (Defensive) Qi are as: Firstly, it functions to warm and nourish the body. Secondly, it functions to regulate the body temperature. Thirdly, it functions to prevent the invasion of the exogenous pathogens. To warm the body implies to warm the body surface, as the particular manifestation of the warming function of the Wei (Defensive) Yang Qi distributing in the body surface. To regulate the body temperature is realized through the regulating the sweating volume from the pores by the Wei (Defensive) Qi. To prevent the invasion of the exogenous pathogens is the centralized manifestation of defending function of the Wei (Defensive) Qi. If the Wei (Defensive) Qi is deficient, there may be the symptoms of fear of cold, spontaneous sweating, easily catching cold, etc.

卫气的主要功能,一是温养肌体,二是调节体温,三是防御外邪。其中,温养肌体,尤以温养肌表为主,正是敷布于体表的卫阳之气的温煦功能的体现。调节体温,主要通过卫气调控汗孔出汗量来实现。防御外邪,也正是卫表之气抗邪机能的集中体现。若卫气虚弱,就可能出现畏寒、自汗、易感冒等表现。

Section 2   Blood

1   Concept of blood

The blood is a kind of red and thick liquid, composed of the Ying (Nutrient) Qi and body fluid and circulating inside the vessels. The blood possesses the nourishing and moisturizing functions and the important significance in maintaining the human life.

The blood is closely related to the five zang organs. The five zang organs can realize their normal physiological functions on the basis the nourishing and moisturizing functions of the blood, while the blood can be transformed and produced continu-

第 2 节   血

1   血的概念

血主要由营气和津液所组成,运行于脉道之中,是色红质稠的液体。血具有营养和滋润作用,对于维持人的生命具有极重要意义。

血与五脏的关系非常密切。五脏需要血的营养和滋润作用,才能发挥其正常的功能,而血也需要五脏功能的共同作用,才能源源不断

ously on the basis of the common functions of the five zang organs.

2　Formation of blood

The substantial foundation of the blood is the essence, including the congenital essence (the kidney essence) and the acquired essence (the food essence). The congenital essence is the initial condition of the blood formation, while the acquired essence has to combine with the congenital essence so as to produce the blood. Therefore, if the congenital kidney essence is not sufficient, the blood is lack of substantial source. However, after birth, the acquired essence has the most decisive function. Therefore, the function of the spleen and stomach has the decisive function in the formation of the blood. If the functions of the spleen and stomach are normal, they may absorb sufficient essence and body fluid from the food to transform into the blood. If the functions of the spleen and stomach decrease, they fail to absorb sufficient essence and body fluid, the blood is lack of necessarily productive source.

The process that the essence transforms into blood is a transforming process of qi, depending upon the functions of qi. The organs involved in the transforming process of qi are the heart and lung. The transforming function of the heart in the process of blood formation is called "to transform into red color" in Huang Di Nei Jing. It is believed that when the function of the heart dominating the blood and vessels is normal, the blood can be transformed into red color. The Qing (Clear) Qi inhaled by the lung participates in the production of the

地得以化生。

2　血的生成

血液生成的物质基础主要是精，包括先天之精（肾精）和后天之精（水谷之精）。其中，先天之精是血液生成的首要条件，后天之精必须与先天之精结合，才能生成血液。因此，先天之肾精不足，血液生化之源匮乏。然而，人出生以后，后天之精就起着决定性的作用。所以在一般情况下，对血液生成有决定性影响的是脾胃的功能。脾胃功能正常，能从饮食中吸收足够的精微物质和津液，从而化生血液。若脾胃功能减弱，吸收精微物质和津液不足，血液也就缺乏必要的生化来源。

精化生血的过程，是一个气化过程，必须在气的作用下才能完成。参与这一气化过程的内脏主要是心肺。心在血液生成过程中的气化作用，《黄帝内经》称其为"化赤"，认为只有在"心主血脉"的特殊作用下，血液才能变成红色。肺通过吸入自然之清气参与营气的生成，而营气是血液的主要组成部分，

Ying (Nutrient) Qi, which is one of the component parts of the blood. Therefore, it may directly influence the formation of blood if the lung's function is normal or not.

3　Functions of blood

The blood circulates inside the vessels, infusing into the five zang organs and six fu organs and reaching the skin, muscles, tendons and bones, in a circular movement constantly, for the purpose to nourish and moisturize the zang-fu organs, tissues, sense organs and orifices, to maintain their normal physiological activities. It is said in Nan Jing that "the blood dominates the nourishment and moisture", the brief summarization of the nourishing and moisturizing functions of the blood.

The physiological functions are as follows:

(1) Nourish and moisturize the zang-fu organs, tissues, sense organs and orifices of the human body

The existence and functional movements of all parts of the human body rely on the nourishment and moisture of the blood. If the blood is sufficient, the complexion is red and lustrous, the skin is soft and moist, the hair is moist and lustrous, the tendons and bones are strong, the muscles are full-grown, and the zang-fu organs are peaceful and harmonious. If the blood is deficient, the complexion is sallow and yellow, the skin is dull and dry, the hair is dry and withered, the tendons and bones are atrophic and flaccid, the muscles are thin, and the zang-fu organs are frail and weak. Therefore, it is said that "the body is sufficient if the blood is sufficient, while the body is depleted if the blood is deficient".

所以肺的功能正常与否，可直接影响血液的生成。

3　血的作用

血行脉中，内注五脏六腑，外达皮肉筋骨，如环无端，运行不息，不断地对全身的脏腑、形体、官窍等组织器官，起着营养和滋润作用，以维持其正常的生理活动。《难经》所说的"血主濡之"，就是对血的营养和滋润作用的简要概括。

血的生理作用大体有以下三方面。

（1）濡润人体脏腑、形体、官窍等组织器官

人体各个部分的生存及其功能活动均依赖于血的濡养滋润。血液充盈，则面色红润，皮肤柔润，毛发润泽，筋骨强健，肌肉丰满，脏腑安和。若血液亏虚，则面色萎黄，皮肤枯燥，毛发枯槁，筋骨萎软，或见拘急，肌肉瘦削，脏腑脆弱。故古人有"血盛则形盛，血弱则形衰"之说。

(2) Maintain the normal movement and sensation of the body

It is said in Huang Di Nei Jing that "the liver gives rise to vision when it obtains the blood, the feet are capable of walking when they obtain the blood, the palms are capable of holding when they obtain the blood, and the fingers are capable of grasping when they obtain the blood". It shows that the vision, walking, holding and grasping movements and sensation rely on the nourishment of the blood. If the blood is sufficient, the sensation and movement are normal. If the blood is deficient, there can be dizziness, blurring of vision, night blindness, tinnitus, numbness and motor impairment of four limbs, and spasm or atrophy and paralysis of tendons and bones.

(3) Function as the substantial foundation to support the spiritual activities of the body

It is said in Huang Di Nei Jing that "the blood and qi are the foundation of human spiritual activities". If the blood is sufficient and the vessels are harmonious, there can be high spirit, clear mind, agile sensation and facile movement. If the blood is deficient, there can be low spirit, failure of thinking, dull reaction, poor memory or insomnia, and palpitation. If the pathogenic heat enters the Xue (Blood) Phase (heat in blood), there can be the pathological manifestations of mental disorders as insomnia, dream-disturbed sleep, restlessness, even delirium and coma. Furthermore, the blood is the major substantial foundation of the spiritual and mental activities, so overstrain of spirit may consume the yin blood, especially the heart blood. Therefore, overstrain of spirit is one of the common

（2）维持机体的正常运动和感觉

《黄帝内经》指出："肝受血而能视，足受血而能步，掌受血而能握，指受血而能摄。"说明视、步、握、摄等运动和感觉对血液营养的依赖关系。血液充盈，则感觉与运动正常；血液虚少，则常见头晕，目花，夜盲，耳鸣，四肢麻木，运动无力，筋骨拘挛，甚至萎废不用。

（3）提供机体精神活动的主要物质基础

《黄帝内经》有"血气者，人之神"之说。若血液充盛，血脉和调，则表现为精神充沛，神志清晰，感觉灵敏，活动自如。若血虚，都可出现精神衰退，不耐思考，反应迟钝，健忘或失眠，惊悸等症；若热入血分（血热），则多见失眠多梦，烦躁不安，甚至谵妄、昏迷等神志失常的病理表现。此外，正是因为血是神志活动的主要物质基础，所以劳神过度可耗伤阴血，尤其是心血。因此，临床上劳神过度是心血不足的常见原因之一。

causes of the heart blood insufficiency pattern.

4   Circulation of blood

The blood circulates inside the blood vessels, distributing all over the body in a circular movement. The blood pertains to yin, so the constantly-circulating blood relies on the promoting function of qi. Therefore, the normal circulation of blood is determined by the harmonious balance between the promoting and checking functions of qi.

In particular, the blood circulation is related to the functions of zang-fu organs and factors as follows:

(1) The heart dominates the blood circulation. It is said in Huang Di Nei Jing that "all types of blood belong to the heart". The heart functions to dominate the blood of the whole body, and to promote the blood circulating inside the vessels normally as well. The promoting function of the blood is realized by the heart qi. Therefore, the strength of the heart qi is the key to maintaining the force and speed of the blood circulation. If the heart qi is weak and deficient, the blood flow will be slow and weak. If the heart yang is hyperactive, the blood flow will be fast and reckless.

(2) The lung dominates qi and governs dispersing and descending. The lung dominates qi of the whole body. The blood circulation relies on the promoting function of qi, while the lung, through its dispersing and descending functions, assists the heart to dominate the blood circulation. The dispersing function of the lung is helpful to make the

4   血的运行

血液循脉运行,流布全身,循环不已。属阴的血,其运行不息,主要靠气的推动作用,即所谓"血非气不运"。血运行于脉中而不致逸脱,主要依赖于气的固摄作用。所以说血液的正常运行,取决于气的推动和固摄作用的协调平衡。

具体地说,血液运行与以下脏腑功能及因素有关。

(1)心主行血:《黄帝内经》有"诸血者,皆属于心"之论。心有主宰一身之血的作用,并能推动血液在脉中正常运行。对血的推动作用主要由心气来完成。所以,心气的强弱,是维持血行力量和血流速度的关键。心气虚弱则血流迟缓而无力,心阳过亢则血流薄疾而妄行。

(2)肺主气司宣降:肺主一身之气。血的运行靠气的推动,肺通过宣发和肃降作用协助心主行血。肺气宣发的运动状态,有助于血向外向上布散;肺气肃降的运动状态,有利于血向内向下运

blood flow outwards and upwards, while the descending function of the lung to make the blood flow inwards and downwards. The above functions of the lung is termed "to assist the heart to circulate the blood" in TCM. Clinically, if the lung qi fails to disperse and descend, causing the lung qi blockage, so as to lead to the heart blood stagnation pattern. Such a pathological progress is another evidence of that the lung assist the heart to circulate the blood.

(3) The liver dominates dredging and draining, and stores the blood. The dredging and draining function of the liver refers to its regulating function on qi activities. The blood can flow only when qi flows, therefore, the liver qi maintains the smooth flow of the blood. The blood-storing function of the liver refers that the liver stores the blood, regulates the blood volume and prevents bleeding. When the human body is quiet, the surplus blood in the peripheral circulation is stored in the liver. When the human body is in movement, the liver regulates the distribution of the blood volume according to the various necessities of all parts of human body. If the liver fails to dominate dredging and draining or fails to store the blood, the normal blood circulation will be influenced, leading to blood stagnation or bleeding.

(4) The spleen controls the blood. The spleen functions to control and check the blood, so as to make the blood to flow inside the vessels without spilling out, as it is said in Nan Jing that the spleen "dominates controlling the blood". If the spleen qi is weak and deficient, it fails to control the blood, leading to the pathological phenomena as bloody feces, metrorrhagia or metrostaxis. The spleen function "to control the blood" and the liver function

行。肺的上述功能,中医学称之为"助心行血"。临床上常见由肺失宣肃,肺气壅塞,日久不愈,而渐致心血瘀阻的病理传变过程,正是肺助心行血的佐证。

(3) 肝主疏泄而藏血:肝的疏泄功能重在调畅气机,因气行则血行,故随之亦保持了血行的通畅。肝主藏血,有贮藏血液、调节血量和防止出血三方面意义。人在安静时,外周循环中多余的血贮藏于肝;人在活动时,根据人体各处的不同需要,肝能调节血量的分布。若肝失疏泄或肝不藏血,均有可能影响血液的正常运行,而导致瘀血或出血。

(4) 脾主统血:脾气具有统摄血液,使其行于脉中不致外溢的生理功能。《难经》所说的脾"主裹血",即是此意。若脾气虚损,无力摄血,则可引起便血、崩漏等脾不统血的病理现象。脾的"统血"功能,与肝的"藏血"功能是相互协调的。临床上

"to store the blood" are mutually coordinated. Clinically, the pathogenesis of some bleeding diseases involves both the spleen and liver, as "failure to store and control".

(5) Whether or not the vessels are unblocked and whether or not the temperature is proper are also the factors to directly influence the normal circulation of the blood. The unblocked vessel is one of the prerequisites for the normal circulation of the blood. Clinically, the blockage of vessels (due to phlegm or stagnant blood) may cause the slow flow of blood or even blood stagnation. The cold or heat may also influence the blood flow. If the yin and yang in the body is in equilibrium, the body temperature is constant, so the blood circulation is normal. If yin and yang are disharmonious, there can be heat due to yang excess or yin deficiency, or cold due to yin excess or yang deficiency. The heat may accelerate the blood flow, dilate the vessels, or even make the blood flow reckless. The cold may slow down the blood flow, contract the vessels, or even cause the blood stagnation. The kidney, as the basis of yin and yang of the whole body, influences the blood circulation indirectly through regulating yin and yang of the whole body.

In summary, the heart is the primary motive power to promote the blood circulation, the lung and liver assist to circulate the blood and regulate the blood volume in distribution, while the liver and spleen control and store the blood to prevent bleeding. Besides, whether or not the vessels are unblocked and whether or not the temperature is proper are also the factors to influence the normal circulation of the blood.

某些出血,其病机涉及脾与肝两脏,即所谓"藏统失司"。

(5) 此外,脉道是否通利,寒热是否适度,也是直接影响血液运行是否正常的因素。脉道通利与否,是血液正常运行的前提条件之一。临床上因脉道不利(如痰浊、瘀血阻脉)而致血行迟涩甚至血瘀状态也并非少见。至于寒热对血行的影响更是显而易见。人体阴阳平衡,体温恒定,则血行正常。若阴阳失调,阴虚则热,阳虚则寒。热则血行加速,脉管扩张甚者迫血妄行;寒则血行迟缓,脉络蜷缩甚至引起血瘀。肾为一身阴阳之根本,肾通过调节全身阴阳而间接地影响着血液运行。

综上所述,推动血液运行的原动力在心;协助行血,调节血量分布的是肺与肝;贮藏、统摄血液,防止出血的是肝与脾;脉道通利与否,寒热适度与否,也是影响血行是否正常的常见因素。

Section 3   Body Fluid

1   Basic concept of body fluid

The body fluid, one of the fundamental substances to form up the human body and to maintain the human vital activities, is composed of water and essential materials. The body fluid inside the blood vessels is the component part of the blood, while the body fluid outside the vessels distributes everywhere of the body, including the zang-fu organs, orifices and tissues. The body fluid secreting or excreting from the five sense organs and nine orifices, becoming the urine, sweat, tear, snivel, Tuo (Thick) Saliva and Xian (Thin) Saliva.

The body fluid is a general term of the Jin (Thin-Light) Fluid and Ye (Thick-Heavy) Fluid, which are different in properties, distributions and functions. Generally, the Jin (Thin-Light) Fluid, with a clear and thin property and a high liquidity, distributes in the skin, muscles and orifices to function to moisturize them, while the Ye (Thick-Heavy) Fluid, with a thick and heavy property and a low liquidity, infuses into the zang-fu organs, brain marrows and joints to function to nourish them.

The Jin (Thin-Light) Fluid and Ye (Thick-Heavy) Fluid have some differences, but both of them originate from the food essence transformed by the spleen and stomach, distribute outside the meridians, and mutually permeate and support. Therefore, they are not strictly distinguished physiologically, just referred "the body fluid" in general. But pathologically, "the injury of Jin (Thin-Light)

第 3 节   津液

1   津液的基本概念

津液,也是构成人体和维持人体生命活动的基本物质之一,其主要成分是水,其中也含有精微物质。津液在血脉中,成为血液的组成部分;津液在血脉外,则遍布于脏腑形体各处。若津液从五官九窍中分泌或排泄,就成为尿、汗、泪、涕、唾、涎等。

津液是津与液的合称,而津与液在性状、分布和功能等方面均有一定区别。一般而言,性状较清稀,流动性较大,布散于皮肤、肌肉和孔窍之中,起滋润作用的,总称为津;性状较稠厚,流动性较小,灌注于脏腑、脑髓、骨节之中,起濡养作用的,总称为液。

津与液虽有一定区别,但两者同源于水谷,生成于脾胃,流布于经脉之外,能相互渗透、补充,所以通常在生理上不予严格区别,而并称为"津液",只是在病理上,"伤津"与"脱液"有程度的不同。一般来讲,伤津在前,程

Fluid" is distinguished from "the loss of Ye (Thick-Heavy) Fluid". Generally, the injury of Jin (Thin-Light) Fluid is primary with a mild condition, while the loss of Ye (Thick-Heavy) Fluid is secondary with a severe condition.

2   Formation of body fluid

The body fluid is produced from the digestive and absorptive functions of the stomach, spleen, large intestine and small intestine. The body fluid originates from the food, especially the liquid food. The formation process of the body fluid is as follows.

The stomach dominates the acceptance, while the spleen the transportation and transformation. The stomach, called the sea of water and grain, accepts and decomposes the food, and absorbs some essence including the body fluid. Based on the transporting and transforming function of the spleen and the spleen qi's function in lifting the clear, the body fluid absorbed by the stomach is sent upwards to the heart and lung, and then to the whole body.

The small intestine dominates the Ye (Thick-Heavy) Fluid. The small intestine functions to separate the clear from the turbid, absorb the most nutrients and water in the food, and send them upwards to the spleen, and then to the whole body. At the same time, it sends the metabolic products downwards to the bladder through the kidney and to the large intestine. The small intestine involves in the formation of the body fluid based on its function "to dominate the Ye (Thci-Heavy) Fluid".

The large intestine dominates the Jin (Thin-Light) Fluid. The large intestine receives the food

度较轻,脱液在后,程度较重。

2   津液的生成

津液是通过胃、脾及大小肠的消化吸收功能而化生的。津液来源于饮食物,尤以水饮流汁食物为主。其大体生成过程如下。

胃主受纳,脾主运化:胃为水谷之海,饮食物首先入胃,经胃受纳腐熟后,吸收包括津液在内的部分精微。经脾的运化功能,并赖于脾气的升清作用,将胃肠吸收的津液上输于心肺,而后输布于全身。

小肠主液:小肠泌别清浊,吸收饮食物中大部分的营养物质和水分,上输于脾,而布散全身;并将水液代谢产物经肾输入膀胱,将糟粕下输于大肠。小肠通过"主液"的功能参与人体内津液的生成。

大肠主津:大肠接受小肠下注的饮食物残渣和剩余

waste and rest water transported from the small intestine, reabsorbs some water, and transforms the food waste into feces to discharge. The large intestine involves in the formation of the body fluid based on its function "to dominate the Jin (Thin-Light) Fluid".

In general, the formation of the body fluid is determined by two factors: Firstly, the sufficient liquid food is the primary substantial foundation to produce the body fluid. Secondly, the functions of the zang-fu organs, especially the functions of the spleen, stomach, large intestine and small intestine, should be normal. The abnormality of any of the links may cause lack of body fluid formation, leading to the pathological changes of the body fluid deficiency.

3   Distribution and metabolism of body fluid

The distribution and metabolism is a very complicated process, involving a series of physiological functions of many zang-fu organs. The distribution and metabolism of body fluid are realized upon the synthetic efficacy of the physiological functions of the spleen, lung, kidney, liver and triple energizer.

The spleen qi spreads the essence. The spleen dominates the transportation and transformation of the food essence. Through its transporting function, the spleen sends the body fluid upwards to the lung, while the lung distributes the body fluid to the whole body to irrigate the zang-fu organs, body, limbs and all orifices through its dispersing and descending functions. Besides, the spleen also sends the body fluid directly to the whole body, as it is

水分后,将其中部分水液重新吸收,使残渣形成粪便而排出体外。大肠通过其"主津"功能参与人体内津液的生成。

总之,津液的生成取决于两个方面的因素:一是充足的水饮类食物,这是生成津液的原始物质基础;二是脏腑功能正常,特别是脾胃、大小肠的功能正常,其中任何一个环节的异常,均可导致津液生成不足,引起津液亏虚的病理变化。

3   津液的输布代谢

津液的输布代谢是一个极其复杂的过程,它涉及到多个脏腑的一系列生理活动。津液的输布代谢主要依靠脾、肺、肾、肝和三焦等脏腑生理功能的综合作用而完成的。

脾气散精:脾主运化水谷精微,通过其转输作用,一方面将津液上输于肺,由肺的宣发和肃降,使津液输布全身而灌溉脏腑、形体和诸窍。另一方面,又可直接将津液布散至全身,即《黄帝内经》所说的脾有"灌溉四旁"的功能。

said that in Huang Di Nei Jing that the spleen functions "to irrigate the all parts".

The lung dominates to circulate the water. The lung functions to circulate the water and regulate the water passage, as the upper source of water. The lung accepts the body fluid transported from the spleen, it then distributes the body fluid to the upper part and surface of the body through its dispersing function, so as to moisturize the skin and to discharge the surplus water in a sweating way. Furthermore, it sends the body fluid to the kidney, bladder and lower part of body through its descending function, while the kidney and bladder transform the surplus water into urine to discharge through their transforming function.

The kidney dominates the body fluid. It is said in Huang Di Nei Jing that "the kidney as the water organ dominates the body fluid". The kidney possesses the dominating function in the distribution of the body fluid. Firstly, the transpiring and transforming function of the yang qi in the kidney is the primary motive power of the stomach yang "spreading the Jing (Essence) Qi", the spleen transporting and transforming the essence, the lung unblocking and regulating the water passage and the small intestine separating the clear from the turbid. The yang qi in the kidney thus promotes the distribution of the body fluid. Secondly, based on the transforming function of kidney qi, the body fluid transferred from the lung to the kidney is divided into the clear and the turbid. The clear is sent upwards to the lung and then to the whole body through the triple energizer, while the turbid is transformed into urine and infused into the bladder. The productive volume

肺主行水：肺主行水，通调水道，为水之上源。肺接受从脾转输而来的津液之后，一方面通过宣发作用将津液输布至人体上部和体表，以润泽肌肤，并将多余水分发为汗液而排出体外。另一方面通过肃降作用，将津液输布至肾和膀胱以及人体下部，经肾与膀胱的气化作用，将多余水分化为尿液而排出体外。

肾主津液：《黄帝内经》说："肾者水脏，主津液。"肾对津液输布起着主宰作用。主要表现在两个方面。一是肾中阳气的蒸腾气化作用，是胃阳"游溢精气"、脾的运化散精、肺的通调水道以及小肠的泌别清浊等的原动力，推动着津液的输布。二是由肺下输至肾的津液，在肾的气化作用下，清者蒸腾，经三焦上输于肺而布散全身，浊者化为尿液注入膀胱，而尿液的生成量和排泄量的多少对整个水液代谢的平衡至关重要。

and excreting volume of urine are very important to the balance of the whole water metabolism.

The liver dominates dredging and draining. The liver functions to dominate dredging and draining, so as to make the qi activities of zang-fu organs normal. If qi moves smoothly, the body fluid flows normally, and the metabolism is also normal as well, so as to promote the circular distribution of body fluid. Besides, the Liver Meridian runs around the external genitalia and reaches the lower abdomen. If the liver qi flows smoothly, it may promote urination, so as to assist the relative balance of the water metabolism.

In terms of excretion of body fluid, such as sweating, exhaling, urination, etc. it is also closely related to the physiological functions of other zang-fu organs.

The lung dominates dispersing, to spread the body fluid to the skin and hair of body surface and transform it into sweat through the yang qi's transpiration, then to discharge it through the sweating pores. The lung dominates respiration, so the lung also excretes some water during exhaling. The urine is the final product of body fluid metabolism. Its formation is related to the functions of the lung, spleen, kidney, etc., especially the kidney. The transforming function of the kidney qi and bladder qi acts to produce the urine and discharge it. Besides, the large intestine also discharges a little water through defecation. Therefore, in diarrhea, the water in feces increases, so the large amount of water is taken away, leading to the pathological manifestation of injury of Jin (Thin-Light) Fluid.

肝主疏泄:肝主疏泄,使脏腑气机调肠,气化有权,气行则津液通达,气化则代谢正常,由此促进津液的输布环流。此外,肝经绕阴器抵少腹,肝气通达,可疏利尿窍,以助开合,从而协助水液代谢的相对平衡。

就出汗、呼气、排尿等等津液的排泄而言,其也与相关脏腑的功能密切有关。

肺气宣发,将津液输布到体表皮毛,被阳气蒸腾而形成汗液,由汗孔排出体外。肺主呼吸,肺在呼气时也带走部分水分。尿液为津液代谢的最终产物,其形成虽与肺、脾、肾等脏腑功能相关,但尤与肾的关系最为密切。肾的气化功能与膀胱的气化作用相配合,共同形成尿液并排出体外。此外,大肠排出的水谷糟粕所形成的粪便中亦带出少许津液。腹泻时,大便中含水量增多,带走大量津液,易引起伤津的病理表现。

4   Functions of Body Fluid

The body fluid is very important to maintain the normal vital activities of human body. Generally, the body fluid functions to moisturize and nourish, to transform and produce the blood, to regulate yin and yang and to discharge the wastes. When the body fluid is deficient, the related functions of body fluid decrease, leading to various clinical manifestations.

4.1   Moisturize and nourish

The body fluid is composed mainly of water, functioning to moisturize. The body fluid contains various necessary substances for the life, functioning to nourish. The Jin (Thin-Light) Fluid is different from the Ye (Thick-Heavy) Fluid. The Jin (Thin-Light) Fluid, with property of clearance and thinness, is light and mobile, while the Ye (Thick-Heavy) Fluid, with property of thickness and glittering, is thick and quiet. The zang-fu oranges, tendons and bones inside the body, and the skin and hair on body surface all rely on the moisture and nourishment of the body fluid. The body fluid locating on body surface functions to moisturize the skin, to nourish the muscles, and to make the skin and hair lustrous, and the muscles full-grown, while the body fluid infusing inside the body functions to moisturize and nourish the zang-fu organs and to lubricate the meridians, so as to maintain their normal physiological functions. If the body fluid is not sufficient, its moisturizing and nourishing function deceases, leading to a series of symptoms of dryness, such as dry lips and tongue, dry eyes, dry throat, constipation, scanty urine, dry and with-

4   津液的作用

津液对人体生命活动的正常维持具有十分重要的作用。概括起来,津液的功能主要包括滋润濡养、化生血液、调节阴阳、排泄废物等方面。当津液亏虚时,津液有关功能势必减退而见种种临床表现。

4.1   滋润濡养

津液以水分为主体,故有很强的滋润作用,津液又富含各种生命必需物质,故有一定的营养功能。津、液有别,津质地清稀,轻而流动;液稠而晶莹,厚而凝静。内而脏腑筋骨,外而皮肤毫毛,莫不赖于津液的滋润濡养。分布于体表的津液,能滋润皮肤,濡养肌肉,使皮毛光泽、肌肉丰满;流注于体内的津液能滋养脏腑、滑利经脉,维持其正常生理功能。如津液不足,滋润濡养功能减退,势必出现一系列干燥失润之象,如唇舌干燥,两目干涩,咽喉干燥,大便干结,小便短少,皮肤干枯等。甚至可因阴液亏虚,无力制约阳热,而致火热内生,出现潮热、升火、颧红、盗汗、五心烦热等症。

ered skin, etc. If the yin fluid is deficient, it fails to inhibit the yang heat, leading to the symptoms of endogenous fire, such as tidal fever, feverish sensation, flushed cheeks, nocturnal sweats, feverish sensation in five centers, etc.

4.2 Transform and produce the blood

The body fluid permeates into the vessels to combine with the Ying (Nutrient) Qi, becoming the basic component part of the blood. If the blood decreases suddenly due to some factors, the body fluid permeates into the vessels to complement the insufficient blood. The body fluid makes the blood more plentiful and functions to moisturize and nourish the vessels as well. If the body fluid is consumed suddenly due to profuse sweating, severe vomiting, severe diarrhea or high fever, the blood also decreases at the same time when the body fluid is lost. It is the so-called "the fluid exhaustion leading to blood deficiency" or "the fluid loss leading to blood failure" in the ancient classics. On the contrary, the blood deficiency may also cause the fluid depletion, leading to the pattern of fluid and blood deficiency as a result.

4.3 Regulate yin and yang

In normal situation, yin and yang of the human body stay in a relatively equilibrium state. As the component part of the yin essence, the body fluid is important to regulate the yin-yang equilibrium of the body. It is closely related to the sufficiency or deficiency of the body fluid if the yin-yang equilibrium is normal or not. In the seasons when it is very cold, if one wears too little, the sweating pores of the skin will close to prevent the body fluid discharge, so as to decrease the rejection of heat, for

4.2　化生血液

津液渗入血脉之中,与营气相合,成为化生血液的基本成分。若血液因故而骤减,津液亦可渗入脉内,以补充血液的不足。津液使血液充盈,并濡养和滑利血脉。因大汗、大吐、大泻或高热等而使津液急剧耗伤,在伤津脱液的同时,脉中血液亦可随之而减少,古医籍中称之为"津枯血少"或"津脱血竭"。反之亦然,血虚亦可导致津亏,从而导致津血两亏之证。

4.3　调节阴阳

在正常情况下,人体阴阳之间处于相对平衡的状态。津液作为阴精的组成部分,对调节机体的阴阳平衡起着重要作用。人体阴阳的正常与否,与津液的盛衰密切相关。如寒冷季节,或穿戴太少,皮肤汗孔闭合,津液不致外泄而减少散热,有利于保温御寒;温热季节,或穿

the purpose to preserve the thermal and to keep out the cold. In the seasons when it is warm, if one wears too much, the sweating pores of the skin will open to discharge the body fluid through sweating, for the purpose to reject the heat. Such a process is to regulate the body temperature constancy and yin-yang equilibrium, so as to maintain the normal vital activities of human body. If the body fluid is severely insufficient, it fails to make sweating, so the functions to regulate the body temperature and yin-yang equilibrium decrease as the result.

4.4   Discharge the wastes

During its metabolic process, the body fluid continuously discharges the metabolic products through sweating and urination, so as to make the qi activities of zang-fu organs normal. If this function is injured or disturbed, the metabolic products or toxins will be laid inside the body. Clinically, if the body fluid is consumed due to severe vomiting, severe diarrhea or high fever, and the body fails to be supported by the yin fluid, the body can be poisoned, even to death due to sudden decrease of urine volume or anuria.

Section 4   Relationships among Qi, Blood and Body Fluid

Qi, blood and body fluid are fundamental substances to maintain the vital activities of the human body, and closely related.

着太多,皮肤腠理开张,津液借出汗形式以散发热量。由此调节体温恒定和阴阳平衡,从而维持人体正常的生命活动。若津液严重不足,无源作汗,以致体温调节、阴阳调和能力势必下降。

4.4   排泄废物

津液在其自身的代谢过程中,将机体的代谢产物通过出汗、排尿等方式,不断地排出体外,使机体各脏腑的气化活动正常。若这一作用受到损害或发生障碍,就会使代谢产物或毒性物质潴留于体内。临床上因严重吐泻、高热不退而耗伤津液,若不能及时补充阴液即可因尿量急剧减少,甚或无尿,而致毒性物质无法随尿排出而自身中毒,重则甚可危及生命。

第4节   气血津液 之间的关系

气、血、津液都是维持人体生命活动的基本物质,三者之间存在着密切关系。

1　Relationship between qi and blood

Qi is featured of motion, pertaining to yang, while the blood is featured of quietness, pertaining to yin. Therefore, the relationship between qi and blood can be illustrated by the mutual depending and mutual functioning relations between yin and yang. It is said in TCM that qi is the commander of the blood, while the blood is the mother of qi.

1.1　Qi produces the blood

During the process of the blood formation, the transforming function of qi is very important. Qi of zang-fu organs acts to digest and absorb the food to transform it into the food essence, which further is to produce the Wei (Defensive) Qi, Ying (Nutrient) Qi, body fluid, etc. The Ying (Nutrient) Qi and body fluid enters in the vessels, transforming into the red-colored blood. The Ying (Nutrient) Qi is not only the component part of the blood, but also the important factor to promote the blood production as well. The blood is formed from a series of transforming function of qi, acted by the spleen-stomach qi and Ying (Nutrient) Qi. Therefore, it is said that qi produces the blood. If qi is sufficient, the blood is also sufficient. If qi is deficient, the blood is also deficient. Clinically, in the treatment of the blood deficiency pattern, it is necessary to add the qi-reinforcing herbs at the same time when reinforcing the blood, for the purpose to increase the therapeutic effects. This is the practical application of the theory that qi produces the blood.

1.2　Qi moves the blood

The blood is quiet, pertaining to yin. The blood circulation relies on the promoting function of

1　气与血的关系

由于气性动而属阳,血性静而属阴,所以气与血之间的关系,可以从阴阳的互根互用关系来认识。中医学将其概括为:气为血之帅,血为气之母。

1.1　气能生血

在血的生成过程中,气化作用十分重要。在脏腑之气的作用下,饮食物被消化吸收而化生水谷精微,水谷精微又分别生成卫气、营气、津液等。营气和津液进入脉中,变化而赤为血。营气不只是血的主要组成部分,而且是促进血液生成的重要因素。血是在脾胃之气和营气的作用下,发生一系列气化过程而生成的,因此说气能生血。气旺则血充,气衰则血虚。临床上治疗血虚病证,在补血的同时,每加补气药以提高疗效,便是气能生血理论在实践中的应用。

1.2　气能行血

血属阴而静,血的运行,必须依赖于运行不息的气的

constantly-moveable qi. In details, the normal blood circulation is based upon the promoting function of the heart qi, the dispersing and descending function of the lung qi, the dredging and draining function of the liver qi, and the checking function of the spleen qi. The deficiency of the heart qi which fails to promote, or the deficiency of the lung qi which fails to disperse and descend, or the stagnation of the liver qi which fails to promote smooth qi activity, may lead to unsmooth circulation of blood. Besides, the derangement of qi activity or abnormal up-flow, down-flow, outflow and inflow of qi may also cause the abnormality of blood circulation. In the condition of up-reverse flow of qi, the blood may up-flow excessively along with qi to lead to red complexion, red eyes, distension in head, headache, even spitting blood, coma, etc. In the condition of qi sinking, the blood may down-flow excessively along with qi to cause weighty and distending sensation in lower abdomen, bloody feces, bloody urine, metrorrhagia, metrostaxis, etc.

1.3 Qi checks the blood

Checking implies controlling and restraining. That qi checks the blood refers that qi functions to control and restrain the blood to circulate inside the vessels without spilling. That qi checks the blood is the concrete manifestation of the qi's checking function. Theoretically speaking, that qi checks the blood is same as that the spleen controls the blood. The spleen is regarded as the source to produce qi and blood. If the spleen qi is sufficient, it is strong enough to produce qi, which can check the blood normally. If the spleen qi is deficient, it is weak and fails to check the blood, leading to various

推动。具体地说,血的正常运行,有赖于心气的推动,肺气的宣降,肝气的疏泄,脾气的固摄。若心气虚损则推动无力,肺气不足则宣降失司,肝气郁结则气机阻滞,均会引起血行不畅。此外,气机的逆乱,升降出入的异常,也常导致血运失常。气逆,血随气升,可见面红目赤、头胀头痛,甚则吐衄、昏厥;气陷,血随气下,可见少腹坠胀同时伴有便血、尿血、崩漏等症。

1.3 气能摄血

摄,即统摄、固摄。气能摄血,是指气能统摄、控制血液循脉道而行,不溢出脉外。气能摄血,正是气的固摄作用的具体体现。从理论上说,气能摄血与脾能统血是统一的。脾为气血生化之源,脾气健旺,生气有源,气的摄血功能正常;脾虚生气无源,气虚无力摄血,就会出现各种出血倾向,临床上称为"气不摄血",或"脾不统

kinds of bleeding conditions. It is the so-called "qi failing to check the blood" or "the spleen failing to control the blood" clinically. In the condition of qi failing to check the blood, there are symptoms of qi and blood deficiency pattern, such as thin-natured and light-colored blood, or purple-colored blood, lusterless complexion, tiredness, shortness of breath, pale tongue, weak pulse, etc.

1.4　Blood carries qi

Qi is featured of being intangible and moveable. So it should be attached to the tangible blood, so as to flow inside the vessels without scattering. It is said that the blood is the carrier of qi. Clinically, in the condition of severe bleeding, qi is also lost along with bleeding, the so-called "qi losing along with bleeding". That "the blood carries qi" is the theoretical basis of such a pathological state. In the treatment of qi losing along with bleeding, it is necessary to reinforce qi to prevent the collapse besides to reinforce the blood to stop bleeding.

1.5　Blood nourishes qi

All parts of the body, including the five zang organs, six fu organs, four limbs and all bones, rely on the nourishment of the blood, for the purpose to maintain the normal physiological functions of the human body. If the tissues and organs of human body cannot be nourished by the blood, their functional activities cannot be maintained, and qi cannot be produced. The physiological functions of any parts of the human body rely on the promoting function of qi, while qi relies on the nourishment of the blood, for the purpose to realize its normal physiological efficacy. Therefore, the patient of blood deficiency also has the manifestations of the

血"。气不摄血,一般多见血色稀淡或紫暗,并伴有面色不华,倦怠气短,舌淡脉虚等气血虚损之象。

1.4　血能载气

气无形而动,必须附着于有形之血,才能行于脉中而不致散失,即血为气的载体。临床上见大量出血的病人,其气亦常随之而逸脱,即所谓"气随血脱"其理论根据即在于此。临床上治疗气随血脱时,除补血止血外,还需益气固脱以急救之。

1.5　血能养气

人体各部,内至五脏六腑,外至四肢百骸,无不有赖于血的濡养,才能维持正常的生理功能。机体的组织器官若得不到血的供养,其功能活动也就无法维持,气亦无由化生。人体任何部位的生理功能,虽然均来源于气的推动,但气亦须依赖于血的濡养,才能发挥其正常的生理效应。故临床上血虚之人,皆有气虚的表现。

qi deficiency clinically.

2　Relationship between qi and body fluid

The body fluid, similar to the blood, is a kind of tangible substance of liquid. Therefore, the relationships between qi and body fluid are quite similar to those between qi and blood.

2.1　Qi produces the body fluid

The body fluid originates from the food. The food, after acceptance and decomposition by the stomach and transportation and transformation by the spleen, disintegrates into the essence and waste, while the liquid part in the essence is the body fluid. The body fluid is distributed all over the body through the transportation and transformation of the spleen. Besides the spleen and stomach, the small intestine absorbs some water when it "separates the clear from the turbid", and the large intestine also absorbs some water when it "transports the waste". Thus there is such a theory of "the small intestine dominating the Ye (Thick-Heavy) Fluid" and "the large intestine dominates the Jin (Thin-Light) Fluid". It can be seen that the whole process that the food is transformed into the body fluid that is distributed all over the body is actually a series of transforming process of qi acted by qi of zang-fu organs of the spleen, stomach, intestines, etc. If the spleen-stomach qi is sufficient, it is strong in transforming and producing the body fluid, and then the body fluid is sufficient as a result. If the spleen-stomach qi is deficient, it is weak in transforming and producing the body fluid, and then the body fluid is deficient as a result.

2.2　Qi moves the body fluid

The body fluid is tangible and quiet, so its dis-

2　气与津液的关系

津液与血相类,也是有形的液态物质。故气与津液的关系,与气和血的关系颇为相似。

2.1　气能生津

津液来源于饮食物。饮食物经过脾胃的受纳腐熟、运化而被分化为精微和糟粕,其精微物质的液体部分,即是津液。津液通过脾的运化转输而布散于全身。除脾胃而外,小肠在"泌别清浊"、大肠在"传导糟粕"的同时,均要吸收水分,故有"小肠主液""大肠主津"的理论。可见饮食物化生成津液,并输布于全身,都是在脾、胃、肠等脏腑之气的作用下进行的一系列气化过程。脾胃之气健旺,化生津液之力就强,人体的津液就充足。若脾胃之气虚弱,则化生津液之力就弱,则易致津液不足。

2.2　气能行津

津液有形而静,津液的

tribution, mutation and discharge rely on the promoting and transforming functions of qi. In the distribution of body fluid, firstly the spleen transport the body fluid to the whole body, and at the same time the spleen "spreads the fluid" to send the body fluid "upwards to the lung". Secondly, the lung qi, sends the body fluid outwards through its dispersing function, and sends the body fluid downwards to the kidney and bladder through its descending function. The transforming function of the Jing (Essence) Qi in the kidney is the important link to metabolize the body fluid into the urine. Qi of the spleen, lung, kidney and triple energizer functions to up-flow, down-flow, outflow and inflow in the constant movement and transformation, so as to promote the distribution, metabolism and mutation of the body fluid inside the body, for the purpose to nourish and moisturize all the zang-fu organs, tissues and organs of the human body. At the same time, the surplus water is metabolized into the sweat and urine to be discharged, so as to maintain the equilibrium of water metabolism in the human body. If qi is deficient, its promoting and transforming functions decrease. If qi does not move smoothly, there can be qi stagnation. These are the causes of disturbance of body fluid movement and distribution, leading to the pathological products of water retention, dampness, phlegm and rheum.

2.3　Qi checks the body fluid

　　Qi functions to check the body fluid, to prevent loss of body fluid. The Wei (Defensive) Qi functions to control the opening and closure of the sweating pores, to prevent the over-discharge of sweat (transformed from the body fluid). The kidney qi functions to check the urine, to prevent its over-dis-

输布、变化和排泄,全赖于气的推动和气化作用。津液的输布,首先依靠脾的转输将其散布全身,同时通过脾"散津"而将津液"上归于肺"。肺气通过宣发,将津液向上向外散布;通过肃降,把津液下输到肾与膀胱。肾中精气的气化作用,是将津液代谢为尿液的极其重要的环节。由于脾、肺、肾及三焦之气的升降出入,不断地运行和气化,推动着津液在体内的运行输布、代谢变化,对全身各脏腑组织器官起着滋润、濡养作用,多余的水分则代谢化为汗液、尿液等排出体外,以保持人体水液代谢的平衡。如果气虚,气的推动与气化无力,或因气滞而流通不畅,均可引起津液运行输布的障碍,进而形成水、湿、痰、饮等病理产物。

2.3　气能摄津

　　气对津液具有固摄作用,以防止津液无故流失。如卫气控制汗孔之开合,不使汗液(由津液所化)过多外泄。肾气固摄尿液,不使其过多排泄。肾气虚则膀胱不

charge. If the kidney qi is deficient and the bladder is in dysfunction, there can be excessive urine, frequent urination, enuresis, even urine incontinence. The spleen qi functions to check the saliva, to prevent its over-secretion. If the spleen qi is deficient, it fails to check the saliva, leading to constant salivation. In the clinic of TCM, there are common therapeutic methods to reinforce the Wei (Defensive) Qi to treat spontaneous sweating, to reinforce the kidney qi to treat excessive urine, while to reinforce the spleen qi to treat salivation.

2.4　The body fluid carries qi

Qi is featured of being intangible and moveable. So it should be attached to the tangible body fluid, so as to flow inside the body without scattering. Pathologically, when the body fluid is lost severely, qi is also lost along with it, the so-called "qi losing along with body fluid loss" in TCM. In the ancient classics, there are descriptions that "profuse sweating consumes yang", and "qi is perfect any more after vomiting and diarrhea", which theoretical basis is that "the body fluid carries qi".

3　Relationship between blood and body fluid

The blood and body fluid, with same sources and similar functions, are mutually produced and transformed. Therefore, both are closely related in the physiological links and pathological influences.

From the source, both blood and body fluid are transformed and produced from the food essence acted by the transportation and transformation of the spleen and stomach. Therefore, it is said that "the body fluid and blood share a same source". In terms of the properties and functions, both the blood and

约,常见多尿、尿频、遗尿,甚至小便失禁。脾气固摄涎液,不使其过多外流。脾气虚失于固摄,出现流涎不止。在中医临床上,补卫气以治自汗,补肾气以治多尿,补脾气以治流涎,均为常用之法。

2.4　津能载气

气无形而动,必须附着于有形之津液,才能存在于人体内。所以,在病理上,当津液大量外泄时,气亦随之而丧失,中医学称之为"气随津脱"。古代医籍有"汗多亡阳""吐泻之余,定无完气"之说,其理论根据即是"津能载气"。

3　血与津液的关系

血与津液,来源相同,功能相似,又能相互资生转化,所以两者在生理上的联系和病理上的影响均较为密切。

就来源而论,血与津液均由脾胃运化而生成的水谷精气化生而来,故有"津血同源"之说。就性状和功能而论,血与津液皆有形而属阴,且都具有滋润和濡养的作

body fluid are tangible, pertaining to yin, and possess the moisturizing and nourishing functions. The blood is inside the vessels, while the body fluid outside the vessels. When the body fluid permeates into the vessels, it combines with the Ying (Nutrient) Qi to form up the blood. When the body fluid spills out of the vessels, it separates from the Ying (Nutrient) Qi to become the body fluid. They integrate and separate, enter and exit, so the blood and body fluid are transformed mutually.

The pathological relationship between the blood and body fluid is also significant. Firstly, both the blood and body fluid originate from the Jing (Essence) Qi of water and grain acted by the transportation and transformation of spleen and stomach. If the food intake is not sufficient or the spleen and stomach are weak, the Jing (Essence) Qi of water and grain is deficient, and the blood and body fluid fail to be transformed and produced, leading to not only the blood deficiency pattern, but also the body fluid insufficiency pattern. Secondly, the body fluid and blood are mutually transformed. In the condition of severe bleeding, the blood in the vessels decreases suddenly, and then the body fluid outside the vessels permeates into the vessels to support the insufficient blood, leading to the body fluid deficiency as well. Clinically, the patient of severe bleeding has the manifestations of dry mouth and thirst. On the contrary, in the condition of profuse sweating, severe vomiting or diarrhea, the body fluid is lost heavily, and then the blood inside the vessels permeates out of vessels, leading to increase of blood viscosity or blood stagnation due to unsmooth flow of blood. Clinically, the patient of chronic

用。血在脉中,津液在脉外。津液渗入脉中,与营气结合,便是血;渗出脉外,与营气分离,即是津液。有分有合,有进有出,津血是相互转化的。

　　血与津液在病理上的影响也较突出。首先,由于血与津液均来源于脾胃运化而生成的水谷精气,故当饮食不足或脾胃虚弱时,水谷精气衰少,血与津液的化源均匮乏,不但可致血虚,也可致津液不足。其次,由于津与血相互转化,所以在大出血时,脉中血液骤减,脉外津液大量渗入脉中,以补充血量的不足,以致津液也显亏虚。临床上大出血的病人,多有口干渴的表现。反之,因大汗、大吐泻等引起津液大量丢失时,血中的津液成分也会渗出脉外,血液的粘稠度增高,也易导致血行不利的血瘀状态。临床上另有阴液慢性耗损,而致血液日渐干枯的,如肺痨患者后期见津亏血枯,俗称"干血痨",便属此列。有鉴于此,古代医家一再强调:失血的病人,慎用

consumption of the yin fluid, the blood is also getting deficient. For example, in the condition of late phase of pulmonary tuberculosis, there present the deficiency of blood and body fluid pattern, the so-called "dry-blood tuberculosis". Therefore, it is stressed by the ancient physicians that it is well-advised not to apply the sweating method for the patient of bleeding, while the blood-letting method for the patient of body fluid loss.

发汗之法；津液丢失之人，慎用放血疗法。

A Brief Chinese Chronology 中国历史年代表

Xia Dynasty (c. 21st-c.16th century B.C.)	夏朝
Shang Dynasty (c.16th-c.11th century B.C.)	商朝
Zhou Dynasty (c.11th century-221 B.C.)	周朝
Qin Dynasty (221 B.C.-206 B.C.)	秦朝
Han Dynasty (206 B.C.-220 A.D.)	汉朝
Three Kingdoms (220-280)	三国
Western Jin Dynasty (265-316)	西晋
Eastern Jin Dynasty (317-420)	东晋
Northern and Southern Dynasties (420-581)	南北朝
Sui Dynasty (581-618)	隋朝
Tang Dynasty (618-907)	唐朝
Five Dynasties (907-960)	五代
Song Dynasty (960-1279)	宋朝
Liao Dynasty (916-1125)	辽国
Jin Dynasty (1115-1234)	金国
Yuan Dynasty (1271-1368)	元朝
Ming Dynasty (1368-1644)	明朝
Qing Dynasty(1644-1911)	清朝
Republic of China (1912-1949)	中华民国
People's Republic of China (1949-)	中华人民共和国

Chapter 3 Visceral Manifestation

The term "visceral manifestation" was first mentioned in Huang Di Nei Jing. "Visceral" refers to the internal organs stored inside the human body, while "manifestation" refers to the shape and phenomenon. Visceral manifestation refers to the internal organs stored inside the body, and also their outward physiological and pathological manifestations as well. Therefore, "visceral" is the intrinsic basis of "manifestation", while "manifestation" is the extrinsic reflection of "visceral".

The theory of visceral manifestation include three parts: ① the physiological functions and pathological changes of the internal organs; ② the relationships between the five zang organs and the five body constituents, five sense organs, five blooms, five fluids; ③ the relationships among the zang-fu organs, including the relationships between zang organs, between zang and fu organs and between fu organs.

The theory of visceral manifestation takes the zang-fu organs as its basis, so it is also called "the theory of zang-fu organs". The zang-fu organs are the general terms of the internal organs, including two categories of five zang organs and six fu organs. The five zang organs refer to the heart, liver, spleen, lung and kidney, while the six fu organs refer to the gallbladder, stomach, small intestine,

第3章 藏象

"藏象"一词,首先见于《黄帝内经》。藏,通"脏",指藏居于体内的内脏;象,指形象或现象。藏象,即指藏于体内的内脏及其表现于外的生理、病理现象。可见"藏"是"象"的内在根据,"象"是"藏"的外在反映。

藏象学说的内容主要有三个部分:一是内脏的生理功能和病理变化。二是五脏与五体、五官、五华、五液之间的关系。三是脏腑之间,包括脏与脏、脏与腑、腑与腑之间的联系。

藏象学说,主要以脏腑为基础,所以有时也称"脏腑学说"。脏腑是内脏的总称,主要有五脏与六腑两类。五脏,即心、肝、脾、肺、肾;六腑,即胆、胃、小肠、大肠、膀胱、三焦。此外,还有一类组织器官,由于其功能类似于

large intestine, bladder and triple energizer. Besides, there are another type tissues and organs, with similar function to the zang organs and similar shape to the fu organs, called "the extraordinary organs". The extraordinary organs include the brain, marrow, bone, vessel, gallbladder and uterus.

The five zang organs have the different functions from the six fu organs. The zang organs function to "store the Jing (Essence) Qi", i. e. to store the necessary essential substances to maintain the vital activities of the human body. The six fu organs function to "transport and transform materials", i. e. to accept and digest the food, to absorb the essence and to discharge the waste.

The theory of visceral manifestation, though based upon some ancient anatomical knowledge, mainly stresses on the observing and studying methods of "the internals possessing their outward manifestations", the so-called "theorizing the internal by observing the surface". It is applied to study the physiological functions, pathological changes and mutual relationships of the zang-fu organs inside the human body through observing the outside physiological and pathological phenomena of the human body. This kind of observing and analyzing result, to theorize "visceral" through "manifestation" from outside to inside, greatly surpasses the single category of internal organs in human anatomy, forming a unique theory of the human physiology and pathology. In the theory of visceral manifestation, there are the same terms of the heart, lung, spleen, liver, and kidney as in the modern human anatomy, but their explanations and illustrations in physiology and pathological are totally different. The physio-

脏,形态相似于腑,故称"奇恒之腑"。奇恒之腑包括脑、髓、骨、脉、胆、女子胞。

五脏与六腑各自的功能特点有所不同。五脏共同的功能特点是"藏精气",即贮藏人体维持生命活动所需要的精微物质;六腑共同的功能特点是"传化物",即受纳、消化饮食物,并吸收其精微,排泄其糟粕。

藏象学说虽然也以一定的古代解剖知识为基础,但主要立足于"有诸内必形诸外"的观察研究方法,古称"司外揣内",即主要通过对人体表现于外的生理、病现现象的观察,研究人体各个脏腑的生理功能、病理变化及其相互关系。这种以"象"测"藏"、由表及里的观察分析的结果,必然大大超越人体解剖学的脏器的范围,形成了独特的关于人体生理和病理的理论。藏象学说中的心、肺、脾、肝、肾等脏腑的名称,虽然与现代人体解剖学的脏器名称相同,但对其生理、病理的认识,却不尽相同。藏象学说中一个脏腑的生理功能,可能包含着现代

logical functions of one organ in the theory of visceral manifestation may include the physiological functions of several organs in the modern human anatomy, while the physiological functions of one organ in the modern human anatomy may be diffused in the physiological functions of several organs in the theory of visceral manifestation. It is because that some zang or fu organ in the theory of visceral manifestation does not refer to a single anatomical concept, but more important to the physiology and pathology of a certain system in the human body.

The theory of visceral manifestation centers on the five zang organs, to divided all the tissues and organs of the six fu organs, five body constituents, five sense organs, nine orifices, four limbs and bones into five large-scale systems. The five large-scale systems form up a whole entirety through the connecting-pertaining relation of the meridians and the circulation of qi and blood. The theory of visceral manifestation, is to study the individual physiological functions of the zang-fu organs, meridians and collaterals, forms and structures, sense organs and orifices on one hand, and to exposit the their complicated inner links and activity regulation in general on the other hand. Furthermore, it is also consider the influence of the external environmental factors as the weather, phenological and geographical conditions on the physiological activities of human body, reflecting the conception of entirety in the theory of visceral manifestation of TCM.

解剖生理学中几个脏器的生理功能；而现代解剖学中的一个脏器的生理功能，亦可能分散在藏象学说的几个脏腑生理功能之中。这是因为藏象学说中的某脏某腑，不单纯是一个解剖的概念，更重要的是概括了人体某一系统的生理和病理概念。

藏象学说以五脏为中心，将六腑、五体、五官、九窍、四肢百骸等组织器官分成五大系统。五个系统之间通过经脉的络属、沟通，气血的流注贯通，形成统一的整体。藏象学说一方面研究脏腑、经络、形体、官窍等各自的生理功能，另一方面从总体上揭示它们之间的复杂联系及其活动规律，并注重气象、物候、地理等外界环境因素对人体生理活动的影响，体现了中医藏象学说的整体思想。

Section 1 Five Zang Organs

The five zang organs are the generic term of the heart, lung, liver, spleen and kidney. In this section, it is to introduce the physiological functions of the five zang organs, and their relationships to the five body constituents, five sense organs, five blooms, five emotions and five fluids.

Five body constituents refer to the five kinds of structures of the vessel, skin, tendon, muscle and bone, dominated by the five zang organs respectively.

Five sense organs refer to the five organs of the tongue, nose, eye, mouth and ear. There is another saying of "nine orifices", including the mouth, nose, eye, ear, anterior orifice (the external genitalia and urethral meatus) and posterior orifice (anus). The heart, lung, liver and spleen dominate one sense organ respectively, while the kidney dominates ear, anterior orifice and posterior orifice.

Five blooms refer to the five specific areas on body surface where the Jing (Essence) Qi of five zang organs manifests, i. e. the face, body hair, nail, lip and hair, dominated by five zang organs respectively.

Five emotions refer to five kinds of emotional activities, i. e. the joy, anger, worry, grief and fear, dominated by five zang organs respectively.

Five fluids refer to five kinds of body fluid, i.e. the sweat, snivel, tear, Xian (Thin) Saliva and Tuo (Thick) Saliva, dominated by five zang organs respectively.

1 Heart

The heart locates in the chest, between the two

第 1 节　五脏

五脏,是心、肺、肝、脾、肾的合称。本节主要介绍五脏的生理功能,以及五脏与五体、五官、五华、五志、五液的关系。

五体,即脉、皮、筋、肉、骨五种形体组织,五脏各主其一。

五官,即舌、鼻、目、口、耳五种器官。另有"九窍"之说包括口、鼻、目、耳及二阴。心、肺、肝、脾各主一官窍,肾开窍于耳及二阴。

五华,是五脏精气显露于外的五个特殊部位,即面、毛、爪、唇、发,五脏各主其一。

五志,即喜、怒、思、忧、恐五种精神情志活动,五脏各主其一。

五液,即汗、涕、泪、涎、唾五种人体液体,五脏各主其一。

1　心

心位于胸中,居两肺叶

lobes of lung. The heart, taking the position of top prominence, possesses the dominating function on the vital activities of whole body, so it is called in Huang Di Nei Jing "the organ severed as the Monarch".

1.1 Physiological functions of the heart

The major physiological functions of the heart are: first, dominating the blood and vessels and second dominating the spirit and mind.

1.1.1 Heart dominates the blood and vessels

This function of the heart includes that heart dominates the blood and heart dominates the vessels. The function of the heart in dominating the blood refers to the blood circulation all over the body through the heart's pulsation, and also refers to the relation between the heart and blood production. The function of the heart in dominating the vessels refers that the heart links with the vessels of the whole body. Therefore, the heart, blood and vessels form up an airtight circulative system.

The blood circulates inside the vessels. The heart links with the vessels, so the heart's pulsation functions to inspire the blood circulation. Therefore, the heart is the motive power to promote the blood to circulate inside the vessels. Under the comprehensive actions of heart's pulsation and vessels' restraint, the blood can circulate all over the body normally. The heart's pulsation is the key to maintaining the blood circulation, playing a leading role.

That the reason why the heart can promote the blood to circulate inside the vessels is because of the promoting and warming functions of the heart qi and heart yang, and also the nourishing and mois-

之间。心在五脏六腑中居于首要地位,对全身生命活动起着主宰作用,故《黄帝内经》称其为"君主之官"。

1.1 心的生理功能

心的主要生理功能,一是主血脉,二是主神志。

1.1.1 心主血脉

心主血脉,包括心主血与心主脉的功能。心主血,是指血液通过心的搏动而运行全身,也指心与血液的生成有关。心主脉,是指心与全身的脉道相连,心、血与脉道构成一个密闭的循环系统。

血液运行于脉道之中。由于心与脉道相连,心的搏动具有鼓动血液运行的能力,所以心是推动血液在脉道中运行的动力所在。血液只有在心的搏动与脉道约束的共同作用下,才能正常地运行于周身,而其中心脏的搏动是维持血液运行的关键,起着主导作用。

心之所以能够推动血液在脉道内运行,是依赖于心气、心阳的推动和温煦作用,以及心阴、心血的营养和滋

turizing functions of the heart yin and heart blood as well. If the qi, blood, yin and yang of the heart is sufficient, the heart's pulsation will be normal, and the blood circulation of human body will be continuous to nourish the five zang organs, six fu organs, four limbs and all bones, to maintain the normal physiological functions of all tissues and organs, so as to show the manifestations of energetic vigor, reddish, moist and lustrous complexion, and moderate and strong pulse. If the qi, blood, yin or yang of the heart is insufficient or disturbed, there will be a series of pathological manifestations due to dysfunction of the heart to dominate the blood and vessels, such as pale complexion, thready and weak pulse in the heart qi deficiency pattern, or purple complexion, choppy or irregular pulse in the heart blood stagnation pattern.

At the same time, the heart has the "reddening function" on the production of blood. The spleen and stomach digest the food and absorb the food essence, and then send the essential substance upwards to the heart and lung. Combined with the Qing(Clear) Qi inhaled by the lung from the nature, the essential substance is transformed into the red-colored blood under the warming and transpiring function of the heart yang.

1.1.2　Heart dominates the spirit and mind

The function of the heart to dominate the spirit and mind is also called "the heart housing the spirit". The spirit is divided into two kinds in broad sense and narrow sense. The spirit in broad sense refers to the supreme dominator of the whole vital activities of human body. The spirit in narrow sense refers to the general term of the spiritual activities

润作用。心之气血阴阳充足，心的搏动就正常，人体的血液循环不息，营养周身五脏六腑、四肢百骸，使各组织器官的生理功能正常，从而表现出精力充沛、面色红润光泽、脉象和缓有力等现象。如心之气血阴阳不足或失调，就会影响心主血脉的功能而出现一系列病理表现，如心气不足，可见面色苍白、脉细弱无力；心血瘀阻，可见面色青紫、脉涩结代等。

同时，心对血液的生成具有"化赤"的作用。饮食物经过脾胃的消化吸收之后，将其中的精微物质上输于心肺，在肺部结合自然界之清气，又在心阳的温煦蒸腾作用下，化生为红色的血液。

1.1.2　心主神志

心主神志的功能，又称"心藏神"。神有广义和狭义之分。广义之神，是指整个人体生命活动的最高主宰。狭义之神，是对人的认知、思维、意识、情志等精神活动的总称。心主神志，主要指心

including cognition, thinking, consciousness and e-motion. That the heart dominates the spirit and mind refers to the function of heart in dominating the spiritual activities of human body.

The spiritual activities of human body are related to the function of the brain in responding to the outward objects and some immanent functional activities of the brain. In the theory of visceral manifestations in TCM, it centers on the five zang organs, so the spiritual activities pertain to the functional scope of the heart. Therefore, the function of heart in dominating the spirit and mind actually generalizes some functional activities of the brain.

The normal function of the heart in dominating the spirit and mind mainly relies on the nourishing and moisturizing functions of the heart blood or heart yin on the spirit of the heart. The heart blood is the important substantial foundation of the spiritual activities. Besides, the enhancing and inspiring function of the heart qi or heart yang on the spirit of the heart is also related. If the heart is normal in dominating the spirit and mind, there can be the manifestations of high spirit, clear consciousness, quick thinking and sensitive reaction. If the qi, blood, yin or yang of the heart is insufficient or disturbed, there will be dysfunction of heart function in dominating the spirit and mind, leading to the symptoms of palpitation, insomnia, dream-disturbed sleep, poor memory, even loss of consciousness, delirium, coma, etc.

有主管人的精神活动的功能。

人的精神活动,与大脑对客观外界事物的反映及其固有的某些功能活动有关,但中医藏象学从以五脏为中心的理论出发,把精神活动主要归属于心的功能范畴。因此,心主神志,实际上概括了大脑的某些功能活动。

心主神志功能的正常发挥,主要依赖心血、心阴对心神的营养及滋润作用,这是精神活动的重要物质基础,其次也与心气、心阳对心神的鼓舞及振奋作用有关。心主神志功能正常,则人的精神振奋,神志清晰,思维敏捷,反应灵敏。若心之气血阴阳不足或失调,使心主神明的功能异常,可出现心悸、失眠、多梦、健忘,甚至神昏、谵语、不省人事等症。

1.2 Relationships between the heart and its body constituent, bloom, orifice, emotion and fluid

1.2.1 Have its body constituent in vessel, and its bloom on the face

The vessels are the passage of the blood circulation. The heart has its body constituent in vessel, implying that the heart is closely related to the vessel structurally, functionally and pathologically. Structurally, the heart links with the vessels directly. Functionally, the heart's pulsation promotes the blood to circulate inside the vessels normally. Therefore, if the function of the heart is normal and the vessels are unblocked, the blood can flow smoothly, and the pulse is moderate and forceful. If the function of the heart is abnormal or the vessels are blocked, the blood circulation will be disturbed, and the pulse becomes abnormal as well. For example, if the heart blood is insufficient, the vessels will be vacuous, leading to thready and weak pulse. If the heart yang is insufficient, it fails to inspire the blood circulation, leading to deep and weak pulse.

The heart has its bloom on the face. It implies that the qi, blood, yin or yang of the heart may be shown specifically on the face. From observing the color, luster and form of face, it is possible to determine if the qi, blood, yin or yang of the heart is normal or not. If the heart blood is sufficient and flows smoothly, the complexion is red, moist and lustrous. If the heart qi is insufficient or the heart blood is deficient, there can be pale and lusterless complexion. If the heart blood is stagnant, there can be purple complexion.

1.2 心与体、华、窍、志、液的关系

1.2.1 在体合脉,其华在面

脉道是血液流通的道路。心在体合脉,是指心与脉在结构、功能以及病理上都有着密切的关系。在结构上,心与脉道直接相连;在功能上,心的搏动推动着血液在脉道中的正常运行。因此,心的功能正常,脉道通利,则血液流畅,脉象和缓而有力;心的功能异常,或脉道不利,则血行障碍,脉象也会出现相应的异常反应。如心血不足,血脉空虚,可出现脉细弱;心阳不足,鼓动无力,可出现脉象沉微等。

心其华在面,是说心的气血阴阳,可特异性地表露于面部,观察面部的色泽形态,可以判断心的气血阴阳正常与否。如心血充足,运行通畅,则面部红润有光泽;如心气不足,心血亏少,可见面白而无华;心血瘀阻,又可见面色青紫等。

1.2.2 Open into the tongue

That the heart opens into the tongue implies that the heart has some specific relation to the tongue, and that the pathological manifestations of the heart can be reflected on the tongue. The collateral of the Heart Meridian of Hand-Shaoyin runs upwards to connect with the tongue. It can be exposed to the tongue if the heart blood is sufficient or not, while the heart spirit also influence directly the sensation and movement of the tongue. Therefore, no matter which function of the heart in dominating the blood and vessels or in dominating the spirit and mind is normal or not, it can be reflected from the color, luster and form of the tongue. Therefore, there is such a saying that "the tongue is the mirror of the heart". If the qi, blood, yin and yang of the heart are normal, the tongue is red and moist, the tongue body is soft and flexible, the tasting sensation is fine, and the speech is fluent. If the heart blood is insufficient, the tongue body is pale, and the food intake is found tasteless. If the heart fire is flaring-up, the tongue body is red or scarlet, and ulcers occur on the tongue. If the heart spirit is deranged, there can be symptoms of tongue flaccidity, tongue rigidity, or dysphasia.

1.2.3 Have its emotion as the joy

The emotion of the heart is the joy. The joy is the only benign emotional reaction among the five emotions or seven emotions. It is believed in Huang Di Nei Jing that the proper joyful and happy emotion may harmonize the blood and qi, smoothen the Ying (Nutrient) Qi and Wei (Defensive) Qi, and the mood is pleasurable, so as to benefit the sound mind and body. But over joy or happiness may dam-

1.2.2 开窍于舌

心开窍于舌,是指心与舌有着某种特定的联系,心的病理表现也可通过舌得以反映。手少阴心经的别络上行联系到舌,心血的充足与否显露于舌,心神也直接影响着舌的感觉与运动。因此,无论是心主血脉还是心主神志的功能正常与否,每可从舌的色泽形态上反映出来,故又有"舌为心之苗"之说。如心的气血阴阳正常,则舌质红润,舌体柔软灵活,味觉灵敏,语言流利。若心血不足,可见舌质淡白,食不知味;心火上炎,可见舌质红绛,或舌上生疮;心神失常,可见舌卷、舌强、语言謇涩等。

1.2.3 在志为喜

心,在志为喜。喜,是五志、七情中惟一的属于良性的情绪反映。早在《黄帝内经》就认为:适度的喜乐,能使血气调和,营卫通利,心情舒畅,有益于心身健康。但过度的喜乐,则可损伤心神,即所谓过喜伤心,以致心气

age the heart spirit, the so-called "over-joy dama-ging the heart", so as to lead to distraction of the heart qi and sorrow turned by excessive joy. On the contrary, if the heart spirit is hyperactive, the heart fire is flaring-up, so as to lead to the disease state of unceasing laugh and play.

1.2.4   Its fluid as the sweat

The sweat originates from the body fluid. Why the body fluid can transform into sweat to discharge outwards, is because of the result of the transpiring function of the yang qi. The heart pertains to the fire of the five elements. The heart fire transforms into the yang qi which functions to transpire the body fluid into sweat, flowing outwards to the body surface. Therefore, the sweat is regarded as the flu-id of the heart. Clinically, profuse sweating may damage and consume the qi and blood of the heart, leading to palpitation and fearful throbbing. If the heart qi is deficient or the heart yang declines, there can be the symptom of spontaneous sweating or sweating all over the body.

Appendix: Pericardium

The pericardium, also called "the Pericardium Collateral", is a membrane surrounding the heart and functions to protect the heart. In the theory of meridian and collateral, the Pericardium Meridian of Hand-Jueyin connects with the Triple Energizer Meridian of Hand-Shaoyang in an exterior-interior relation. Therefore, the pericardium pertains to the zang organ. It is believed by the ancient physicians that the heart, served as the monarch of the human body, cannot be attacked by the Xie (Pathogenic) Qi. When the exogenous pathogen attacks the heart, the pericardium takes the place of the heart to be attacked, so the pericardium functions

涣散,乐极生悲。反之,若心神过亢,心火亢盛,亦可出现喜笑不休的病态。

1.2.4   在液为汗

汗来源于津液。津液之所以能形成汗液而排出体外,主要是阳气蒸腾作用的结果。心在五行属火,心火化为阳气而能蒸化其津液,外出于肌肤便形成汗,所以汗为心之液。中医临床上,汗出过多,可耗伤心之气血,易见心悸、怔忡等。反之,心气虚损、心阳衰惫之人,自汗不止,甚则大汗淋漓,亦为常见之症。

附:心包

心包,又称"心包络",为心的外围结构,有保护心脏的作用。在经络学说中,手厥阴心包经与手少阳三焦经相为表里,故心包络属于脏。古代医家认为,心为人身之君主,不得受邪,所以若外邪侵心,则心包络当先受病,故心包有"代心受邪"之功用。后世温病学派就将外感热病中出现的高热、神昏、谵语等症,称为"热入心包"或"痰热

to "substitute the heart to be attacked by the Xie (Pathogenic) Qi)". It is said in the School of Febrile Diseases that the symptoms of high fever, loss of consciousness and delirium in the febrile disease due to exogenous pathogens are diagnosed as "heat entering pericardium" or "phlegm-heat hoodwinking pericardium". Actually, the diseases and patterns of the pericardium are exactly those of the heart. Same as other zang organs, the heart can also be attacked by the Xie (Pathogenic) Qi.

2　Lung

The lung locates in the chest, in a highest position of the body, so it is called "the canopy". The lobes of lung are tender and delicate, and unendurable to cold or heat, so the lung is easy to be attacked by the Xie (Pathogenic) Qi to cause diseases. Therefore, the lung is also called "the delicate zang organ".

The movement of the lung qi is featured of dispersing and descending actions. The dispersing movement refers to the up-flow and outflow of lung qi, while the descending movement refers to the down-flow and inflow of lung qi. These two features are reflected in the physiological functions of the lung.

The lung functions to assist the heart to move the blood, so the lung is called "the organs served as a premiere" in Huang Di Nei Jing.

2.1　Physiological functions of the lung

The major physiological functions of the lung are: first to dominate qi, and second to dredge and regulate the water passage.

蒙蔽心包"。实际上，心包受邪所出现的病证，即是心的病证，心和其他脏器一样，皆可受邪气之侵。

2　肺

肺位于胸中，居位最高，故有"华盖"之称。又因为肺叶娇嫩，不耐寒热，易被邪气侵犯而发病，故又称"娇脏"。

肺气的运动特点有宣发和肃降两方面。宣发，是指向上向外的宣通发散；肃降，是指向下向内的清肃下行。这两方面的特点都体现在肺的生理功能之中。

由于肺具有助心行血的作用，所以《黄帝内经》称肺为"相傅之官"。

2.1　肺的生理功能

肺具有主气和主通调水道两方面的生理功能。

2.1.1　Lung dominates qi

The function that the lung dominates qi includes that the lung dominates qi of respiration and qi of whole body.

That the lung dominates qi of respiration implies that the lung functions to govern the respiratory movement. The lung is the major organ of respiratory movement of the human body, as the place of the air exchange *in vivo* and *in vitro*. Through its respiratory movement, the lung inhales the Qing (Clear) Qi in the nature and exhales the Zhuo (Turbid) Qi inside the body. Such a circular movement of taking in the fresh and getting rid of the stale maintains the normal vital activities of the human body.

The normal function of the lung in dominating respiration relies on the moisturizing function of the lung yin, and also on the dispersing and descending function of the lung qi as well. The lung exhales the Zhuo (Turbid) Qi inside the body through its dispersing function, and inhales the Qing (Clear) Qi in the nature through is descending function. Therefore, the dispersing function and descending function of the lung qi are mutually restrained and also mutually dependent as well, for the purpose to maintain the normal respiratory movement of the human body. Physiologically, the dispersing function and descending function of the lung qi are harmonious, so the qi passage is unblocked and the respiration is regular. Pathologically, the lung fails to dominate dispersing and descending, so the respiration is disturbed, leading to the symptoms of stuffy chest, cough, panting, breathing difficulty, etc.

That the lung dominates qi of the whole body

2.1.1　肺主气

肺主气的功能,包括主呼吸之气和主一身之气。

肺主呼吸之气,是指肺具有主持呼吸运动的功能。肺是人体呼吸运动的主要器官,是体内外气体交换的场所。通过肺的呼吸运动,吸入自然界清气,呼出体内浊气,由此而不断地吐故纳新,维持人体生命活动的正常进行。

肺司呼吸功能的正常发挥,除了肺阴的滋润作用以外,主要依赖于肺气的宣发和肃降。通过肺气向上向外的宣通发散,呼出体内浊气;通过肺气向下向内的清肃下行,吸入自然界清气。因此,肺气的宣发和肃降,既相互制约,又相互依存,共同维持人体正常的呼吸功能。在生理情况下,肺气的宣降保持协调,则气道通畅,呼吸调匀。在病理情况下,如肺失宣降,影响其呼吸功能,则出现胸闷、咳嗽、气喘等呼吸不利的症状。

肺主一身之气,是指肺

implies that the lung functions to govern and regulate the qi of the whole body, including three aspects as follows:

Firstly, it refers to the formation of the Zong (Pectoral) Qi. The Zong (Pectoral) Qi, one component part of qi of human body, originates from the Jing (Essence) Qi of water and grain through the transportation and transformation of the spleen, and the Qing (Clear) Qi in the nature inhaled by the lung. After its formation, the Zong (Pectoral) Qi is distributed to the whole body through the function of lung in dispersing and descending, and the function of the heart in dominating the blood circulation, for the purpose to warm and nourish all the zang-fu organs and tissues, to maintain their normal physiological functions. The Qing (Clear) Qi in the nature is the necessary condition to produce the Zong (Pectoral) Qi, and it is inhaled by the respiratory function of the lung. Therefore, if the function of lung in dominating respiration is normal or not directly influences the formation of the Zong (Pectoral) Qi of human body, and also influences the formation of qi of the whole body as well.

Secondly, it refers to the regulation of the qi activities. The lung possesses the dispersing and descending functions, which directly influence the qi activities of the whole body. Besides, the respiration of the lung reflects the features of qi movement in up-flow, down-flow, outflow and inflow, so as to influence the qi activities of the whole body. Therefore, the smooth qi activity of the whole body relies on the respiratory function of the lung. If the respiratory function is normal, the qi of all the zang-fu organs, meridians and collaterals in the whole

有主持、调节周身之气的功能。其具体体现在如下三个方面：

一是宗气的生成。宗气是人体之气的一部分，它是由脾通过消化饮食物，吸收其中的精微物质而上输于胸中，与肺吸入的自然界之清气互相结合而生成的。宗气生成后，又通过肺的宣发肃降及心主行血的功能而布散于全身，以温养各脏腑组织，维持其正常的生理功能。由于自然界清气是生成宗气的必要条件，而其又是有赖肺的呼吸功能吸入，所以肺司呼吸功能正常与否，直接影响着人体宗气的生成，也影响着全身之气的生成。

二是气机的调节。肺具有宣发肃降的功能，直接影响着全身的气机运动，而肺之呼吸也体现出升降出入的特点，对全身之气的运动有重要影响。所以，全身之气的运行调畅与否，与肺的呼吸功能密切有关。如呼吸功能正常，则周身各脏腑经络之气就随着肺气的运动而能正常地升降出入。可见，肺

body can normally up-flow, down-flow, outflow and inflow along with the movements of the lung qi. It is thus clear that the lung functions to regulate the up-flow, down-flow, outflow and inflow of qi of the whole body.

Thirdly, it refers to its function to assist the heart to move the blood. The heart dominates the blood and vessels, while the heart's pulsation is the basic motive power to promote the blood circulation. The lung functions to assist the heart to move the blood, because the blood of the whole body converges in the lung through vessels on one hand, and the blood distributes to the whole body from the lung on the other hand. Therefore, it is said in Huang Di Nei Jing that "the lung collects all the vessels".

2.1.2 Lung dredges and regulates the water passage

The water passage refers to the passage from where the water distributes and discharges. The function of the lung in dredging and regulating the water passage implies that the lung functions to promote and regulate the distribution and discharge of water.

The taken-in water inside the body is absorbed by the function of the spleen in transportation and transformation, is then sent upwards to the lung. The lung qi, through its dispersing function in up-flow and outflow, sends the water to the body surface, transforms it into sweat to discharge, and also discharges some water through lung's respiration. The lung qi, through its descending function in down-flow and inflow, sends the water inwards to the internal organs and downwards to the kidney,

对全身气的升降出入运动起着重要的调节作用。

三是助心行血。心主血脉,心脏的搏动是推动血液运行的基本动力。肺助心行血,体现在一方面血液通过脉道从全身会聚于肺,另一方面血液又通过脉道从肺散行于全身,所以《黄帝内经》有"肺朝百脉"之论。

2.1.2 肺主通调水道

通调,是疏通、调节的意思。水道,指水液输布和排泄的通道。肺主通调水道,即指肺具有推动、调节水液输布和排泄的功能。

摄入体内的水液,经脾的运化功能吸收后,上输于肺。肺气一方面通过其向上向外的宣发作用,将水液输布到体表,经利用后化为汗液而排出体外,同时呼气中也排出了部分水分;另一方面通过其向下向内的肃降作用,将水液输布至内脏,经利用后下行于肾,在肾的气化

which transforms the water into urine, and sends it downwards to the bladder to discharge. The lung, termed as the canopy in the highest position in the body, involves in the water metabolism of the body, so the lung is also called "the upper source of water". If the lung qi fails to disperse and descend, its function in dredging and regulating water passage is abnormal and then influences the distribution and discharge of water, leading to the diseases and symptoms of phlegm, rheum, edema and abnormal urination.

2.2 Relationships between the lung and its body constituent, bloom, orifice, emotion and fluid

2.2.1 Have its body constituent in skin, and its bloom on the body hair.

The skin functions to protect the body, excretes the sweat and regulates the body temperature. It may be illustrate the relation between the lung and skin in two aspects as follows: Firstly, the lung possesses the dispersing function to distribute the Wei (Defensive) Qi and body fluid to the skin, so as to warm, nourish and moisturize the skin, for the purpose to maintain the normal physiological functions of the skin. Secondly, the normal opening and closing function of the sweating pores on skin can not only excrete the sweat and regulate the body temperature, but also assist the lung's respiratory function to discharge some part of Zhuo (Turbid) Qi as well. Therefore, the sweating pores are also called "the gate of qi". If the lung functions normally, the skin can be nourished to be fine and close, the discharge of sweat is proper, and the defending ability against the exogenous pathogens is strong. If the lung

作用下生成尿液，下输膀胱而排出体外。由于肺为华盖，位置最高，而肺又参与了体内水液代谢，所以肺又称为"水之上源"。如果肺失宣降，导致肺主通调水道的功能失常，影响水液的输布和排泄，便可出现痰饮、水肿及小便异常等病症。

2.2 肺与体、华、窍、志、液的关系

2.2.1 在体合皮，其华在毛

皮，即皮肤，具有保护人体、排泄汗液及调节体温等功能。肺与皮肤的关系，可从两方面来理解：一是肺可以宣发输布卫气和津液至皮肤，以温养、滋润皮肤，维持皮肤正常的生理功能。二是皮肤汗孔开合有度，既可排泄汗液，调节体温，又可协助肺呼吸功能，排出部分浊气，所以汗孔又称为"气门"。如肺的功能正常，皮肤得养，则皮肤致密，汗液排泄适度，抵御外邪的能力亦强。如肺之气阴不足，皮肤失养，可见皮肤干燥枯槁、多汗而易于感冒；而外邪侵袭人体，也常从皮肤影响及肺，引起肺气不

qi or yin is not sufficient, the skin fails to be nourished, leading to dry and withered skin, profuse sweating and easiness to catch cold. If the exogenous pathogens attack the human body, they affect the skin first and then the lung, leading to dysfunction of lung in dispersing, with the symptoms of aversion to cold, fever, nasal obstruction and cough.

The lung has its bloom on the body hair. The lung dominates the skin, so the Wei (Defensive) Qi and body fluid distributed by the lung qi may moisturize and nourish the body hair, to make the body hair lustrous and not easily lose. So from observing the condition of the body hair, it is able to determine if the lung's function is normal or not. If the lung qi or yin is not sufficient, the body hair fails to be nourished, leading to dry and withered hair, which are easy to be broken or lost. Since the skin is closely related to the body hair, it is also said that "the lung dominates the skin and hair".

2.2.2 Open into the nose

The nose is the olfactory organ and the passage of the respiratory qi to outflow and inflow, while the lung dominates the respiration and qi of the whole body, so it is said that "the lung opens into the nose". The smelling and respiratory functions of the nose are closely related to the function of the lung qi. If the lung qi is harmonious, the respiration is smooth, and the sense of smell is sensitive. If the lung qi fails to disperse, there can be nasal obstruction, running nose and hyposmia. If the lung qi is not sufficient, there can be difficult respiration.

2.2.3 Have its emotion as the grief

The lung has its emotion as the grief. The grief is not an emotional activity of benign emotional

宣,出现恶寒、发热、鼻塞、咳嗽等症状。

肺,其华在毛。由于肺主皮肤,肺宣发的卫气和津液可以通过皮肤而滋养毫毛,使毫毛具有光泽而不易脱落,故毫毛的荣枯可反映出肺的功能正常与否。如肺之气阴不足,毫毛失养,则出现毫毛干燥枯槁,并容易折断或脱落等。由于皮肤与毫毛密切相关,故也习称"肺主皮毛"。

2.2.2 开窍于鼻

鼻是嗅觉器官,为呼吸之气出入的通道,而肺司呼吸,主一身之气,故称"肺开窍于鼻"。鼻的嗅觉和通气功能与肺气的作用紧密相关。肺气调和,呼吸通畅,嗅觉才能灵敏。如肺气不宣,可见鼻塞流涕,嗅觉减退;如肺气不足,可致鼻息不利等。

2.2.3 在志为忧

肺,在志为忧。忧愁为非良性刺激的情志活动,尤

stimulation, so over-grief may damage the normal physiological activities of human body. "The grief make qi vanish", it implies that the grief may consume qi of the human body. The lung dominates qi, so over-grief may damage the lung. If the lung qi is deficient, the body's tolerance to the unhealthy stimulation from the external decreases, so as to cause emotional change of grief. It can be clearly seen that there is a reciprocal causation and vicious circle between the lung deficiency and grief.

2.2.4 Have its fluid as the snivel

The snivel is a kind of mucus secreted in the nose, functioning to moisturize the nostrils. The nose is the orifice of the lung, so the snivel is the fluid of the lung. If the lung qi fails to disperse, there can be nasal obstruction and running nose. If the heat in the lung damages the body fluid, the nose becomes dry with scanty snivel.

3 Spleen

The spleen locates in the abdominal cavity, dominates the digestion and absorption, is the source to transform and produce qi, blood and body fluid, and functions to maintain the vital activities. This kind of function occurs after birth of human body, so the spleen is called "the acquired basis" and "the source to transform and produce qi and blood". In Huang Di Nei Jing, the spleen and stomach are called "the organs served as a warehouse".

3.1 Physiological functions of the spleen

The major physiological functions of the spleen are: first to dominate the transportation and transformation, and second to control the blood.

其是在过度忧伤的情况下,颇易损伤机体正常的生理活动。"悲则气消",悲忧对人体的影响,主要是损耗人体之气。因肺主气,故悲忧过度易于伤肺。在肺气虚弱时,机体对外来不良刺激的耐受能力下降,容易产生忧愁悲伤的情志变化。可见,肺虚与悲忧之间,存在着互为因果、恶性循环的关系。

2.2.4 在液为涕

涕是鼻中分泌的粘液,能滋润鼻孔。鼻为肺之窍,所以涕为肺之液。肺气失宣则鼻塞而流涕,肺热伤津则鼻干而涕少。

3 脾

脾位于腹中,主管消化吸收,是气血津液化生的源泉,对维持生命活动起着根本的作用,而这种作用是人体出生以后才体现出来的,所以称脾为"后天之本""气血生化之源",《黄帝内经》将脾与胃合称为"仓廪之官"。

3.1 脾的生理功能

脾的生理功能包括主化和主统血两方面。

3.1.1　Spleen dominates the transportation and transformation

That the spleen dominates the transportation and transformation implies that the spleen functions to digest the food, absorbs the essential substance and water from the food, and then sends them to the heart and lung.

The stomach accepts the food, while the digestion and absorption of food are carried out by the stomach and small intestine, but they should rely on the spleen's transforming function to transform the water and grain into essence, and rely on the spleen's transporting function to transport and distribute the essence of water and grain to the whole body simultaneously. Furthermore, the spleen functions to transport the surplus water absorbed from the food essence to the lung and kidney, which transform the water respectively into the sweat and urine to discharge through the transforming function of the lung qi and kidney qi respectively. Therefore, the spleen's function in dominating the transportation and transformation includes to transport and transform the essence and to transport and transform the water. During the process of digestion, absorption and transportation of the spleen, the action to transport and transform the essence and the action to transport and transform the water are carried out simultaneously, so the two functions are closely related physiologically and mutually influenced pathologically.

The spleen's function in dominating transportation and transformation relies on the promoting function of the spleen qi. In the movement of the spleen qi, the major form is up-flow, so it is said

3.1.1　脾主运化

脾主运化,是指脾能够消化饮食,吸收其中的精微物质和水液,然后再转输至心肺的功能。

饮食入胃后,对饮食物的消化和吸收,实际上是在胃和小肠内进行的。但是,必须依赖于脾的运化功能,才能将水谷化为精微。同样,也有赖于脾的转输和散精功能,才能把水谷精微布散至全身。另一方面,对被吸收的水谷精微中多余水分,能及时转输至肺和肾,通过肺、肾的气化功能,化为汗和尿排出体外。因此一般将脾主运化的功能分为运化精微和运化水液两个方面。但是,由于在脾的消化、吸收和转输过程中,运化精微和运化水液是同时进行的,所以,这两方面的功能有着密切联系,病理上也多相互影响。

脾主运化的功能,主要依赖于脾气的推动作用。脾气的运动特点,是以上升为主,故有"脾主升清"之说。

that "the spleen dominates to elevate the clear". "To elevate" implies to the up-flow and distribution, while "the clear" refers to the essential substance in the food. That the spleen dominates to elevate the clear implies that the spleen sends the essential substance in the food upwards to the heart and lung through the function of the spleen qi. Therefore, if the spleen's function in dominating to elevate the clear is normal, and the source to produce qi and blood is sufficient, the vital activities of human body will be vigorous. Furthermore, "to elevate" also implies to lift and support as well, so that the up-flow of the spleen qi can maintain the internal organs in their constant positions without prolapse.

If the spleen's transporting and transforming function is abnormal, there can be decrease of digestion and absorption, with the symptoms of poor appetite, abdominal distension, abdominal pain and constipation, and disturbance of water metabolism that causes internal retention of water and dampness, with the diseases of phlegm, rheum and edema. If the spleen fails to elevate the clear, there can be sinking of the spleen qi, with the symptoms of prolapse of internal organs, chronic diarrhea and prolapse of rectum.

3.1.2 Spleen controls the blood

That the spleen controls the blood implies that the spleen can control and check the blood to circulate inside the vessels, preventing its spilling out of the vessels.

That the spleen controls the blood relies on the checking function of the spleen qi. If the spleen qi is sufficient, it can control the blood of whole body

升,指上升和输布;清,指饮食中的精微物质。脾主升清,即通过脾气的作用将饮食中的精微物质上输于心肺。因此,脾主升清功能正常,气血化生充足,人体的生命活动就能保持旺盛的生机。另一方面,"升"还具有升提、托举之意。脾气上升,还能维持内脏恒定的位置而不致下垂。

脾的运化功能失常,其临床表现主要有:消化吸收功能减弱,表现为食欲不振、腹胀、腹痛、便溏等症;水液代谢障碍,引起水湿内停,可出现痰饮、水肿等症;如脾不升清,可见头晕目眩、神疲乏力;如脾气下陷,可见内脏下垂、久泻脱肛等。

3.1.2 脾主统血

统,是统摄、控制的意思。脾主统血,指脾能够统摄血液在脉道中运行,使其不致逸出脉外。

脾统血,主要依赖于脾气对血液的固摄作用。脾气充足,就能将周身血液控制、

to restrain it inside the vessels to circulate, so as to prevent its spilling out of the vessels. If the spleen qi is deficient, its function in controlling the blood is abnormal, so the blood fails to circulate inside the vessels, leading to various bleeding diseases, such as bloody feces, bloody urine, uterine bleeding, subcutaneous bleeding, etc.

3.2 Relationships between the spleen and its body constituent, bloom, orifice, emotion and fluid

3.2.1 Its body constituent in muscle, and its bloom on the lip

The function that the spleen dominates the muscles and four limbs implies that the nourishment of the muscles and four limbs comes from the essence of water and grain transported and transformed by the spleen. If the spleen's transporting and transforming function is normal, the essence of water and grain can be transformed into sufficient qi and blood, which nourish the muscles and four limbs, so as to make the muscles full and strong and the four limbs strong and forceful. If the spleen fails to transport and transform normally, the absorption of essence of water and grain absorbed decreases, resulting in failure to transform and produce sufficient qi and blood, which fail to nourish the muscles and four limbs, so as to cause thin and weak muscles, tiredness of four limbs, and even atrophy and paralysis.

The spleen has its bloom on the lip. The lips are the external part of the mouth. The spleen is the source to transform and produce qi and blood, so it is possible to determine if the qi and blood of human body are sufficient or not by observing the color,

约束在脉道中循行,从而防止其逸出于脉外。脾气虚弱,可致统血功能失常,血液不循常道,就会出现便血、尿血、崩漏、皮下紫斑等多种出血倾向。

3.2 脾与体、华、窍、志、液的关系

3.2.1 在体合肉,其华在唇

脾主肌肉、四肢,是指肌肉与四肢的营养均来自脾运化的水谷精微。脾气健运,水谷精微化生气血充足,肌肉四肢得其营养,则肌肉丰满壮实,四肢强劲有力。若脾失健运,水谷精微吸收减少,气血化生不足,肌肉四肢失养,则肌肉消瘦软弱、四肢倦怠乏力,甚至痿废不用。

脾其华在唇,唇为口之外露部分。脾为气血生化之源,而人体气血盛衰的状况,可从唇的色泽、形态反映出来。如脾气健运,气血充足,

shape and form of lips. If the spleen's transporting and transforming function is normal, qi and blood are sufficient, so the lips are red, moist and lustrous. If the spleen fails to transport and transform normally, the lips are pale, lusterless, or sallow and yellow, or even withered.

3.2.2 Open into the mouth

The mouth is the beginning of the digestive tract. The digestive function is dominated by the spleen, so the mouth is termed as "the orifice" of the spleen. The so-called "mouth" here refers to the appetite and taste. If the spleen's transporting and transforming function is normal, the appetite is good and the taste is normal. If the spleen fails to transport and transform normally, there can be symptoms of poor appetite, tastelessness in mouth, or sticky or sweet taste in mouth.

3.2.3 Have its emotion as the worry

The spleen has its emotion as the worry. Worry here refers to thinking and worry, a kind of state of spiritual, conscious and thinking activities. The normal thinking activity has no any harmful influence on the physiological activities of human body. But over-thinking or melancholy due to failing to realize desire is harmful for health. If the spleen qi is vigorous, it may transform and produce sufficient qi and blood, so the thinking activity is agile, and absence of tiredness after long-term thinking. If the spleen is deficient, the thinking activity cannot last long. And over-thinking may make the spleen qi stagnant and cause failure in transportation and transformation, with the symptoms of poor appetite, epigastric and abdominal distension in the beginning, and the heart and spleen deficiency pattern

口唇红润而有光泽；如脾失健运，气血衰少，则口唇淡白无华，或萎黄不泽。

3.2.2 脾开窍于口

口为消化道的开端。由于消化功能由脾所主，所以口成为脾之"开窍"。这里所言"口"，主要指食欲与口味。如脾运强健，则食欲旺盛，口味正常；如脾运失健，可见食欲减退，口淡乏味，或口腻、口甜等。

3.2.3 在志为思

脾，在志为思。思，即思考、思虑，是人的精神意识思维活动的一种状态。正常的思考，对机体的生理活动并无不良的影响。但若思虑过度，或所思不遂，就有可能不利健康。脾气健旺，化源充足，气血旺盛，则思维敏捷，久思不疲。脾虚则不耐思虑。而思虑太过，可使脾气壅滞，运化失司，初则饭茶不香，脘腹胀闷，久则易致面色萎黄，头目眩晕，心悸健忘等心脾两虚之证。

with the symptoms of sallow-yellow complexion, dizziness, blurring of vision, palpitation, poor memory, etc.

3.2.4 Have its fluid as the Xian (Thin-Light) Fluid

The Xian (Thin-Light) Fluid, a kind of thin body fluid in mouth, functions to assist to take in food. The mouth is the orifice of the spleen, so the Xian (Thin-Light) Fluid is termed as the fluid of the spleen. If the spleen is deficient, it fails to check the saliva to cause salivation. If the spleen yin is not sufficient, there can be dry mouth due to lack of saliva.

4 Liver

The liver locates under the diaphragm, inside the right hypochondria. The physiological features of the liver are described as "pertaining to yin as an organ while to yang in its function". "Pertaining to yin as an organ" implies that the liver is a zang organ and stores the yin blood. "Pertaining to yang in its function" implies that the yang qi of the liver is easy to up-flow and move, so the liver is called "the fierce organ", and "the organ served as a general" in Huang Di Nei Jing.

4.1 Physiological functions of the liver

The major physiological functions of the liver are: first to dominate dredging and draining, and second to store the blood.

4.1.1 Liver dominates dredging and draining

Dredging and draining mean to circulate smoothly. That the liver dominates dredging and draining implies that the liver functions to smoothen and regulate the qi activities of human body. The

3.2.4 在液为涎

涎为口中津液之清稀者,能帮助进食。口为脾之窍,所以涎为脾之液。脾虚失于固摄则涎多而外溢,脾阴不足则涎少而口干。

4 肝

肝位于横膈之下,右胁之内。肝的生理特性是"体阴而用阳"。"体阴",是指肝为阴脏而内藏阴血。"用阳",是指肝之阳气易升易动,故肝为"刚脏",《黄帝内经》则称其为"将军之官"。

4.1 肝的生理功能

肝具有主疏泄和主藏血两方面的功能。

4.1.1 肝主疏泄

疏泄,即疏通畅达的意思。肝主疏泄,是指肝具有疏通、调节人体气机运动的功能。气的运动,称为"气

movement of qi is called "the qi activity". The physiological functions of all zang-fu organs and tissues of human body rely on the normal movement of qi. The liver dominates dredging and draining, so as to smoothen and regulate the qi activities, so as to play an important role in the regulation of the physiological functions of all zang-fu organs and tissues. The function of liver to dominate dredging and draining so as to regulate the qi activities is mainly reflected in the four aspects as follows.

Firstly, it promotes the blood circulation and body fluid metabolism. The blood circulation and body fluid metabolism rely on the promoting function of qi in zang-fu organs, while the normal movement of qi of zang-fu organs relies on the liver qi that keeps in smooth flow. If the liver fails to dominate dredging and draining, the blood circulation or body fluid metabolism may be influenced, resulting in relative diseases. If the liver is hypoactive in dredging and draining, there can be liver qi stagnation, causing unsmooth flow of blood to form up the stagnant blood. If the liver is hyperactive in dredging and draining and up-flows excessively, the blood flows upwards along with the up-reverse flow of qi, leading to spitting blood. If the qi activity is stagnant, the water cannot flow smoothly, leading to phlegm, rheum, edema, etc.

Secondly, it assists the spleen and stomach in digestion. The digestion and absorption of food are carried out by the spleen and stomach, but the liver's function in dredging and draining plays an important assisting role in the whole digestive process. On one hand, the liver regulates the qi activities of the spleen and stomach through its dred-

机"。人体各脏腑组织的生理活动,都有赖于气的正常运动。肝主疏泄,能够调畅气机,从而对各脏腑组织的生理功能发挥着重要的调节作用。肝主疏泄,调节气机的功能,主要表现在以下四个方面。

一是促进血液运行和津液代谢。血液的运行和津液的代谢,都有赖于有关脏腑之气的推动作用,而脏腑之气的正常运行,又必须依靠肝气的疏通才能保持调畅。若肝失疏泄,气的运行失常,就可影响血液运行和津液代谢,出现相应的病变。如肝疏泄不及而气机郁结,血行不畅,可形成瘀血;或肝疏泄太过而升发无制,血随气逆,可出现吐血;或气机阻滞,水道不利,则产生痰饮、水肿等。

二是协助脾胃消化。人体对饮食物的消化吸收,是由脾胃来完成的,而肝的疏泄功能对消化过程起着十分重要的协助作用。这种协助作用主要表现在,肝通过疏泄来调畅脾胃的气机运动,

ging and draining function, to coordinate the spleen qi in elevating the clear and the stomach in subduing the turbid, so as to guarantee the normal digestive process. On the other hand, the bile is formed by the surplus of the liver qi, stored in the gallbladder, and infuses into the small intestine to carry out its assisting function in digestion. The normal secretion and excretion of the bile are closely related to the liver's function in dredging and draining. If the liver fails to dominate dredging and draining, the qi activities of the spleen, stomach and small intestine are influenced, so as to cause the disturbance in food digestion and absorption. If the liver qi attacks the spleen, there can be the symptoms of abdominal distension, abdominal pain, diarrhea, etc. If the liver qi attacks the stomach, there can be the symptoms of epigastric distension, stomach pain, vomiting, belching, etc. If the liver fails to dominate dredging and draining and influences the secretion and excretion of the bile, there can be the symptoms of the liver and gallbladder disharmony pattern as hypochondriac pain, jaundice, poor appetite, etc.

Thirdly, it regulates the emotional activities. The emotional activities refer to the psychological activities of joy, anger, worry, thinking, etc. The emotional activities are a part of the spiritual activities, related to the heart's function in dominating the spirit and mind, and also related to the liver's function in dredging and draining as well. The normal emotional activities rely on the sufficient and smooth qi and blood. The liver functions to regulate the qi activity, to promote the blood circulation, and to harmonize qi and blood, thus mani-

使脾气之升清与胃气之降浊得以协调配合,从而保证消化过程的正常进行。同时,由于胆汁是肝之余气积聚而成,贮存于胆,并排出于小肠而发挥其帮助消化的作用,而胆汁的正常分泌与排泄,与肝的疏泄功能有密切关系。如果肝失疏泄,影响到脾、胃、胆的气机,必会引起饮食的消化吸收障碍。若肝气犯脾,可出现腹胀、腹痛、腹泻等症。若肝气犯胃可出现胃部胀痛、呕吐、嗳气等症。若肝失疏泄,影响到胆汁的分泌与排泄,还可出现胁痛、黄疸、食欲不振等肝胆不和的症状。

三是调畅情志活动。情志,是指人的喜、怒、忧、思等心理活动。情志活动是精神活动的一部分,其与心主神志功能有关外,也与肝的疏泄功能密切相关。因为正常的情志活动有赖于气血的充足、调畅,而肝能疏通气机,促进血行,使气血调和,表现为精神愉快、心情舒畅、乐观开朗等情绪反应。如肝失疏

fested by the emotional reactions as mentally happiness, pleasurable mind and optimistic and elastic spirit. If the liver fails to dominate dredging and draining, the qi activities are disturbed, so manifested by the symptoms of bad mood, melancholy thoughtfulness, sentimentality, belching, sighing, etc. If the liver qi is stagnant and further transforms into fire, there are symptoms and signs of restlessness, anger, red complexion, red eyes, head distension, headache, etc.

Fourthly, it regulates the menstruation. In women, the blood is the important substance in their physiological process, as blood flow in menstruation, need of blood to nourish the fetus in pregnancy and blood flow in delivery, which are closely related to the volume and circulation of the blood. The liver functions to dominate dredging and draining, so as to regulate the qi activities, to smoothen the blood flow in vessels, making the blood downward infuse into the uterus and playing an important role in the physiological activities of menstruation and reproduction. Therefore, it is said by the ancients that "the liver is taken as the acquired basis in women". If the liver's function in dredging and draining is disturbed, there can be various gynecological and obstetric diseases, such as irregular menstruation, dysmenorrheal, amenorrhea, sterility or infertility.

4.1.2 Liver stores the blood

That the liver stores the blood implies that the liver functions to store the blood and to regulate the volume of the blood.

The liver's function in storing the blood is physiological significant, i. e. the liver blood may mois-

泄而气机不畅,可表现为心情不舒、郁郁寡欢、多愁善虑、嗳气太息等证候;若肝气横逆而气郁化火,可表现为性情急躁、容易发怒、面红目赤、头胀头痛等证候。

四是调理妇女月经。妇女的生理特点是以血为用,如行经耗血、妊娠血聚养胎、分娩出血等,都与血液的充盈及运行密切有关。而肝主疏泄,调畅气机,使血脉流通,下注胞宫,对维持妇女月经、生育等特殊的生理活动起着非常重要的作用,所以古人有"女子以肝为先天"的说法。如肝的疏泄功能失常,临床上可出现多种妇产科病症,如月经不调、痛经、闭经、不孕、不育等。

4.1.2 肝主藏血

肝主藏血,是指肝具有贮藏血液和调节血量的功能。

肝藏血的生理意义在于,肝血可以濡养自身,肝得

turize and nourish the liver itself, so the yin fluid in the liver is sufficient to restrain the liver yang to prevent its hyperactivity. At the same time when the liver regulates the volume of blood, the liver blood may moisturize and nourish all the tissues and organs in the whole body for the purpose to meet the demand of their physiological activities.

Physiologically, the volume of blood varies in all parts of body in the different states of physiological activities. Generally speaking, in the quiet state, the need for blood volume of tissues and organs of human body is small, so the surplus blood flows back to the liver. In the severely active state or activation emotion, the need for blood volume of tissues and organs is large, so the liver transfers its stored blood to tissues and organs so as to meet the demand of the physiological activities of the body. Therefore, along with the variation of the physiological activities, the blood redistributes to various tissues and organs, relying on the liver's function in storing the blood.

If the liver's function in storing the blood is disturbed, there can be two types of diseases. The first one is the liver blood insufficiency pattern, in which the blood fails to nourish the body, leading to the symptoms of dizziness, blurring of vision, tiredness in body and limbs, scanty volume and light color of blood in menstruation, or amenorrhea. The second is the pattern of liver failing to store the blood, in which the blood fails to be sent back to the liver and stored inside, leading to spitting blood, nasal bleeding, bloody feces, heavy flow of blood in menstruation, even constant hematemesis, metrorrhagia, metrostaxis, etc. in severe conditions.

血养则阴液充足,肝阴足则能制约肝阳而不致过亢;同时在调节血量的过程中,肝血能滋养全身组织器官以适应其生理活动的需要。

在生理状态下,人体各部分的血液量随着其生理活动的不同状态而有所不同。一般地说,安静状态下人体各器官血液的需要量较小,其有余部分回流入肝。当人体在剧烈活动或情绪激动时,各器官血液的需要量就较大,肝可将其贮藏的血液输送出来,以满足机体生理活动的需要。因此,随着生理活动的变化,血液在各组织器官之间重新分配,与肝藏血的功能密切相关。

肝主藏血功能失常,可引起两方面的病变。一是肝血不足,周身失养,可出现头昏、目眩、肢体乏力、妇女月经量少色淡或闭经等症状。二是肝不藏血,血液不能归藏于肝而妄行,可出现吐血、衄血、便血、妇女月经量多等症,严重时可导致呕血不止,或崩漏下血量多等症。

4.2 Relationships between the liver and its body constituent, bloom, orifice, emotion and fluid

4.2.1 Have its body constituent in tendon, and its bloom on the nail.

The tendon is a kind of body constituent to bind the muscle, bone and joint. The contraction and extension of the tendon maintain the flexion, extension and latroduction of the joint movements in human body.

The liver's function in dominating the tendon implies that the tendon can function normally on the basis of the nourishment of the liver blood and moisture of the liver yin. If the liver blood and liver yin are sufficient, the tendon can be nourished, so the joint movement is active and strong. If the liver yin or blood is not sufficient, it fails to nourish the tendon, leading to the symptoms of motor impairment of joint, tremor of hand and foot, numbness or tiredness of body and limbs, etc.

The nail includes the fingernail and toenail. The nail is the external continuation of the tendon, so it is said that "the nail is the surplus of the tendon". Both the nail and tendon rely on the moisture and nourishment of the liver blood, so the volume of blood determines the property of the nail. If the liver blood is sufficient, the nail is firm, bright, red and lustrous. If the liver blood is not sufficient, the nail will become soft, thin, even deformed and fragile and cracking.

4.2.2 Open into the eye.

The eye is also called "jingming". The Liver Meridian runs upwards to link with the eye, and the liver's function in dredging and draining regulates

4.2 肝与体、华、窍、志、液的关系

4.2.1 在体合筋,其华在爪

筋,是联结肌肉、骨骼和关节的一种组织。筋的收缩和弛张,维持着人体关节运动的屈伸或转侧。

肝主筋,是指筋有赖于肝血的营养和肝阴的滋润,才能保持正常的功能。肝阴肝血充足,筋得其养,关节运动便灵活而有力。如果肝之阴血不足,血不养筋,可出现关节活动不利、手足震颤、肢体麻木或容易疲劳等症状。

爪即爪甲,包括手指甲和脚趾甲。爪是筋延续在外的部分,故称"爪为筋之余"。爪与筋均依赖肝血的濡养,所以肝血的盈亏,往往可以影响爪甲的荣枯。如肝血充足,则爪甲坚韧明亮,红润而有光泽;若肝血不足,则爪甲软薄,甚至变形或脆裂。

4.2.2 开窍于目

眼睛,又称"精明"。由于肝的经脉上连于目,肝之阴血营养于目,肝之疏泄调

the eye activity, so the vision is closely related to the liver. However, it can be reflected from the eye if the liver's function is normal or not. Therefore, it is said that "the liver opens into the eye". If the liver yin or blood is not sufficient, there can be the symptoms of dryness of eyes and blurring of vision. If the liver fails to dominate dredging and draining to cause liver fire hyperactivity, there can be the symptoms of redness, swelling and pain of eyes, cloudy eyes, etc.

Furthermore, the Jing (Essence) Qi of five zang organs and six fu organs upward infuses into the eye, so the eye has the intrinsic relation to the other zang-fu organs, besides to the liver. The white part of the eye (sclera) pertain to the lung, while the lung dominates qi, so the sclera is called "the ocular part of qi". The black part of the eye (cornea) pertain to the liver, while the liver dominates the wind, so the cornea is called "the ocular part of wind". The outer and inner canthi pertain to the heart, while the heart dominates the blood, so the outer and inner canthi are called "the ocular part of blood". The upper and lower eyelids pertain to the spleen, while the spleen dominates the muscle, so the upper and lower eyelids are called "the ocular part of muscle". The pupil pertains to the kidney, while the kidney dominates the water, so the pupil is called "the ocular part of water". These are the so-called "five ocular parts".

4.2.3 Have its emotion as the anger.

The anger is a kind of emotional change in the agitation. When feel angry, be angry, because a proper anger is not harmful. But the incontinent anger is a kind of bad stimulation to the physiological

节于目,故目的视觉功能与肝密切相关,而肝的功能正常与否,也往往从目反映出来,所以说"肝开窍于目"。如肝阴肝血不足,可见两目干涩、视物模糊;肝失疏泄,肝火上炎,可见目赤肿痛、目睛生翳等。

另外,由于五脏六腑之精气皆上注于目,所以目不仅与肝有关,而且与其他脏腑都有内在的联系。如白睛属肺,因肺主气,故称白睛为气轮;黑睛属肝,因肝主风,故称黑睛为风轮;内、外眦属心,因心主血,故称内、外眦为血轮;上、下眼胞属脾,因脾主肉,故称上、下眼胞为肉轮;瞳孔属肾,因肾主水,故称瞳孔为水轮。以上合称"五轮"。

4.2.3 在志为怒

肝,在志为怒。怒是人在情绪激动时的一种情志变化。一般说来,当怒则怒,怒而有度,尚不为害。若怒而

activities of human body, leading to the derangement of qi and blood, and harmful to the body. The liver is a fierce organ, so its qi is easy to move and to up-flow. The big anger may make the liver qi up-flow, even both qi and blood up-flow, leading to the symptoms of red complexion, head distension and headache. Therefore, the anger is the emotion of the liver, while the big anger is easy to damage the liver. On the contrary, the liver fire flaring-up or the liver yang hyperactivity may lead to emotional irritability, and a minor stimulation may cause a anger.

4.2.4 Have its fluid as the tear

The tear is secreted from the eye, functioning to moisturize the eye. The eye is the orifice of the liver, so the tear is the fluid of the liver. The wind-heat in liver may cause incessant lacrimation, while the liver yin insufficiency may lead to lack of tear and dryness of eye.

5 Kidney

The kidney locates in the lumbus, so it is said that "the lumbus is the house of the kidney". The kidney functions to store the essence, being the basis of yin and yang of human body. The kidney essence accepted from the parents, a kind of congenital primitive substance to form up the human body, to maintain the life and to multiply the offspring. Therefore, the kidney is called "the congenital basis". The kidney dominates the bones and produces marrows, dominates the growth, development and reproduction. If the kidney qi is sufficient, the tendon and bone are strong and active, the movements are sensitive, the energy is vigorous, and the repro-

无节,则对于机体的生理活动是一种不良刺激,可使气血逆乱,有害身体。肝为刚脏,其气易动易升。盛怒之时,每致肝气勃发甚则气血并走于上,出现面红目赤、头胀头痛诸症。故怒为肝志,大怒极易伤肝。反之,肝火上炎,肝阳偏亢,也易致情绪急躁,稍有刺激,便易发怒。

4.2.4 在液为泪

泪出于目,能滋润眼睛。目为肝之窍,所以泪为肝之液。肝有风热则流泪不止,肝阴不足则泪少目干。

5 肾

肾位于腰部,故有"腰为肾之府"之说。肾藏精,肾为人体阴阳之根本。肾精禀受于父母,来源于先天,是构成人体、维持生命及繁衍后代的原始物质,所以又称肾为"先天之本"。肾主骨生髓,主生长、发育与生殖。肾气充盛则筋骨强健,动作敏捷,精力充沛,生殖机能正常,胎孕得以化生,故《黄帝内经》称其为"作强之官"。

ductive ability is normal, capable to produce the fetus. So the kidney is called "the organ served as a giant" in Huang Di Nei Jing.

5.1　Physiological functions of the kidney

The major physiological functions of the kidney are: first to store the essence, second, dominate the water, and third to accept qi.

5.1.1　Kidney stores essence, dominates the growth, development and reproduction.

That the kidney stores the essence implies that the kidney functions to accept, store and seal up the Jing (Essence) Qi, so as to prevent its gratuitous loss. The physiological significance of the kidney's function in storing and sealing up the Jing (Essence) Qi is to promote the constant abundance of the Jing (Essence) Qi in the kidney, to prevent the gratuitous loss of the Jing (Essence) Qi, and to create the necessary conditions for the kidney to fully realize its physiological efficacy. If the kidney's function in storing and sealing up the essence decreases, it may cause the gratuitous loss of the Jing (Essence) Qi in the kidney, so as not only to present the diseases due to the unstable pass of essence, as seminal emission, premature ejaculation, etc., but also to present the diseases due to the insufficiency of the Jing (Essence) Qi, as poor growth, slow development or reproductive decrease.

The essence is one of the fundamental substances to form up the human body and to maintain the vital activities of human body. The so-called "Jing (Essence) Qi in the kidney" refers to the major substantial foundation to promote the growth, development and reproduction of human body.

The Jing (Essence) Qi in the kidney originates

5.1　肾的生理功能

肾具有主藏精、主水液、主纳气等方面的功能。

5.1.1　肾藏精,主生长、发育与生殖

肾主藏精,是指肾具有摄纳、贮存、封藏精气而不致无故流失的生理功能。肾主封藏精气的主要生理意义在于其能促进肾中精气的不断充盈,防止精气无故流失,为精气在体内充分发挥生理效应创造必要条件。若肾主封藏功能减退,则可导致肾中精气的无故流失,不仅可出现精关不固的遗精、滑泄等病症,还可因精气不足而影响机体的生长、发育及生殖功能。

精,是构成人体和维持人体生命活动的基本物质之一。所谓"肾中精气",是指具有促进机体生长、发育和生殖机能的主要物质基础。

肾中精气的来源有二:

from two parts. First, it originates from the parents' essence of reproduction. It is inherent, so called "the congenital essence", which actually is the primitive substance to form up the embryo. Second it, after birth, originates from the nutrients absorbed from food and the surplus part of the essential substances produced in the physiological activity process of the zang-fu organs after the self-metabolism and equilibrium.

"The congenital essence" and "the acquired essence" are mutually dependent and functioned. The congenital essence relies on the constant cultivation and supply of the acquired essence, so as to fully realize its physiological efficacy. The acquired essence relies on the active support of the congenital essence, so as to work to accept, transform and produce itself constantly. The two merge closely to become the Jing (Essence) Qi in the kidney, to maintain the vital activities and reproductive ability of the human body.

If one is born congenitally deficient, or if one is lack of proper care after his birth, or if other zang-fu organs are deficient for long time without recovery, or if the kidney fails to store and seal up the essence, there can be the pathological conditions of the Jing (Essence) Qi in the kidney.

The major function of the Jing (Essence) Qi in the kidney is to promote the growth, development and reproduction of human body. The Jing (Essence) Qi possesses a self-process that it grows from juvenile to abundant gradually, and from abundant to recessionary even to exhausted gradually. This process of the Jing (Essence) Qi in the kidney di-

一是来源于父母的生殖之精。因其与身俱来，常先身生，故称为"先天之精"，实际上即是构成人体胚胎发育的原始物质。二是来源于人出生以后，机体从饮食中摄取的营养成分，以及脏腑生理活动过程中化生的精微物质经自身代谢平衡后的剩余部分。

"先天之精"和"后天之精"，两者相互依存，相互为用。先天之精须赖后天之精的不断培育和补充，才能充分发挥其生理效应；后天之精须赖先天之精的活力资助，才能不断摄入和化生。两者在肾中密切结合组成肾中精气，以维持机体的生命活动和生殖能力。

凡先天禀赋不足，或后天脾胃失调，或其他脏腑久虚不复，或肾主封藏功能失职等，均可形成肾中精气的病理状态。

肾中精气的主要作用是促进机体的生长发育和逐步具备生殖能力。肾中精气自身存在着一个由未充盛到逐步充盛，由充盛到逐步衰少而耗竭的过程。而肾中精气的盛衰，直接决定着机体的

rectly determines the birth, growth, development, ageing and death.

From the juvenile stage of a person, the Jing (Essence) Qi in the kidney starts to be abundant gradually, manifested by the phenomena of rapid growth, as change of teeth and growth of hair. Along with the constant abundance of the Jing (Essence) Qi in the kidney, a kind of substance called "Tian Gui" (gonadotropin) occurs. The so-called Tian Gui (gonadotropin) refers to the substance that is directly related to the reproductive ability occurred in the certain stage when the Jing (Essence) Qi in the kidney fully develops. The Tian Gui (gonadotropin) acts to promote the gonadal development of body that enters the adolescence stage, when the phenomena of menstruation in females and spermiation in males occur, indicating that the sexual ability is gradually matured and the reproductive ability is possessed. After the middle-aged stage, along with the gradual decrease of the Jing (Essence) Qi in the kidney, the Tian Gui (gonadotropin) decreases to be exhausted, so that the reproductive ability is gradually disappearing and the sexual ability is gradually declining, and the body is gradually senescent to enter the ageing stage.

If the Jing (Essence) Qi is not sufficient, "the five retardation pattern" (retarded standing, retarded walking, retarded growth of teeth, retarded growth of hair and retarded speaking) and "five flaccidity pattern" (flaccid head and nape, flaccid mouth, flaccid hands, flaccid feet and flaccid muscle) due to poor growth and slow development in infants may occur. In the young and middle-aged persons, the diseases of sexual or reproductive disabili-

生、长、壮、老、已。

人自幼年开始,随着肾中精气的逐步充盛,出现齿更发长等迅速生长的现象。以后又随着肾中精气的不断充盛而产生一种称为"天癸"的物质。所谓天癸,是指肾中精气发展到一定阶段所产生的与生殖机能直接有关的物质。在天癸的作用下,促使机体的性腺发育而进入青春期,在女子则出现"月事以时下",在男子则出现"精气溢泻"的排精现象,说明性机能逐步成熟而具备了生殖能力。人至中年以后,随着肾中精气的逐渐衰少,天癸也随之衰少直至耗竭,出现生殖机能的逐步消失和性机能的逐步衰退,形体亦日趋衰弱而至老年。

若肾中精气不足,婴幼儿可出现"五迟"证(迟立、迟行、迟齿、迟发、迟语)和"五软"证(头项软、口软、手软、足软、肌肉软)生长发育不良的表现;青壮年可出现性机能或生殖机能减退的病症;老年人可出现牙齿松动、头发枯萎、骨骼疏松等老衰现

ty may occur. In the old-aged person, the aging phenomena as loosening of tooth, withered hair and osteoporosis may occur.

5.1.2　Kidney dominates the water

That the kidney dominates the water implies that the kidney functions to dominate and regulate the water metabolism, so the kidney is also called "the water organ". The kidney plays an important role in the water metabolism of human body, which is realized by the transforming function of the kidney qi. The transforming function of the kidney qi carries from the beginning to the end in the whole physiological process of water metabolism.

Firstly, the functions of all the zang-fu organs that are involved in the water metabolism rely on the inspiring and promoting function of the Jing (Essence) Qi in the kidney. All the functions, such as the stomach's acceptance and decomposition, the lung's dispersing and descending, the spleen's transportation and transformation and distribution of essence, the triple energizer's unobstructed state, the bladder's opening and closure, etc., are unable to carry out without the transpiration and transformation of the kidney qi. If the kidney is weak, especially if the yang qi in the kidney is deficient, the functions of all the zang-fu organs involved in the water metabolism will decrease due to lack of the transpiring and promoting function of the kidney yang, so as to disturb the normal distribution and discharge of water.

Secondly, the transpiring and transforming function of the kidney qi is directly related to the productive volume and discharge volume of urine, while the production and discharge of urine are of

象。

5.1.2　肾主水液

肾主水液,是指肾有主持和调节水液代谢的生理功能,故肾又有"水脏"之称。肾在机体水液代谢中的重要作用,主要是依赖于肾的气化作用来实现的。肾的气化作用,在水液代谢的整个生理过程中贯穿始终。

首先,一切参与水液代谢的脏腑功能均有赖于肾中精气的激发推动。如胃的受纳、游溢,肺的宣发、肃降,脾的运化、散精,三焦的通利,膀胱的开合等功能的正常发挥,均离不开肾的蒸腾气化。一旦肾虚,尤其是肾的阳气虚损时,参与水液代谢的其它脏腑功能也容易因缺乏肾阳的蒸腾推动而减退,从而影响水液的正常输布和排泄。

其次,是因为肾的蒸腾气化作用与尿液的生成量和排泄量直接有关,而尿液的生成和排泄,对于维持整个

the utmost importance in maintaining the equilibrium of whole water metabolism. If the transpiring and transforming function of the kidney qi is abnormal, there can be the pathological phenomena of metabolic disturbance, such as scanty urine, edema, etc., or the pathological phenomena of kidney qi failure, such as clear and excessive urine, obvious increase of urine volume, etc.

5.1.3 Kidney accepts qi.

The kidney accepts qi. "Accept" means receive and collect. That the kidney accepts qi is a component part of the kidney's function in storing and sealing up the essence, implying that the kidney functions to accept the Qing (Clear) Qi inhaled by the lung and to prevent the superficial respiration. In other words, the kidney's function in accepting qi can assist the lung qi to down-flow, and the depth of lung's inhalation is maintained by the kidney's function in accepting qi, while the exhalation is realized by the lung's function in dispersing. It is clear that the respiratory movement of human body is realized by the close cooperation of the lung and kidney.

The kidney's function in accepting qi is actually the concrete manifestation of the kidney's function in storing and sealing up essence in the respiratory movement, which takes the Jing (Essence) Qi in the kidney as its substantial foundation. If the Jing (Essence) Qi in the kidney is not sufficient, the kidney is too weak to accept qi, so that the Qing (Clear) Qi inhaled by the lung cannot be sent down but flow upwards instead, causing the pathological phenomena of superficial respiration, or more exhalation than inhalation and shortness of breath on exertion. It is called "the kidney failing to accept qi" clinically.

水液代谢的平衡起着至关重要的作用。若肾中精气的蒸腾气化失常,则既可引起尿少、浮肿等尿液代谢障碍的病理现象,又可引起小便清长、尿量明显增多等肾气不固的病理现象。

5.1.3 肾主纳气

肾主纳气。纳,有接纳、摄纳之义。肾主纳气是肾主封藏功能的一个组成部分,是指肾具有摄纳肺吸入的清气,防止呼吸表浅的作用。亦即说,肾气的摄纳有助于肺气的降纳,肺吸气的深度主要靠肾的摄纳作用来维持,呼气则主要靠肺的宣发作用来实现。可见,人体的呼吸运动是由肺肾两脏密切配合来完成的。

肾的纳气功能,实际上是肾主封藏在呼吸运动中的具体体现,也是以肾中精气为其物质基础。若肾中精气不足,则摄纳无力,由肺气吸入的清气不能归于下元而上浮,因而出现呼吸表浅,或呼多吸少,动辄气喘的病理现象,临床称之为"肾不纳气"。

5.2 Relationships between the kidney and its body constituent, bloom, orifice, emotion and fluid

5.2.1 Have its body constituent in bone, and its bloom on the head hair

That the kidney dominates the bone implies that the normal growth, development and function of bones rely on the nourishment of the kidney essence. The kidney stores the essence, the essence acts to transform and produce the bone marrows, while the bone marrows act to nourish the bones to promote the growth and recovery of bones, so as to make the bones stronger and more stable. If the kidney essence is deficient, the bone marrows are not enough to nourish the bones, leading to weakness of bones and delayed growth in children, and frail bones and easy fracture in the old persons.

The tooth is the surplus of the bone, and both the tooth and bone need to be nourished by the kidney essence. If the kidney essence is sufficient, the teeth are firm and not easy to lose. If the kidney essence is deficient, the tooth growth is delayed in children, and the tooth is loosened and even lost in adults.

The kidney has its bloom on the hair. The hair is nourished by the blood, so it is said that "the hair is the surplus of the blood". The kidney stores the essence, while the kidney essence acts to transform and produce the blood. If the essence and blood are sufficient, the hair can be nourished to be dense and lustrous. If the kidney essence is not sufficient, the blood will be deficient and fail to nourish the hair, causing sparse hair, withered hair, grey hair, even loss of hair.

5.2 肾与体、华、窍、志、液的关系

5.2.1 在体合骨,其华在发

肾主骨,是指骨骼的生长发育和功能的发挥,都有赖于肾精的充养。肾藏精,精可以化生骨髓,骨髓可以滋养骨骼,促进骨骼的生长、修复,使骨骼强劲而坚固。如果肾精亏少,骨髓空虚,骨骼失去营养,则出现小儿骨骼软弱无力,发育迟缓,以及老年人骨质脆弱,易于骨折等。

齿为骨之余,齿与骨都需要得到肾精的滋养。肾精充盛,则牙齿坚固而不易脱落。肾精亏虚,则小儿牙齿生长缓慢,成人牙齿易于松动,甚至早脱。

肾其华在发。头发的营养来源于血液,故称"发为血之余"。由于肾藏精,肾精可化生血液,精血旺盛,头发得养,则生长浓密而有光泽。如肾精不足,血液亏虚,头发失养,则头发稀疏、枯槁、易白,并容易脱落。

5.2.2 Open into the ear and anterior and posterior orifices

The kidney essence acts to produce the marrows, while the brain is the sea of marrows and the ears are interlinked with the brain. Therefore, it is closely related to the kidney essence whether the ear function is normal or not. If the kidney essence is sufficient, the sea of marrows will be full and the ears can be nourished, so the hearing is sensitive. If the kidney essence is not sufficient, the sea of marrows will be empty and the ears fail to be nourished, so that the hearing is decreased, or the symptom of tinnitus or deafness occurs. The hearing is often decreased in the old persons, because of the natural decline of the kidney essence.

Two orifices are anterior and posterior orifices. The anterior orifice refers to the urethra and external genitalia, while the posterior orifice to the anus. The discharge of urine relies on the transforming function of the kidney qi, so the diseases as frequency of urination, enuresis, incontinence of urine, retention of urine, etc. are related to the disturbance of the kidney's function in dominating the water. The kidney dominates the reproduction, including the functions of the external genitalia. If the kidney's function in dominating the reproduction is abnormal, there can be the diseases of impotence, premature ejaculation and seminal emission in males, and excessive leucorrhea in females.

The relationship between the kidney and the posterior orifice implies that the kidney, through its yin and yang, functions to influence the spleen and large intestine, so as to determine the defecation state. The kidney yang possesses the warming and

5.2.2 开窍于耳及二阴

由于肾精生髓,脑为髓海,耳与脑髓相通,故耳的功能正常与否,也与肾精有密切关系。肾精充足,髓海满盈,耳窍得养,则听觉灵敏;反之,肾精不足,髓海空虚,耳窍失养,则听力减退,或出现耳鸣、耳聋等。人到老年听力每多下降,就是因为肾精自然衰减的缘故。

二阴,即前阴和后阴。前阴包括尿道和外生殖器,后阴指肛门。如尿液的排泄,必须依赖于肾的气化作用,因此尿频、遗尿、尿失禁、尿闭等病变,大多与肾主水的功能失常有关。肾主生殖,也涵盖了外生殖器的功能,所以肾主生殖的功能失常,可出现男子阳痿、早泄、遗精,或女子白带过多等病变。

肾与后阴的关系,主要是指肾通过其阴、阳来影响脾、大肠及肛门的功能,从而决定大便的排泄状况。肾阳的作用是通过温化而吸收水

transforming function to absorb the water, so as to promote the formation of feces. The kidney yin functions to moisturize the large intestine and anus, so as to smoothen the defecation. Therefore, the insufficiency of kidney yin or kidney yang may cause abnormal defecation. If the kidney yin is deficient, the fluid in the large intestine dries up, so constipation occurs. If the kidney yang is deficient, the spleen yang will be insufficient, leading to diarrhea due to disturbed transportation and transformation.

5.2.3 Have its emotion as the fear

The kidney has its emotion as the fear. The fear is a kind of spiritual state when one is afraid of something and becoming timid. Over-fear may cause the kidney fail to be consolidated, but downflows instead. For example, If an infant is scared, there can be enuresis. If a young man is threatened suddenly, there can be seminal emission. If a pregnant woman is frightened, there can miscarriage.

5.2.4 Have its fluid as the Tuo (Thick-Heavy) Fluid

The Tuo (Thick-Heavy) Fluid can moisturize the mouth and tongue. The Tuo (Thick-Heavy) Fluid is produced from the sublingual part, where the Kidney Meridian connects with, so the Tuo (Thick-Heavy) Fluid is termed as the fluid of the kidney. In the theory of life preservation of TCM, it is believed that the Tuo (Thick-Heavy) Fluid is transformed from the kidney essence. Therefore, it is proposed to swallow the Tuo (Thick-Heavy) Fluid in the mouth, so as to assist the kidney to reproduce the essence, for the purpose to strengthen the body. If the yin essence in the kidney is not sufficient, the

液,促使大便成形;肾阴的作用是滋润肠腑及肛门,使大便排出顺畅。故肾阴肾阳不足,都可引起大便的排泄异常。如肾阴亏虚,可导致肠液枯涸而发生便秘;肾阳虚弱,可导致脾阳不足,运化失常而产生腹泻等症。

5.2.3 在志为恐

肾,在志为恐。恐,即恐惧、恐吓,是人对事物惧怕、胆怯时的一种精神状态。恐惧过度,易使肾气不固,气泄于下。如小儿经受恐惧,可致尿床;青年男子突受恐吓,可致遗泄;怀孕女子遭受恐慌,可致流产。

5.2.4 在液为唾

唾为口中津液之稠厚者,能滋润口舌。唾生于舌下,而舌下为肾脉所系,所以唾为肾之液。中医养生理论认为唾为肾精所化,养生家主张常吞口中津液(唾)以达肾生精,从而达到健身的目的。若肾之阴精不足,则唾少而口干。

saliva in the mouth is deficient, causing dry mouth.

Appendix: Ming Men (Vital Gate)

The Ming Men (Vital Gate) originally refers to the key or basis to the life. In terms of the location and function of the Ming Men (Vital Gate), there are many different explanations, but it mostly believed that the Ming Men (Vital Gate) is closely related to the kidney. The kidney is the foundation of the five zang organs and the root of yin and yang of whole body as well. The Jing (Essence) Qi stored in the kidney is the foundation of the life occurrence, growth and development, and also the key to the control of the ageing process. This is the implication of the Ming Men (Vital Gate). In other words, it is to extract the most important part of the various functions of the kidney in TCM, and this part is termed as the Ming Men (Vital Gate), which actually pertain to the scope of "the kidney". The Ming Men (Vital Gate) is divided into two parts of water and fire. The water of the Ming Men (Vital Gate) actually refers to the kidney yin, while the fire of the Ming Men (Vital Gate) actually refers to the kidney yang. Clinically, the so-called Ming Men (Vital Gate) fire deficiency pattern is same as the kidney yang insufficiency pattern basically, therefore the method to reinforce the fire of the Ming Men (Vital Gate) is nothing different from that to reinforce the kidney yang.

Section 2　Six Fu Organs

The six fu organs refer to the gallbladder, stomach, small intestine, large intestine, bladder and triple energizer. The six fu organs function to "transport and transform materials", i.e. to accept and digest the food, to absorb the essence and to

---

附：命门

命门，本意指生命的关键、根本。关于命门的部位和功能，历来有许多不同的见解，但大多认为命门与肾有密切关系。由于肾为五脏之本、阴阳之根。肾中所藏的精气是生命产生、发育成长的根本，也是控制衰老进程的关键，这一意义本身就具有"命门"的含义。也就是说，中医学把肾的各种功能作用中最重要的一部分单独提出，取名为"命门"，而实际上命门仍属于"肾"的范畴。命门之中有水、火之分。命门之水，实际上就是肾阴；命门之火，实际上就是肾阳。从临床运用看，多强调命门火衰，而实际上其与肾阳不足基本一致，补命门之火与补肾阳也没有根本的差别。

第2节　六腑

六腑，是指胆、胃、小肠、大肠、膀胱和三焦。六腑的共同生理功能是"传化物"，即受纳、消化饮食物，吸收其精微、排泄其糟粕。由于六

discharge the waste. The process to transport and transform materials downwards is based upon the unblocked state of the six fu organs. Therefore, it is said that the six fu organs "are smooth in descending" and "are normal in unblocking".

1　Gallbladder

The gallbladder is attached to the liver and stores the bile. The bile originates from the liver, is formed by the surplus of liver qi that infuses into the gallbladder. The bile, in bitter taste and yellow color, plays an important role in assisting the digestion of food. The bile is clear and clean, so in TCM the bile is called "the essential juice" or "the clear juice", while the gallbladder is called "the fu organ of the central essential juice" or "the fu organ of the central clear juice".

The major physiological functions of the gallbladder are to store and discharge the bile. The gallbladder is a cavity where the bile is stored after its formation from the liver. Under the action of the liver qi in dredging and draining, the bile enters the small intestine to involve in the digestive and absorptive process, so as to promote the normal function of the small intestine in separating the clear from the turbid.

The normal discharge of the bile is related to the liver's function in dredging and draining on one hand, and also to the smooth state of the gallbladder on the other hand. If the liver qi fails to keep dredging and draining, or if the gallbladder is blocked, the gallbladder will fail to keep dredging and draining. In such a condition, the digestive and absorptive function is disturbed, leading to the

腑传化水谷,须保持通畅下行,故有六腑"以降为顺""以通为用"的说法。

1　胆

胆与肝相连,附于肝下,内贮胆汁。胆汁来源于肝,是肝之余气溢入于胆积聚而成。胆汁味苦色黄,对帮助某些食物的消化起了重要的生理作用。由于胆汁清净,所以中医学又将胆汁称为"精汁""清汁",而将胆称为"中精之腑""中清之腑"。

胆的生理功能是贮存胆汁和排泄胆汁。胆腑中空,胆汁由肝生成后贮存于胆,然后在肝气疏泄的作用下排泄入小肠,参与消化吸收过程,并促进小肠分别清浊功能的正常进行。

胆汁排泄正常与否,一方面与肝气的疏泄有关;另一方面与胆腑的通畅与否有关。肝气疏泄失职,或胆腑失于畅通,都会使胆失于疏泄。若胆失疏泄,胆汁排泄不畅,引起消化吸收功能障碍,可出现食欲不振、腹胀、

symptoms of poor appetite, abdominal distension, vomiting, hypochondriac pain, etc. If the bile overflows to the muscle and skin, there can be jaundice.

2   Stomach

The stomach, also called the epigastria, connects with the esophagus above, and with the small intestine below. The stomach is divided into three parts of the upper stomach, middle stomach and lower stomach. The upper part of stomach and cardia are called the upper stomach, the middle part of stomach is called the middle stomach, while the lower part of stomach and pylorus are called the lower stomach.

The major physiological function of the stomach is to accept and decompose the food. This function implies that the stomach digests the food preliminarily and makes the food into the chyme. The food enters the mouth, passes through the esophagus and goes into the stomach. The stomach accepts the food, digests it preliminarily and makes it into chyme, and then transmits the chyme downwards to the small intestine. The stomach can contain large amount of food, so it is called "the sea of water and grain".

The function of the stomach relies on the promoting function of the stomach qi. The movement form of the stomach is mainly to down-flow. Besides, the passage between the stomach and small intestine should be kept unblocked, so as to maintain the basic condition in "down-flowing". Only when both the unblocked state and down-flowing movement are kept normal, can the chyme enter the small intestine and large intestine successively.

呕吐、胁痛等症状,若胆汁泛溢于肌肤,则出现黄疸。

2   胃

胃又称为胃脘,上连食道,下通小肠。胃脘分为上脘、中脘、下脘三个部分,胃的上部及贲门部分称上脘,胃的中部称中脘,胃的下部及幽门部分称下脘。

胃的生理功能是受纳和腐熟水谷,指对饮食物进行初步消化并形成食糜的作用。饮食经口,下入于胃中。胃接受容纳了饮食物之后,经过初步的腐熟消化,形成食糜,然后向下传入小肠。由于胃内容纳较多饮食物,故称胃为"水谷之海"。

胃的功能主要依赖于胃气的推动。胃气的运动特点是以降为主。同时,胃与小肠之间的道路必须保持畅通,这是维持"降"的基本条件,只有通降无阻,形成食糜状的饮食才能依次进入小肠、大肠。所以中医学又有"胃主通降"之说。胃的功能

Therefore it is said that "the stomach dominates the unblocked and descending" in TCM. The abnormal function of the stomach may cause stomach qi disharmony pattern, with the symptoms of epigastric distension and pain, poor appetite, etc., or cause up-reverse flow of stomach qi instead of normally down-flowing movement, with the symptoms of belching, nausea, vomiting, hiccup, etc.

3　Small intestine

The small intestine settles in the abdominal cavity, connecting with the pylorus above through the stomach and with the large intestine below through the ileocecum. The small intestine has two major physiological functions of to accept and transform the materials, and to separate the clear from the turbid.

The function to accept and transform the materials implies that the small intestine accepts the chyme transported from the stomach, stores it for a rather long period of time, and further digests it adequately.

In terms of the function to separate the clear from the turbid, the clear refers to the essence of water and grain, while the turbid refers to the food dregs. The small intestine digests adequately the chyme transported from the stomach, absorbs the essential substance and some part of water inside, and then transports the food dregs further downwards to the large intestine.

Actually, the small intestine's functions to accept and transform materials and to separate the clear from the turbid are the two aspects in the same digestive process. To accept and transform materials

失常,可引起胃气不和,出现胃脘胀痛、食少等症;亦可导致胃气不降或上逆,出现嗳气、恶心、呕吐、呃逆等症。

3　小肠

小肠盘踞于腹中,上经幽门与胃连接,下经阑门与大肠相通。小肠的生理功能有两个方面:一是受盛化物;二是泌别清浊。

受盛化物指小肠接受由胃初步消化而下输的食糜,贮盛容纳相当长的时间,以进行充分的消化。

泌别清浊,清指水谷精微,浊指食物糟粕。小肠在对由胃传来的饮食物进行充分消化的基础上,吸收其中的精微物质及部分水液,并将食物残渣继续向下传送至大肠。

实际上,小肠受盛化物和分别清浊的功能,是同一消化吸收过程的两个方面,受盛化物是分别清浊的前

is the precondition of separate the clear from the turbid, while separate the clear from the turbid is the result of to accept and transform materials. The two functions have a close intrinsic relation.

The theory of visceral manifestation is centered in the five zang organs, so the digestive and absorptive function of the small intestine often pertains to the spleen's function in dominating transportation and transformation in TCM. Therefore, the small intestine diseases in abnormal digestion and absorption, such as poor appetite, abdominal distension, loose feces, are diagnosed as "the spleen failing to transport and transform pattern" and treated by treating the spleen.

4   Large intestine

The large intestine connects with the small intestine above through the ileocecum, and with the rectum below, and its lower end is the anus. The major physiological functions of the large intestine are transport the waste and absorb the water.

The large intestine accepts the food dregs transported from the small intestine, and reabsorbs some part of water inside, it is said that "the large intestine dominates the Jin (Thin-Light) Fluid". Thus it can be speculated that the too long or short time when the food dregs stay in the large intestine is the direct cause of constipation or diarrhea. The large intestine transforms the food dregs into feces and discharges the feces from the anus.

If the transporting function of the large intestine is disturbed, there can be constipation or diarrhea. The transporting function of the large intestine is closely related to the body fluid, the stomach

提,分别清浊是受盛化物的结果,两者有着密切的内在联系。

由于藏象学强调以五脏为中心,所以中医学往往把小肠消化吸收的功能归属于脾主运化的范畴。因此,临床上常将小肠消化吸收失常的病变,如食欲不佳、腹胀、便溏等,辨证为"脾失健运"而从脾治疗。

4   大肠

大肠上端接小肠,连接处称阑门,下端为直肠,末端外口即为肛门。大肠的主要生理功能是传导糟粕和吸收水分。

大肠接受小肠下注的食物残渣,再吸收其中的部分水分,故说"大肠主津"。由此可以推测食物残渣在大肠中停留时间的过长或过短,是导致便秘或腹泻的直接原因。大肠形成粪便,经直肠由肛门排出。

大肠传导失司,可致便秘或腹泻。大肠的传导变化,与机体津液的盈亏和胃气、肺气的通降有密切关系。

qi and the lung qi. If the body fluid is consumed to be deficient, it is impossible to sail a boat without water in the river, leading to constipation. If the water-dampness is accumulated in the large intestine, it inundates the large intestine to cause diarrhea. The normal transporting function of the large intestine is actually the extension of the stomach's function in subduing the turbid. If the stomach fails to subdue the turbid, the transporting function of the large intestine is also disturbed.

5 Bladder

The bladder, locating in the lower abdomen, is an organ to store the urine. Its major function is to store and discharge the urine.

The water and the Zhuo (Turbid) Qi formed in the metabolic process of human body are transformed into urine through the transforming function of the kidney qi, and then the urine is transmitted downwards to the bladder to be stored temporarily. When the urine is accumulated to a certain mount, it is discharged naturally through the transforming function of the kidney qi. The checking and transforming functions of the kidney qi are the decisive factors of the bladder's function in storing and discharging the urine. Generally speaking, if the kidney qi is deficient, and its checking and transforming functions are disturbed, there can be abnormal urination. If the bladder is attacked by the exogenous pathogens that disturb the transforming function of the bladder qi, there can be abnormal urination as well. The former is regarded as a deficiency pattern, while the latter as the excess pattern. The bladder diseases due to qi deficiency are as frequen-

津液亏耗,无水行舟,易致便秘;水湿内停,渍于大肠,易致濡泄。大肠的正常传导,又是胃的降浊功能的延伸。胃失和降,大肠传导之职亦易受影响。

5 膀胱

膀胱位于小腹部,为贮尿的器官,其功能是贮存尿液和排泄小便。

人体在新陈代谢过程中形成的水液及浊气,经肾的气化作用而生成小便,下输于膀胱暂时贮存,当膀胱内小便积存到一定量时,就通过气化作用而自然地排出体外。肾气的固摄和气化作用是膀胱贮存和排泄小便的决定性因素。一般来说,肾气虚而固摄、气化失常时,可导致膀胱排尿异常;若膀胱本身感受外邪,使气化不利,也会导致排尿异常。但前者形成的是虚证,后者形成的是实证。凡膀胱气虚不固,可见尿多、遗尿、尿失禁等症;若膀胱气化不利,可见小便不利、淋漓不爽、尿闭等症。

cy of urination, enuresis, incontinence of urine, etc., while the bladder diseases due to abnormal transforming function are as difficult urination, dribbling of urine after urination, retention of u-rine, etc.

6　Triple energizer (Sanjiao)

6.1　Concept of triple energize

Triple energizer is a specific fu organ. It acts to partition the chest and abdomen and their internal organs inside the human body, and also to generalize some functional systems of the human body.

The triple energizer is divided into three parts of the upper energizer, middle energizer and lower energizer. Usually, the diaphragm and umbilicus are taken as the partition materials. The part above the diaphragm is taken as the upper energizer, the part below the diaphragm and above the umbilicus is taken as the middle energizer, while the part below the umbilicus as the lower energizer. The upper energizer includes the chest, heart and lung; the middle energizer includes the upper abdomen, spleen, stomach, liver, gallbladder and small intestine; while the lower energizer includes the lower abdomen, kidney, bladder and large intestine.

6.2　Physiological functions of triple energizer

As an independently functional system, the triple energizer based upon the form and structure of all zang-fu organs and tissues of human body, is the high generalization of the physiological functions of all zang-fu organs. The physiological functions of the triple energizer are as follows.

6　三焦

6.1　三焦的概念

三焦是一个特殊的腑，它既是对人体胸腹部位及其所藏脏腑器官的划分，又是对人体某些功能系统的概括。

三焦，可分为上焦、中焦、下焦三部。对于三焦部位的划分，通常以横膈和脐为界线，横膈以上为上焦，膈下脐上为中焦，脐以下为下焦。上焦主要包括胸部和心、肺，中焦主要包括上腹部和脾、胃、肝、胆、小肠，下焦主要包括下腹部和肾、膀胱、大肠等。

6.2　三焦的生理功能

三焦作为一个独立的功能系统，是以人体各脏腑组织的形态结构为基础的，因而它实际上是对各脏腑生理功能的高度概括。三焦的生理功能可包括如下两个方面。

Firstly, it is the passage of the Yuan (Primary) Qi and water.

The triple energizer is the major drainage system. as the passage of some substances of human body, such as the Yuan (Primary) Qi, water, etc.

The Yuan (Primary) Qi is the fundamental qi of the human body, originating from the congenital and supported and nourished by the acquired, as the primary motive power of the vital activities of the human body. The Yuan (Primary) Qi is rooted in the kidney and distributed all over the body through the triple energizer, to warm and nourish the zang-fu organs and tissues and to inspire and promote the physiological functions of all the zang-fu organs and tissues. If the Yuan (Primary) Qi is deficient, or if the passage of the triple energizer is blocked, there can be the phenomena of qi deficiency in some parts of body.

The water metabolism of human body is mainly related to the lung, spleen and kidney. The lung locates in the upper energizer, the spleen in the middle energizer, and the kidney in the lower energizer. The triple energizer acts to integrate the three organs into a system of water distribution and metabolism, so it is the important passage of the water flow. If the triple energizer is abnormal as the water passage, the related functions of the lung, spleen and kidney will be disturbed, leading to the diseases of scanty urine, edema, etc.

Secondly, it is the generalization of the functional system of zang-fu organs in human body.

The triple energizer is applied to generalize some physiological functions of some internal organs

一是元气和水液运行的通道：

三焦是人体主要的输导系统，人体的某些物质如元气、水液等的运输和传导，是以三焦作为道路的。

元气是人体的根本之气，其来自于先天，充养于后天，是人体生命活动的原动力。元气的根源在于肾，并可通过三焦而输布周身内外上下，温养脏腑组织，以激发和推动各脏腑组织的生理功能。如果元气虚弱，三焦通道运行不畅，便可引起某些部位的气虚现象。

人体的水液代谢，主要与肺、脾、肾有关。其中，肺居上焦，脾居中焦，肾居下焦，正是三焦将肺、脾、肾三脏联结成一个水液输布、代谢的系统，所以说三焦也是水液运行的重要通道。如果三焦水道不利，影响肺、脾、肾等脏的相应功能，就会产生尿少、水肿等病变。

二是对人体脏腑功能系统的概括：

用三焦来概括相应部位的某些内脏的部分生理功

in the related areas, especially the functions in digesting and absorbing the food, distributing the food essence and body fluid metabolism. This process is generalized in Huang Di Nei Jing as that "the upper energizer is like the sprayer", "the middle energizer is like the fermentation vat", and "the lower energizer is like the drainage".

The upper energizer is like the sprayer. The upper energizer is the place where the heart and lung locate. That the upper energizer is like the sprayer implies that the spraying state is applied to describe the functional state of the heart and lung in spreading and distributing qi and blood as the spraying state. That is to say, the heart and lung distribute the essential substances as qi and blood all over the body, like the mist spraying everywhere. If the exogenous pathogens attack the upper energizer, the normal spread and distribution of qi and blood are disturbed, and the symptoms due to dysfunction of the heart and lung may occur, such as irritability, palpitation, cough, stuffy chest, etc.

The middle energizer is like the fermentation vat. The fermentation means dipping. Anything that is dipping is easily decayed. That the middle energizer is like the fermentation vat implies that the fermentation vat is applied to describe the functional state of the spleen and stomach in digesting and absorbing the food. The digesting and absorbing function, not only related to the spleen and stomach, but also related to the liver and gallbladder as well, while all the spleen, stomach, liver and gallbladder locate in the middle energizer. Therefore, that the middle energizer is like the fermentation vat is to generalize the digesting and absorbing

能，主要是针对饮食的消化吸收、水谷精微的输布和津液的代谢而言的，《黄帝内经》把这一过程归纳为："上焦如雾""中焦如沤""下焦如渎"。

上焦如雾。上焦为心、肺两脏所居之处。上焦如雾，是以"雾"的弥漫状态来形容心肺宣发输布气血的功能状态。也就是说，心肺将气血等精微物质输布于周身，状如雾露般弥漫，无处不到。如果外邪侵犯上焦，不但影响气血的正常宣发和输布，还可见心烦、心悸、咳嗽、胸闷等心肺功能失常的病变。

中焦如沤。沤，是浸渍的意思，物质经浸渍则易腐变。中焦如沤，是以"沤"来形容脾胃等对饮食物的消化吸收状态。食物的消化吸收功能，不仅与脾胃有关，与肝胆也密切相关，而脾胃肝胆皆居于中焦。可见中焦如沤，概括了脾胃肝胆在消化吸收方面的功能。如果邪聚中焦，影响消化吸收功能的正常发挥，可见脘腹胀满、呕吐、腹泻、黄疸等脾胃肝胆的

function of the spleen, stomach, liver and gallbladder. If the pathogens attack the middle energizer, the normal digesting and absorbing function is disturbed, leading to the diseases of the spleen, stomach, liver and gallbladder, manifesting symptoms such as epigastric and abdominal distension, vomiting, diarrhea, jaundice, etc.

The lower energizer is like the drainage. That the lower energizer is like the drainage is applied to describe the functional state of the kidney and bladder in draining and discharging the turbid water downwards and outwards. If the pathogens attack the lower energizer, the normal discharge of urine is disturbed, leading to the diseases of the kidney and bladder, manifesting symptoms such as scanty urine, frequency of urination, urgency of urination, painful urination, etc.

Section 3　Extraordinary Fu Organs

The extraordinary fu organs include the brain, marrow, bone, vessel, gallbladder and uterus. The gallbladder is one of the six fu organs, and also one of the extraordinary fu organs as well. The gallbladder functions to secrete the bile to directly assist the digestion of food, so it is taken as one of the six fu organs. The gallbladder does not possess the physiological function to accept, transport and transform the food as other fu organs, but it stores "the essential juice", similar to the storing function of the zang organs, so it is also taken as one of the extraordinary fu organs as well. Except the gallblad-

病变。

下焦如渎。渎，是水道的意思。下焦如渎，是以"渎"来形容肾与膀胱将水浊不断地向下疏通、向外排泄的功能状态。如果邪侵下焦，主要是影响小便的正常排泄，可见尿少、尿频、尿急、尿痛等肾与膀胱的病变。

第3节 奇恒之腑

奇恒之腑，包括脑、髓、骨、脉、胆、女子胞。其中胆既是六腑之一，有属奇恒之腑。因为胆排泄的胆汁直接有助于饮食物的消化，所以为六腑之一。但胆本身并没有受盛和传化水谷的生理功能，且能藏"精汁"，有"藏"的功能，故又属奇恒之腑。奇恒之腑中除胆为六腑之一外，其余的都没有表里配合，也没有五行配属，这是不同

der that pertains to the category of six fu organs, the other extraordinary fu organs have not the exterior-interior relation and the five-element attribution, so it is another feature different from the five zang organs and six fu organs.

The physiological functions of the vessel, marrow, bone and gallbladder have been described in the related chapters and sections, so only the brain and uterus will be illustrated in this section as follows.

1 Brain

The brain locates in the skull and connects with spinal marrow, so it is called "the sea of marrow" in Huang Di Nei Jing. The major physiological functions of the brain are as follows.

Firstly, it is the center of the vital activities. The brain plays a very important role in the vital activities of human body, including the function to dominate the five zang organs and six fu organs and the function to regulate the vital activities of whole body. If the brain is injured, the life is threatened. It is said in Huang Di Nei Jing that "If the head is pierced, one dies immediately when the brain is injured".

Secondly, it dominates the spiritual activities. The brain is the cognitive and thinking organ. All the thinking, conscious and emotional activities of human body are the reflection of the brain to the external objective things. In the theory of visceral manifestation, the spiritual activities dominated by the brain pertain to the heart's function in dominating the spirit, but it is also believed that the brain is also important in the spiritual activities. It is said in Huang Di Nei Jing that "the head is the residence

于五脏六腑的一大特点。

脉、髓、骨、胆的生理,在本章相关内容中已有论述,本节仅对脑与女子胞论述如下。

1 脑

脑位于头颅之内,由髓汇聚而成,所以《黄帝内经》称之为"髓海"。脑的生理功能主要有以下几方面。

一是生命活动的中枢。脑在人体生命活动中具有十分重要的作用,主要表现在主宰五脏六腑的功能、调节一身的生命活动方面。如果脑受到损伤,就会危及生命。所以《黄帝内经》有"刺头中脑户,入脑立死"之说。

二是主管精神活动。脑是认识和思维的器官,人的各种思维意识及情志活动,都是客观外界事物反映到脑的结果。虽然藏象学说将脑主管精神活动的作用归属于心主神明的功能,但也已认识到脑在精神活动方面的重要作用。《黄帝内经》有"头者,精明之府"的说法。明代

of the intelligence". Li Shizhen in the Ming Dynasty (1368-1644) pointed out that "the brain is the house of the Yuan (Primary) Spirit", because the brain is the important organ of the spiritual activities of human body. If the brain's function in dominating the spiritual activities is normal, one has the high spirit, clear consciousness, fluent speaking and good memory. If the brain's function is abnormal, there can be the diseases due to spiritual derangement, such as low spirit, slowness of thought, dizziness, blurring of vision, poor memory, etc.

Thirdly, it dominates the sensation and movement. The various sense organs, such as the eyes, ears, nose, tongue, body (skin) of the human body, can accept the extrinsic stimulations as the sound, light, taste, pain, cold, heat, etc., and then all the stimulations are accepted by the brain through the meridians and collaterals to produce various sensations. The brain is also the dominator of the body movement. If the sensory and motor functions of the brain are disturbed, there can be the symptoms of insensitivity, movement disorder, etc.

Since it is centered on five zang organs in the theory of visceral manifestation, the important functions of the brain are found to belong to the five zang organs in the theoretical system of TCM. The human mental activities are divided into Shen (spirit), Po (soul), Hun (ghost), Yi (willpower) and Zhi (aspiration), which are attributive to the five zang organs respectively as that the heart stores Shen (spirit), the lung stores Po (soul), the liver stores Hun (ghost), the spleen stores Yi (willpower) and the kidney stores Zhi (aspiration). According to clinical practice, the mental activities are the

李时珍曾指出"脑为元神之府",即指脑是人的精神活动的重要器官。脑主管精神活动的功能正常,则精神振奋,意识清楚,语言清晰,记忆力强。若脑的功能失常,则可出现精神委靡,思维迟钝,头晕目眩,记忆力下降等症,或发生精神异常方面的病症。

三是主管感觉和运动。人身有各种感官,如眼、耳、鼻、舌、身(皮肤)等,可分别接受外来的声、光、味以及疼痛、寒热等刺激,脑通过经脉接受这些刺激而产生感觉。脑又是肢体运动的主宰。脑主管感觉和运动的功能失常,就会出现感觉迟钝,运动失调等病变。

由于藏象学说是强调以五脏为中心的,所以在中医学理论体系中,多将脑的这些重要功能分属于五脏。如将人的精神活动分为神、魄、魂、意、志五个方面,而分别归之于五脏,即心藏神,肺藏魄,肝藏魂,脾藏意,肾藏志。但从临床实际来看,精神活动与心、肝、肾三脏的关系最为密切。这是因为心主神明,主管整个精神活动;肝主疏泄,调

most closely related to the heart, liver and kidney. It is because that the heart dominates the spirit and mind and governs the whole mental activities, the liver dominates dredging and draining and regulates the human emotional activities, and the kidney stores the yin essence which transforms into marrows for the purpose to nourish the brain. Therefore, in the treatment of the diseases due to abnormal mental and emotional activities, it is advisable to stress on and deal with the heart, liver and kidney.

2   Uterus

The uterus, locating in the lower abdomen, is a particular organ of women. The uterus possesses two functions in bringing about menstruation and gestating to cultivate fetus.

At the age about fourteen in females, the uterus is mature, to have menstruation. The menstruation is a phenomenon of cyclical bleeding from the uterus. The menstruation, taking a month as its cycle, comes and goes on time as the tides, so it is also called "the menstrual tides".

In pregnancy, the uterus becomes the site to cultivate the fetus. In this moment, the menstruation stops, because a large amount of blood infuses into the uterus constantly to nourish and cultivate the fetus. Along with the growth of the fetus, the uterus is enlarged till delivery. During the lactation period after delivery, the blood transforms into the milk that flow upwards. In such a period, there are still no menstrual tides. After the delactation, the milk dries up and the blood flows downwards, so that the normal cyclical menstruation is recovered.

The uterus' functions in bringing about men-

节人的情志活动；肾藏阴精，可生髓充养于脑。所以，临床上精神情志活动异常的疾病，往往从心、肝、肾三脏论治。

2   女子胞

女子胞，即子宫，位于小腹部，是女性独有的器官。女子胞具有发生月经和孕育胎儿两方面的生理功能。

十四岁左右女子胞发育渐趋成熟，开始有月经来潮。月经，是子宫周期性出血的现象。月经以月为周期，按时而来，按时而去，如同潮汐一样，故称"月经来潮"。

若致受孕，子宫就成了孕育胎儿的场所。这时，月经停止，大量的血液不断地灌注于子宫，以滋养胎儿。随着胎儿的逐渐长大，子宫也日益增大直至分娩。分娩后的哺乳期间，血液化为乳汁而上行，此时仍无月经来潮，要等到断乳之后，乳汁渐收，血液下行，才会恢复正常的月经周期。

女子胞发生月经和孕育

struation and in gestating to cultivate fetus are a very complicated process of physiological activities, relying on the support and coordination of related zang-fu organs as follows.

Firstly, it relies on the function of the Jing (Essence) Qi in the kidney. The kidney contains the essence, qi, yin and yang. When these essence, qi, yin and yang are getting plentiful to a certain degree, the Tian Gui (gonadotropin) occurs. After the formation of the Tian Gui (gonadotropin), it functions to promote the development of the reproductive organs. The uterus, under the action of the Tian Gui (gonadotropin), is mature to possess the condition to bring about menstruation and to gestate to cultivate fetus. In the old age, due to the gradual decrease of the essence, qi, yin and yang in the kidney, the Tian Gui (gonadotropin) is declining, so the menstruation stops gradually and gestating ability is lost in the end.

Secondly, it relies on the functions of the liver qi and liver blood. The liver plays a very important role in regulating the physiological functions of the uterus. On one hand, the liver dominates the dredging and draining, to regulate and smooth the qi activities, for the purpose to maintaining the normal functions of the uterus to bring about menstruation and to make pregnancy. On the other hand, the liver functions to store the blood, so as to store the blood and regulate the volume of blood, to influence the volume and circulation of the blood in the uterus. Therefore, the liver is closely related to the menstrual volume and the function to gestating to cultivate fetus. Since the function of uterus is closely related to the functions of the liver qi and liver

胎儿的功能,是一个复杂的生理活动过程,有赖于相关脏腑的充养与协调。主要有如下三方面因素。

一是肾中精气的作用。肾中藏有精气阴阳,当精气阴阳充盛到一定程度时,就产生天癸。天癸生成后,能促进生殖器官的发育并使之成熟。女子胞在天癸的作用下发育成熟之后,就具备了发生月经和孕育胎儿的条件。到了老年,由于肾中精气阴阳日趋减少,天癸亦随之衰减,因此此月经逐渐停止,并失去了孕育胎儿的能力。

二是肝气,肝血的作用。肝对女子胞的生理功能,起着十分重要的调节作用。一方面肝主疏泄,调畅气机,使女子胞的功能正常,则能发生月经及受孕。另一方面肝主藏血,能贮藏血液和调节血量,影响女子胞血液的充盈和正常运行,从而与月经量的多少和养育胎儿的功能有着紧密的联系。由于女子胞的功能与肝气肝血的作用密切相关,所以前人有"女子以肝为先天"的说法。

blood, it is said "the liver is taken as the congenital basis in females" in the ancient times.

Thirdly, it relies on the functions of the Thoroughfare Vessel and Conception Vessel. Both the Thoroughfare Vessel and Conception Vessel originate in the uterus. The Thoroughfare Vessel, taken as the sea of the blood, functions to regulate qi and blood of the twelve regular meridians. The Conception Vessel manages the uterus, so related to the pregnancy. If the Thoroughfare Vessel and Conception Vessel are unblocked, the blood can flow downwards to the uterus, for the purpose to bring about menstruation and to gestate to cultivate fetus. The functions of the Thoroughfare Vessel and Conception Vessel are regulated by the functions of the kidney and liver. Therefore, the kidney, liver, Thoroughfare Vessel and Conception Vessel are closely related to the female reproductive function and form up an entity of mutual coordination.

Furthermore, the heart dominates the blood and promotes the blood circulation, the lung dominates qi that promotes the blood circulation, while the spleen controls the blood and acts as the source to produce qi and blood due to its transportation and transformation. So that the zang organs of the heart, lung and spleen also possesses some influence on the functions of the uterus.

三是冲任二脉的作用。冲任二脉同起于胞中,在女子即起于女子胞中。冲为血海,能调节十二经脉之气血;任主胞胎,与女子妊娠有关。所以冲任二脉通利,血液下注于女子胞,平时可产生月经,孕时则养育胎儿。冲任二脉的盛衰,又受肾、肝两脏功能的调节,肾、肝、冲任二脉与女子胞是关系女子生殖生理功能并相互协调的统一整体。

此外,由于心主血、能推动血液运行,肺主气、气行则血行,脾统血、主运化而为气血生化之源,所以心、肺、脾三脏对女子胞的功能也有一定的影响。

Section 4　Relationships among Zang-Fu Organs

第 4 节　脏腑之间的关系

The human body is a whole entirety, composed of many tissues and organs as the zang-fu organs,

人体是一个统一的有机整体,由脏腑、经络等许多组

meridians and collaterals, etc. The relationship among the zang-fu organs is one of the integral connections in the theory of the visceral manifestation. All the zang-fu organs are mutually connected structurally through the meridians and collaterals, share out the work and cooperate with one another physiologically, and influence and transfer each other pathologically.

1　Relationships among five zang organs

The five zang organs of the heart, lung, spleen, liver and kidney have their own physiological functions and pathological changes respectively, while there are the closely physiological connections and pathological influences among the five zang organs. In terms of the relationships among the five zang organs, it includes not only the inter-promoting, interacting, overacting and counteracting relations of the five elements, but also the mutual restraining, depending, generating and coordinating relations as well.

1.1　Heart and lung

Both the heart and lung locate in the upper energizer. The heart dominates the blood, while the lung dominates qi. The heart governs the blood circulation, while the lung governs the respiration. The relation between the heart and lung includes the cooperating and coordinating relation in the blood circulation and in the exhalation and inhalation of respiration.

The heart dominates the blood of the whole body, while the lung dominates qi of the whole body. The two zang organs coordinate mutually to guarantee the normal circulation of qi and blood, so

织器官所构成。脏腑之间的关系,是藏象学说中整体性联系的内容之一。人体各脏腑之间,在结构上通过经络而相互沟通,生理功能上既分工又合作,在病理变化上也可互相影响和传变。

1　五脏之间的关系

心、肺、脾、肝、肾五脏有各自的生理功能和特定的病理变化,而五脏之间又存在着密不可分的生理联系和病理影响。对五脏之间关系的认识,不能只局限于五行的生克乘侮范围,更需从五脏生理功能之间的相互制约、依存、资生、协调等方面加以阐述。

1.1　心与肺

心肺同居上焦,心主血而肺主气,心主行血而肺主呼吸。心与肺的关系,主要表现在血液运行与呼吸吐纳之间的协同调节关系。

心主一身之血,肺主一身之气,两者相互协调,保证气血的正常运行,维持机体各脏腑组织的新陈代谢。血

as to maintain the metabolism of all tissues and organs. The normal blood circulation relies on the promoting function of the heart qi, and also on the dispersing function of the lung qi as well. The lung collects all the vessels, to assist the heart to move the blood, as the necessary condition of the normal blood circulation. The normal blood circulation acts to maintain the lung's function in dominating qi. Since the Zong (Pectoral) Qi possesses the physiological functions to infuse into the heart and to govern the respiration, it enhances the coordination and equilibrium between the blood circulation and respiration. Therefore, the Zong (Pectoral) Qi locating in the chest is the central link to integrate the heart's pulsation and lung's respiration. Pathologically, if the lung qi is deficient, it fails to move the blood. If the lung fails to dominate dispersing and descending, the lung qi is stagnant. The lung qi deficiency or stagnation may influence the heart's function in dominating the blood circulation, causing the heart blood stasis pattern. On the contrary, if the heart qi is not sufficient or if the heart yang is not inspired, the blood does not circulate smoothly, so as to influence the lung's function in dominating the respiration, leading to the symptoms of stuffy chest, cough, panting, etc.

1.2 Heart and spleen

The heart dominates the blood, while the spleen produces the blood. The heart dominates the circulation of blood, while the spleen dominates the control of blood. The relation between the heart and spleen includes the mutual dependence in the production of blood and the mutual coordination in the blood circulation.

液的正常运行，必须依赖于心气的推动，亦有赖于肺气的敷布。肺朝百脉，助心行血，是血液正常运行的必要条件。正常的血液循环，又能维持肺主气功能的正常进行。由于宗气具有贯心脉而司呼吸的生理功能，从而加强了血液运行与呼吸吐纳之间的协调平衡。因此，积于胸中的宗气是连结心的搏动和肺的呼吸的中心环节。在病理上，若肺气虚弱，行血无力或肺失宣肃，肺气壅塞，可影响心主行血的功能，易致心血瘀阻；反之，若心气不足，心阳不振，血行不畅，也可影响肺主呼吸的功能，导致胸闷、咳喘等症。

1.2 心与脾

心主血而脾生血，心主行血而脾主统血。心与脾的关系，主要表现在血液生成方面的相互依存及血液运行方面的相互协同。

1.2.1 Production of blood

The heart dominates the blood of the whole body, so the heart blood supports the spleen which thus can maintain its normal transporting and transforming function. The essence of water and grain is sent upwards through the spleen's function in elevating the clear to the heart and lung, and infuse into the heart vessels to transform into the red-colored blood. The spleen which functions to dominate transportation and transformation is the source of qi and blood. If the spleen qi is sufficient and strong, the blood can be transformed, so as to support the heart. Pathologically, if the spleen fails to dominate transportation and transformation, it can not transform sufficient blood. Or if the spleen fails to control the blood, it may cause chronic hemorrhage. All these conditions may lead to the deficiency of blood which fails to nourish the heart. Furthermore, spiritual strain as over-thinking consumes the heart blood, and damage the spleen qi as well, leading to the heart and spleen deficiency pattern.

1.2.2 Circulation of blood

Thenormal circulation of blood inside the vessels relies on the promoting function of the heart qi to prevent too slow movement, and also on the checking function of the spleen qi to prevent spilling out of vessels. If the heart and spleen can be coordinated normally, the blood circulation is normal. Therefore, the normal blood circulation without under-circulation or reckless movement actually relies on the coordination of the heart's function in moving the blood and the spleen's function in controlling the blood. If the heart qi is not sufficient, it fails to move the blood. If the spleen qi is deficient, it fails to control the blood.

1.2.1　血液生成方面

心主一身之血,心血供养脾以维持其正常的运化功能。水谷精微通过脾的转输升清作用,上输于心肺,贯注于心脉而化赤为血。脾主运化而为气血之化源。脾气健旺,血液化生有源,以保证心血充盈。病理上,若脾虚失于健运,化源不足,或统血无权,慢性失血,均可导致血虚而心失所养。此外,劳神思虑过度,既耗心血,又损脾气,亦可形成心脾两虚之候。

1.2.2　血液运行方面

血液在脉中正常运行,既有赖于心气的推动而不致过于迟缓,又依靠脾气的统摄而不致逸出脉外。心脾协同,血液运行正常。血能正常运行而不致脱陷妄行,全赖心主行血与脾主统血的协调。若心气不足,行血无力,或脾气虚损,统摄无权,均可导致血行失常的病理状态。

Both the conditions may cause the pathological states of abnormal blood circulation.

1.3   Heart and liver

The heart dominates the circulation of blood, while the liver dominates the storage of blood. The heart dominates the spirit and mind, while the liver dominates dredging and draining to regulate the emotions. Therefore, the relation between the heart and liver includes the coordination of the blood circulation and storage, and the regulation of the spirit and emotion as well.

1.3.1   Blood circulation

The heart dominates the blood, as the pivot of the blood circulation of whole body. The liver stores the blood, as the important organ to store the blood and regulate the blood volume. The mutual cooperation of the two zang organs maintains the normal circulation of the blood. Therefore, it is said that "the liver stores the blood, while the heart moves it". If the heart blood is sufficient and the heart qi is vigorous, the blood circulation will be normal, and the liver will have blood to store. If the liver stores the sufficient blood and the liver's function in dredging and draining is normal, the volume of blood can be regulated and adjusted according to the moving or quiet state of human body, so as to assist the heart's function in moving the blood. Pathologically, if the blood of whole body is deficient, it will affect all the zang-fu organs, the heart and liver in particular, resulting in the so-called the heart and liver blood deficiency pattern. Besides, the heart blood stasis pattern may involve the liver, and vice versa, leading to the heart and live blood stasis pattern in the end.

1.3   心与肝

心主行血而肝主藏血，心主神志而肝主疏泄以调畅情志。因此，心与肝的关系，主要表现在行血与藏血以及精神情志调节两个方面。

1.3.1   血液运行方面

心主血，心为一身血液运行的枢纽；肝藏血，肝是贮藏血液、调节血量的重要脏器。两者相互配合，共同维持血液的正常运行。所以说"肝藏血，心行之"。心血充盈，心气旺盛，则血行正常，肝有所藏；肝藏血充足，疏泄有度，随人体动静的不同进行血量的调节，也有利于心主行血功能的正常进行。病理上，若全身血液亏虚影响至脏腑，主要表现在心肝两脏，即心肝血虚。此外，心血瘀阻可累及肝，肝血瘀阻也可累及心，最终导致心肝血瘀。

1.3.2 Spirit and emotion

The heart dominates the spirit and mind, governing the spiritual, conscious and thinking activities. The liver dominates dredging and draining, so as to maintain the smooth spirit and emotion. Therefore, the heart and liver, mutually depending and mutually functioning, jointly maintain the normal spiritual and emotional activities. If the heart blood is sufficient and the heart spirit is healthy, it is possible to assist the liver qi in dredging and draining. If the liver is normal in dredging and draining and the emotions are smooth, it is possible to assist the heart in dominating the spirit and mind. Pathologically, the heart spirit derangement pattern and the liver qi stagnation, or the heart fire hyperactivity and the liver fire hyperactivity, may exist together or be induced each other. The former may lead to absent mindedness, emotional depression, etc., while the latter may cause restlessness, insomnia, impatience, anger, etc., the symptoms of the heart and liver fire hyperactivity pattern.

1.4 Heart and kidney

The physiological relation between the heart and kidney is also as "the harmony between the heart and kidney" or "the harmony between the water and fire".

The heart locates in the upper energizer, pertaining to the fire in the five elements, while the kidney locates in the lower energizer, pertaining to the water in the five elements. According to the theory of yin and yang or the water and fire in up-flow and down-flow movements, that locating in the upper tends to down-flow, while that locating in the lower tends to up-flow. That up-flowed already

1.3.2 精神情志方面

心主神志,以主宰精神、意识、思维活动。肝主疏泄,以维护精神情志的调畅。心肝两脏,相互依存,相互为用,共同维持正常的精神情志活动。心血充盈,心神健旺,有助于肝气疏泄;疏泄有度,情志畅快,亦有利于心主神志。病理上,心神不安与肝气郁结,心火亢盛与肝火偏旺,两者可并存或相互引动。前者出现精神恍惚、情绪抑郁等症,后者出现心烦失眠、急躁易怒等心肝火旺之症。

1.4 心与肾

心与肾在生理上的关系,主要表现在"心肾相交",亦称"水火相济"。

心居上焦属阳,在五行属火;肾居下焦属阴,在五行属水。就阴阳水火的升降理论而言,在上者宜降,在下者宜升,升已而降,降已而升。心位居上,故心火(阳)必须下降于肾,使肾水不寒;肾位居下,故肾水(阴)必须上济

tends to down-flow, while that down-flowed already tends to up-flow. The heart locates in the upper, so the heart fire (yang) tends to down-flow to the kidney, so as to prevent the kidney water from being too cold. The kidney locates in the lower, so the kidney water (yin) tends to up-flow to the heart, so as to prevent the heart fire from being hyperactive. The kidney water will be too cold without the heart fire, while the heart fire will be too flaring without the kidney water. The heart needs the moisture from the kidney water, while the kidney water needs the warmth from the heart fire. Physiologically, such the harmony between the water and fire is based upon the dynamic equilibrium of up-flow and down-flow of yin and yang of the heart and kidney. Generally speaking, the harmony between the heart and kidney stress on the harmonious relations between the upper and the lower, the water and fire, the up-flow and down-flow, yin and yang, so as to maintain the integral equilibrium of the physiological functions between the heart and kidney.

Pathologically, if the dynamic equilibrium of the water and fire and of yin and yang between the heart and kidney is disturbed, it is called the disharmony between the heart and kidney, leading to the heart and kidney yin deficiency pattern in which the water fails to moisturize the fire, because the kidney water deficient in the lower, while the heart fire is hyperactive in the upper, or leading to the heart and kidney yang deficiency pattern, in which the kidney yang deficiency and heart yang deficiency are in the reciprocal causation.

1.5 Lung and spleen

The lung dominates the respiration and accepts

于心，使心火不亢。肾无心之火则水寒，心无肾之阴则火炽。心必得肾水以滋润，肾必得心火以温煦。在生理状态下，这种水火既济的关系，是以心肾阴阳升降的动态平衡为其重要条件的。总之，心肾相交是强调上下、水火、升降、阴阳相济，以维持心与肾之间生理功能的协调平衡。

在病理状态下，心与肾之间的水火、阴阳的动态平衡失调，称为心肾不交。表现为水不济火，肾水虚于下而心火亢于上的心肾阴虚之证，或肾阳虚与心阳虚互为因果的心肾阳虚之候。

1.5 肺与脾

肺司呼吸而摄纳清气，

the Qing (Clear) Qi, while the spleen dominates the transportation and transformation and produces the Gu (Grain) Qi. The lung dredges and regulates the water passage, while the spleen dominates the transportation and transformation of water. The relation between the lung and spleen includes the formation of qi and water metabolism.

1.5.1 Formation of qi

The lung dominates the respiration and inhales the fresh air, the Qing (Clear) Qi in the nature, while the spleen dominates the transportation and transformation and absorbs the essence of water and grain, the Gu (Grain) Qi. The Qing (Clear) Qi and the Gu (Grain) Qi are the major substantial foundation to produce qi of the human body, especially the Zong (Pectoral) Qi. The Jing (Essence) Qi of water and grain transformed by the spleen relies on the lung qi's dispersing and descending function, so as to be distributed to the whole body. The body fluid and qi that the lung is applied to maintain its physiological functions is constantly supported by the essence of water and grain gained from the spleen's function in transporting and transforming. Therefore it is said that "the lung is the pivot to dominate qi, while the spleen is the source to produce qi". Only under the integral actions of both the lung and spleen, it is possible to guarantee the formation and distribution of qi in human body, especially the Zong (Pectoral) Qi. Pathologically, the lung qi deficiency may involve the spleen (the son disease involving the mother), or the spleen deficiency involve the lung (the mother disease involving the son), leading to the lung and spleen deficiency pattern in the end.

脾主运化而化生谷气;肺主通调水道,脾主运化水液。肺与脾的关系,主要表现在气的生成与水液代谢两个方面。

1.5.1 气的生成方面

肺主呼吸,吸入自然界空气(清气);脾主运化,吸收水谷之精气(谷气)。清气与谷气是生成人体之气,尤其是宗气的主要物质基础。脾化生的水谷精气,有赖肺气宣降才能敷布全身。肺维持生理活动中所需的津气,又依靠脾运化的水谷精微以充养,故有"肺为主气之枢,脾为生气之源"之说。只有在肺脾两脏的协同作用下,才能保证人体之气,特别是宗气的生成与敷布。在病理上,肺气虚累及脾(子病犯母),脾气虚影响肺(母病及子),终至肺脾两虚之候。

1.5.2 Water metabolism

The body fluid metabolism is related to the physiological functions of several zang-fu organs. As for the two zang organs of the lung and spleen, the lung dominates dispersing and descending as well as dredges and regulates the water passage, so as to make the water distribute and discharge normally, while the spleen dominates the transportation and transformation and moves the body fluid for the stomach, so as to make the water be produced and distribute normally. The water in the human body, is sent upwards by the spleen to the lung, and is spread to the whole body and sent downwards to the bladder through the lung's function in dispersing and descending. The lung and spleen are mutually coordinated and functioned, as the important link to guarantee the normal formation, distribution and discharge of the body fluid. Pathologically, if the spleen fails to dominate the transportation and transformation, the water cannot be distributed, but accumulates into the damp, phlegm, rheum or swelling, which influences the lung which fails to dominate dispersing and descending, leading to sputum, cough, panting, etc. In those conditions, the symptoms are of the lung, while the causes are of the spleen, so it is said that "the spleen is the source to produce the phlegm, while the lung is the organ to store the phlegm".

1.6 Lung and liver

The liver dominates ascending, while the lung dominates descending. The physiological link between the lung and liver embodies the coordinative regulation in up-flow and down-flow of qi activities in human body.

1.5.2 水液代谢方面

津液代谢涉及多个脏腑的生理功能。就肺脾而言，肺主宣降以通调水道，使水液正常地布散与排泄；脾主运化，为胃行其津液，使水液正常地生成与输布。人体的水液，由脾上输于肺，通过肺的宣发肃降而布散周身及下输膀胱。肺脾两脏协调配合，相互为用，是保证津液正常生成、输布与排泄的重要环节。病理上，若脾失健运，水液不化，聚湿生痰，为饮为肿，影响及肺则失其宣降而痰嗽喘咳。是病其标在肺，而其本在脾，故有"脾为生痰之源，肺为贮痰之器"之说。

1.6 肺与肝

肝主升发，肺主肃降。肺与肝的生理联系，主要体现在人体气机升降的协同调节方面。

The liver dominates the up-flow of qi, while the lung dominates the down-flow of qi. The liver qi is appropriate in up-flowing movement, while the lung qi is smooth in down-flowing movement. These are the characteristics of the liver and lung in their qi activities of up-flow and down-flow. The coordinative movement of the up-flow of the liver qi and the down-flow of the lung qi functions to regulate the qi activities and harmonize qi and blood of the whole body. Furthermore, if the lung qi is sufficient, down-flowing normally, it is possible to benefit the liver qi to up-flow. If the liver qi is kept dredging and draining, up-flowing normal, it is possible to benefit the lung qi to down-flow. It can be seen that the up-flow of the liver qi and the down-flow of the lung qi are mutually dependent and mutually acted.

Pathologically, the liver disease and lung disease are affected each other. For example, the liver qi stagnation transforming into the fire, which may damage the lung-metal, there can be the liver fire attacking lung pattern, with the symptoms of cough, chest pain, hemoptysis, etc. It is said that "the wood's fire attacks the metal" or that "the hyperactive wood counter-acts on the metal" in the theory of five elements. If the lung fails to dominate descending, there can be the internal accumulation of dryness and heat, which may damage the liver-wood, leading to the condition of the lung disease involving the liver, with the symptoms of headache, anger, hypochondriac distension and pain, etc.

1.7　Lung and kidney

The lung is termed as the upper source of wa-

肝主升发之气,肺主肃降之气。肝气以升发为宜,肺气以肃降为顺。此为肝肺气机升降的特点所在。肝升肺降,升降协调,对全身气机的调畅,气血的调和,起着重要的调节作用。此外,肺气充足,肃降正常,有利于肝气的升发;肝气疏泄,升发条达,有利于肺气的肃降。可见肝升与肺降,又相互依存,相互为用。

在病理状态下,肝肺病变可相互影响。如肝郁化火,可伤及肺金,而出现咳嗽、胸痛、咯血等肝火犯肺之症,五行理论称为"木火刑金""木旺侮金"。肺失清肃,燥热内盛,也可伤及肝木,而出现头痛、易怒、胁肋胀痛等肺病及肝之候。

1.7　肺与肾

肺为水之上源,肾为主

ter, while the kidney is termed as the organ to dominate the water. The lung dominates the respiration, while the kidney accepts qi. The lung pertains to the metal, while the kidney pertains to the water, so the metal promotes the water. The relation between the lung and kidney includes the water metabolism, respiratory movement and mutual support of the yin fluid.

1.7.1　Water metabolism

　　The lung acts to dredge and regulate the water passage, as the upper source of water, while the kidney dominates the transformation of qi, as the organ to govern the water. The lung's functions in dispersing and descending and in moving the water rely on the transpiring and transforming functions of the kidney qi or kidney yang. On the contrary, the kidney's functions in domination transformation, in elevating and subduing water and in dominating the open and closure also rely on the dispersing and descending function of the lung qi. Only when the lung and kidney act in coordination, can it be possible to guarantee the normal distribution and discharge of water inside the body. Pathologically, the dysfunction of the lung and kidney may cause the disturbance of water metabolism, with the symptoms of scanty urine, edema, etc.

1.7.2　Respiratory movement

　　The lung dominates qi and governs the respiration, while the kidney stores the essence and accepts qi. The respiratory movement of human body, dominated by the lung, is assisted by the kidney's function in accepting qi. If the Jing (Essence) Qi in the kidney is sufficient and the kidney's function in storing the essence is normal, the Qing (Clear) Qi

水之脏；肺主呼吸，肾主纳气；肺属金，肾属水，金水相生。肺与肾的关系，主要表现在水液代谢、呼吸运动及阴液互资三方面。

1.7.1　水液代谢方面

　　肺主通调水道，为水之上源；肾总司气化，为主水之脏。肺宣发肃降而主行水的功能，有赖于肾气肾阳的蒸腾气化；反之，肾司气化而升降水液，主持开阖的功能，也有赖于肺气的宣发肃降。惟有肺肾协同，才能保证体内水液输布与排泄的正常。病理上，因肺与肾功能失调而致水液代谢障碍，容易出现尿少、浮肿等症。

1.7.2　呼吸运动方面

　　肺主气而司呼吸，肾藏精而主纳气。人体的呼吸运动，虽由肺之所主，但亦需肾的纳气功能来协助。只有肾中精气充盛，封藏功能正常，肺吸入的清气才能经过肃降而下纳于肾，以维持呼吸的

inhaled by the lung can down-flow through the lung's function in descending to be stored in the kidney, so as to maintain the depth of respiration. It is clear that during the respiratory movement of human body, the normal down-flow of the lung qi is beneficial for the kidney to accept qi, while the sufficient kidney qi and its normal accepting function are beneficial for the lung to keep its descending function. Therefore, it is said that "the lung is the dominator of qi, while the kidney is the root of qi". Pathologically, the chronic deficiency of the lung qi that fails to descend and the insufficiency of the kidney qi that fails to accept qi are affected each other, leading to the pattern of the kidney failing to accept qi with the symptoms of shortness of breath, superficial respiration, more exhalation than inhalation, etc.

1.7.3 Mutual support of yin fluid

Yin of the lung and yin of the kidney are mutually supported. The lung pertains to the metal, while the kidney pertains to the water. The metal acts to promote the water, while the water acts to moisturize the metal. If the lung yin is sufficient, it may transfer the essence to the kidney to support the kidney yin. The kidney yin is the basis of yin of whole body. If the kidney yin is sufficient, it may be sent upwards to moisturize the lung to support the lung yin. Pathologically, the lung yin insufficiency pattern and the kidney yin insufficiency can be seen simultaneously and in the reciprocal causation, leading to the pattern of lung and kidney yin deficiency and internal heat, with the symptoms of flushed cheeks, nocturnal sweats, tidal fever, seminal emission, dry cough, hoarseness of voice,

深度。可见,在人体呼吸运动中,肺气肃降,有利于肾的纳气;肾气充足,纳摄有权,也有利于肺之肃降。故有"肺为气之主,肾为气之根"之说。病理上,肺气久虚,肃降失司,与肾气不足,摄纳无权,往往互为影响,以致出现气短喘促,呼吸表浅,呼多吸少等肾不纳气之症。

1.7.3 阴液互资方面

肺肾之阴,相互资生。肺属金,肾属水,金能生水,水能润金。肺阴充足,输精于肾,使肾阴充盈;肾阴为诸阴之本,肾阴充盛,上滋于肺,使肺阴充足。病理状态下,肺阴不足与肾阴不足,既可同时出现,亦可互为因果,以致出现颧红、盗汗、潮热、遗泄、干咳音哑、腰膝酸软等肺肾阴虚内热之候。

aching and weakness of low back and knees, etc.

1.8　Liver and spleen

The liver dominates dredging and draining, while the spleen dominates transportation and transformation. The liver stores the blood, while the spleen produces and controls the blood. The physiological relation between the liver and spleen includes the mutual dependence of dredging-draining function and transporting-transforming function and the mutual coordination of storing the blood and controlling the blood.

1.8.1　Digestive function

The liver dominates dredging and draining, regulates the qi activities and transports the bile to the intestines, for the purpose to promote the spleen-stomach's functions in accepting and transporting the food, and to assist the coordination of the up-flow and down-flow of the qi activities in the middle energizer where the spleen and stomach locate. If the spleen qi is sufficient and the spleen is normal in transportation and transformation, the essence of water and grain will be sufficient and qi and blood can be transported and transformed normally, so that the liver can be moisturized and nourished, to function normally in dredging and draining. Pathologically, the liver and spleen are mutually affected. If the liver fails to dominate dredging and draining to cause qi stagnation, the spleen's function in transportation and transformation is disturbed, so as to lead to the pattern of liver and spleen disharmony, with the symptoms of emotional depression, stuffy chest, frequent sighing, poor appetite, abdominal distension, borborygmus, diarrhea, etc. If the spleen fails to dominate transpor-

1.8　肝与脾

肝主疏泄,脾主运化;肝主藏血,脾主生血统血。肝与脾的生理联系,主要表现在疏泄与运化的相互依存、藏血与统血的相互协调关系上。

1.8.1　消化功能方面

肝主疏泄,调畅气机,疏利胆汁,输于肠道,促进脾胃对饮食物的纳运功能,并有助于中焦脾胃气机升降协调。脾气健旺,运化正常,水谷精微充足,气血运化有源,肝体得以濡养而有利于疏泄。病理上,肝脾病变相互影响。若肝失疏泄,气机郁滞,易致脾失健运,形成精神抑郁,胸闷太息,纳呆腹胀,肠鸣泄泻等肝脾不调之候。脾失健运,也可影响肝失疏泄,导致"土壅木郁"之证。或因脾虚生湿化热,湿热郁蒸肝胆,胆热液泄,则可形成黄疸。

tation and transformation, the liver's function in dredging and draining is disturbed, so as to lead to the pattern of "earth blockage and wood stagnation". If the spleen is weak, there can be the dampness that may transform into heat. When the damp-heat fumigates and blocks the liver and gallbladder, the heat in gallbladder may cause overflow of bile, leading to jaundice.

1.8.2　Blood circulation

The normal blood circulation is dominated by the heart, but is also closely related to the liver and spleen as well. The liver stores the blood and regulates the blood volume, while the spleen produces and controls the blood. If the spleen qi is sufficient and vigorous, it produces sufficient blood and controls the blood normally, so that the liver is normal in storing the blood. If the liver blood is sufficient and the liver is normal in storing the blood, the blood volume can be regulated normally, and qi and blood can circulate smoothly. The liver and spleen are mutually coordinated, to jointly maintain the normal blood circulation. Pathologically, the spleen qi deficiency may cause blood deficiency due to the spleen failing to transport and transform normally, while the failure of spleen in controlling the blood may lead to bleeding. These are the major causes of the liver blood insufficiency. Besides, the patterns of the liver failing to store the blood and the spleen failing to control the blood can be seen simultaneously, termed as "failure in storing and controlling" clinically.

1.9　Liver and kidney

The relation between the liver and kidney is described as "the liver and kidney sharing a same

1.8.2　血液运行方面

血的正常运行,虽由心所主持,但与肝、脾也有密切的关系。肝主藏血,调节血量;脾主生血,统摄血液。脾气健旺,生血有源,统血有权,使肝有所藏;肝血充足,藏疏有度,血量得以正常调节,气血才能运行无阻。肝脾相互协同,共同维持血液的正常运行。病理状态下,脾气虚弱,则生化之源匮乏而血虚,或统摄之功无权而出血,均可导致肝血不足。此外,肝不藏血也与脾不统血同时并见,临床称为"藏统失司"。

1.9　肝与肾

肝肾之间的关系,古医籍中多称为"肝肾同源""乙

source" or "Yi-Heavenly Stem 2 and Gui-Heavenly Stem 10 sharing a same source" in many ancient classics. The liver stores the blood, while the kidney stores the essence. The liver dominates dredging and draining, while the kidney dominates storing and sealing up. The liver is the son of the water, while the kidney is the mother of the wood. Therefore, the relation between the liver and kidney includes the essence and blood sharing a same source, the mutual action of storing and draining and the mutual nourishment of the yin fluid.

1.9.1 Essence and blood sharing a same source

The liver stores the blood, while the kidney stores the essence. The essence and blood are generated each other. The formation of the liver blood relies on the sufficiency of the kidney essence, while the Jing (Essence) Qi in the kidney relies on the nourishment of the liver blood. The kidney essence and liver blood are closely related, as it is said that replenish one and you replenish them all, injury one and you injure them all, in weal and woe. The two are mutually generated and transformed, because the essence acts to produce the blood, while the blood acts to produce the essence. Both of them originate from the essence of water and grain transported and transformed by the spleen and stomach, so it is said that the liver and kidney share a same source, or that "the essence and blood share a same source". Pathologically, the liver blood insufficiency and the kidney essence depletion may be influenced each other, leading to the pattern of liver and kidney deficiency or the pattern of essence and blood deficiency, with the symptoms of dizziness, blurring of vision, deafness, tinnitus, aching and

癸同源"(天干配属五行,肝属乙木,肾属癸水。乙、癸分别为肝肾之代称)。因肝主藏血而肾主藏精,肝主疏泄而肾主封藏,肝为水之子而肾为木之母。故肝肾关系,主要表现在精血同源、藏泄互用以及阴液互养等方面。

1.9.1 精血同源

肝藏血,肾藏精,精血相互资生。肝血的化生有赖于肾精的充盛,肾中精气也依赖于肝血的滋养。肾精肝血,一荣俱荣,一损俱损,休戚相关。二者相互资生,相互转化,精能生血,血能生精,且均化源于脾胃运化的水谷精微,故肝肾同源,亦称"精血同源"。病理上肝血不足与肾精亏损多可相互影响,以致出现头昏目眩、耳聋耳鸣、腰膝酸软等肝肾精血两亏之证。

weakness of low back and knees, etc.

1.9.2　Mutual action of storing and draining

The liver dominates dredging and draining, while the kidney dominates storing and sealing up. There exists a mutual action and mutual restraint relation between the two. The normal liver qi in dredging and draining may assist the kidney qi to open and close properly, while the normal kidney qi in storing and sealing up may prevent the liver qi from over dredging and draining. The dredging-draining function and the storing and sealing-up function are contrary, but are supplemented each other, so as to regulate the female menstruation and male spermiation. If the liver and kidney are abnormal in draining and storing, there can be irregular menstruation, heavy flow in menstruation or amenorrhea in females, and seminal emission, nocturnal emission or ultra-erection in males.

1.9.3　Mutual nourishment of yin fluid

The liver pertains to the wood in five elements, while the kidney pertains to the water in five elements, so the water acts to moisturize the wood. If the kidney yin is sufficient, it acts to moisturize and nourish the liver yin. If the liver yin is sufficient, it also acts to moisturize and nourish the kidney yin as well. The liver yin and kidney yin are mutually moisturized and nourished. Yin acts to restrain yang. If the liver yin and kidney yin are sufficient, they act to support each other, but also to restrain the liver yang from being hyperactive, so as to maintain the coordinative equilibrium between yin and yang of the liver and kidney. Pathologically, the liver yin insufficiency may involve the kidney yin, while the kidney yin insufficiency may cause

1.9.2　藏泄互用

肝主疏泄,肾主封藏,二者之间存在着相互为用、相互制约的关系。肝气疏泄可使肾气开合有度,肾气闭藏以制肝气疏泄太过。疏泄与封藏,相反而相成,从而调节女子的月经来潮和男子的排精功能。若肝肾藏泄失调,女子可见月经周期失常,经量过多或闭经,男子可见遗精、滑精或阳强不泄等症。

1.9.3　阴液互养

肝在五行属木,肾在五行属水,水能涵木。肾阴充盛则能滋养肝阴,肝阴充足亦能滋养肾阴,肝肾之阴相互滋养。阴能制阳,肝肾之阴充盈,不仅能相互资生,而且能制约肝阳不使其偏亢,从而保持肝肾阴阳的协调平衡。病理上,肝阴不足,累及肾阴;肾阴不足,水不涵木。肝肾阴虚,又易致虚火内生或肝阳上亢,出现头昏目眩、急躁易怒、面红目赤、耳鸣、遗精、潮热、盗汗等症。

"water failing to moisturize wood". If the liver yin and kidney yin are deficient, there can be endogenous fire or liver yang hyperactivity, with the symptoms of dizziness, blurring of vision, restlessness, anger, red complexion, tinnitus, seminal emission, tidal fever, nocturnal sweats, etc.

1.10　Spleen and kidney

The spleen is termed as the acquired basis, while the kidney is termed as the congenital basis. The first relation between the spleen and kidney is actually the congenital and acquired relation. The spleen dominates the transportation and transformation of water, while the kidney is the organ to dominate the water. The second relation between the spleen and kidney is embodies the water metabolism.

1.10.1　Mutual support between the congenital and acquired bases

The spleen dominates the transportation and transformation of the food essence and produces qi and blood, as the acquired basis. The kidney stores the essence that is termed the True Fire in Vital Gate, as the congenital basis. The transporting and transforming function of the spleen, relying on the warming, transpiring and transforming function of the kidney yang, can be strong and healthy. The Jing (Essence) Qi in the kidney, relying on the constant support from the food essence transported and transformed by the spleen and stomach, can be sufficient. The acquired and congenital bases are mutually supported and promoted, so none is dispensable. The congenital basis acts to warm, nourish and inspire the acquired basis, while the acquired basis acts to support the congenital basis. Pathologically,

1.10　脾与肾

脾为后天之本,肾为先天之本,脾肾两者首先表现在先天与后天的关系;脾主运化水液,肾为主水之脏,脾肾的关系其次表现在水液代谢方面。

1.10.1　先后天相互资生

脾主运化水谷精微,化生气血,为后天之本;肾藏精,寓命门真火,为先天之本。脾的运化,有赖肾阳的温煦蒸化,始能健旺;肾中精气亦赖脾胃运化的水谷精微的不断补充,方能充盛。后天与先天,两者相互资生,相互促进,缺一不可。先天温养激发后天,后天补充培育先天的脾肾关系,反映在病理上,脾虚气弱与肾虚精亏,中阳虚损与命门火衰,常可相互影响,互为因果。前者多表现为腹胀便溏,腰酸耳鸣,或少年生长发育迟缓的

the spleen qi weakness and the kidney essence deficiency, the middle energizer yang deficiency and the vital gate fire decline, are often mutually influenced in the reciprocal causation. The former is diagnosed as the essence and qi deficiency pattern with the symptoms of abdominal distension, diarrhea, aching at low back, tinnitus, or retarded growth and development in children, while the latter is diagnosed as the spleen and kidney yang deficiency with the symptoms of fear of cold, abdominal pain, aching and coldness in low back and knees, diarrhea at dawn, indigested food in feces, etc.

1.10.2 Water metabolism

The normal spleen's function in transporting and transforming the water relies on the warming, transpiring and transforming function of the kidney yang. The kidney dominates the water and governs opening and closing. It maintains the equilibrium of the water metabolism of whole body under the transforming function of the kidney qi or kidney yang. Such a function of the kidney relies on the assistance of the spleen qi, the so-called "the earth restraining the water". The spleen and kidney, in a mutual coordination, jointly act to fulfill the water metabolism. Pathologically, if the spleen is weak and fails to transport and transform the water, there can be the endogenous dampness that may further cause the water overflow due the kidney deficiency. If the kidney is weak and loses its transforming function, there can be endogenous water-dampness that may influence the spleen's function in transporting and transforming the water. As a result, the pattern of spleen and kidney deficiency or

精气不足之证。后者多出现畏寒腹痛,腰膝酸冷,五更泄泻、完谷不化等脾肾阳虚之候。

1.10.2 水液代谢方面

脾主运化水液功能的正常发挥,须赖肾阳的温煦蒸化。肾主水而司开合,在肾气肾阳的气化作用下,主持全身水液代谢的平衡,又须赖脾气的协助,即所谓"土能制水"。脾肾两脏相互协同,共同完成水液的新陈代谢。在病理方面,脾虚失运,水湿内生,经久不愈,可发展至肾虚水泛;而肾虚气化失司,水湿内蕴,也可影响脾的运化功能,最终均可导致尿少浮肿,腹胀便溏,畏寒肢冷,腰膝酸软等脾肾两虚、水湿内停之证。

the pattern of internal accumulation of water-dampness may occur, with the symptoms of scanty urine, edema, abdominal distension, loose feces, fear of cold, chills in limbs, aching and weakness of low back and knees, etc.

2 Relationship among six fu organs

The relationship among the six fu organs embodies their mutual share of work and orderly cooperation in the process of digesting, absorbing and discharging the water and grain. The food enters into the stomach through the mouth, the stomach accepts and decomposes the food and sends it downwards to the small intestine, and then the small intestine accepts the chyme preliminarily digested by the stomach, and further digests and absorbs it through the function to separate the clear from the turbid. Simultaneously, the gallbladder secrets the bile and discharges it into the small intestine to assist the digestion. The small intestine absorbs the essence of water and grain and transfers it upwards to the heart and lung so as to nourish the whole body. The surplus water is transformed into urine and transferred downwards to the bladder through the transforming function of the kidney qi. At last, the small intestine transfers the food dregs downwards to the large intestine, which absorbs some surplus water from the food dregs, transforms the food dregs into feces and discharges the feces. The triple energizer acts to communicate the upper and the lower, as the passage of water, so that it is related to the whole process of digestion, absorption and discharge. In summary, the digestive process of human body is realized by the close cooperation of the

2 六腑之间的关系

六腑之间的关系,主要体现在对水谷的消化、吸收和排泄过程中的分工协作和有序配合。饮食由口入胃,经过胃的受纳腐熟,下传于小肠。小肠接受胃初步消化后形成的食糜,通过分别清浊,进一步消化吸收;同时胆通过把胆汁排泄入小肠以帮助消化。小肠吸收水谷之精微,上输心肺以营养全身;其剩余的水液,经肾的气化作用生成尿液,下归膀胱;最后小肠将食物残渣继续下传于大肠。大肠吸收食物残渣中剩余的部分水分,使大便成形而排出体外。三焦之气化贯通上下,为水液运行之道路,所以与消化、吸收和排泄的过程均有关。归纳起来说,人体的消化过程是由胃、胆、小肠三个器官密切协作而完成的,吸收过程主要在小肠,大肠也吸收了部分水分;排泄则是膀胱和大肠的作用。

stomach, gallbladder and small intestine, the absorptive process is realized by the small intestine, but the large intestine also absorbs some part of water, and the discharging process is realized by the bladder and large intestine.

The six fu organs, transporting and transforming the water and grain, needs to constantly accept, transport and discharge. In the process of food movement from the upper to the lower, the stomach and intestines should be empty and full alternately, so as to keep an unblocked state. Therefore, it is said that "the six fu organs act to be unblocked" and that "the dredging method is taken as a reinforcing method in treating the fu organ diseases". Clinically, the fu organ diseases are affected each other. If the gallbladder fails to be dredging and draining, the stomach will be involved, leading to the coincided disease of gallbladder and stomach, with the symptoms of hypochondriac pain, jaundice, poor appetite, vomiting, etc. If the excess-type heat in stomach burns and consumes the body fluid, the large intestine may be involved, causing the large intestine qi stagnation, with the symptoms of dry feces, constipation, etc.

3　Relationship between five zang organs and six fu organs

There are various complicated relations among the five zang organs and six fu organs, but the major one is called "the match between zang and fu". The Zang organs pertain to yin that dominate the interior, while the fu oxgans pertain to yang that dominate the exterior. Therefore, a zang organ and a fu organ, a yin and a yang, and an exterior and an

由于六腑传化水谷, 需要不断地受纳、传导和排泄, 在水谷自上而下的过程中, 胃与肠之间又必须虚实更替, 保持宜通不宜滞的状态, 所以前人有"六腑以通为用""腑病以通为补"的说法。临床上, 六腑的病变也常常互相影响。如胆失疏泄, 可影响到胃, 出现胁痛、黄疸、食少、呕吐等胆胃同病的症状; 而胃有实热, 消灼津液, 亦可使大肠腑气不通, 出现大便秘结等症。

3　五脏与六腑之间的关系

五脏与六腑之间具有多种复杂的关系, 其主要表现为"脏腑相合"。因为脏属阴, 腑属阳, 阴主里, 阳主表, 所以一脏一腑, 一阴一阳, 一表一里互相配合, 就形成了脏腑相合的特殊联系。

interior are mutually coordinated, to form up a specific link called "the match between zang and fu".

The match between zang and fu includes the exterior-interior relation of five pairs of zang-fu organs, i.e. the heart matching the small intestine, the lung matching the large intestine, the spleen matching the stomach, the liver matching the gallbladder, and the kidney matching the bladder. The triple energizer has no its matched zang organ, so it is called "the solitary fu organ". But it is said in Huang Di Nei Jing that the triple energizer is adopted by the kidney to match, as "the kidney matching the triple energizer and bladder".

The match between zang and fu includes the mutual pertaining and connecting relations by the meridians and collaterals, but also the mutual cooperation physiologically and mutually influence pathologically.

2.1 Heart matching small intestine

The heart dominates the blood and vessels, acting to circulate the blood all over the body, so as to moisturize and nourish the small intestine. The small intestine acts to accept and transform food, absorbing the essence of water and grain to transform into the heart blood and to support and nourish the heart. The two organs are mutually dependent. Pathologically, it is said that "the heart transfers its heat to the small intestine", i.e. if the heart fire is hyperactive, it may be transferred downwards along the meridians to the small intestine, leading to the symptoms of irritability, red tongue, ulcers in mouth and tongue, scanty urine, dark-col-

脏腑相合包括五对表里相合关系,即心合小肠、肺合大肠、脾合胃、肝合胆、肾合膀胱。三焦没有相合的脏,故称为"孤府"。但《黄帝内经》中又把三焦寄合于肾,而提出"肾合三焦、膀胱"的概念。

脏腑相合,既有经脉上的相互络属,也有功能上的相互配合和病理上的相互影响。脏与腑在经脉上的相互络属,可参见"经络"章。以下讨论脏与腑在功能上的相互配合和病理上的相互影响。

2.1 心合小肠

心主血脉,运行血液于周身而能滋养小肠,小肠受盛化物,吸收的水谷精微能化生心血而充养于心,两者存在着相互依赖的关系。在病理方面,历来有"心移热于小肠"的说法,即心火亢盛,可循经下移于小肠,出现心烦、舌红、口舌糜烂及尿少、尿赤、尿痛等症。

ored urine, painful urination, etc.

2.2 Lung matching the large intestine

The lung qi tends to down-flow, while the large intestine dominates the transportation. If the lung qi is normal in down-flowing, the body fluid can be transferred downwards to the large intestine, which is moisturized to perform its downward transportation. If the large intestine's function in transporting is normal and its qi flows smoothly, it is beneficial for the lung qi to down-flow smoothly as well. Therefore, the lung's descending function and the large intestine's transporting function are mutually assisted. Pathologically, the lung failing to descend and the large intestine failing to transport are often influenced each other, leading to the coincided disease of the lung and large intestine, with the symptoms of stuffy chest, cough, panting, dry feces, constipation, etc.

2.3 Spleen matching the stomach

Both the spleen and stomach locate in the middle energizer, and their physiological link embodies in the digestive and absorptive function of the human body. The spleen and stomach are taken as "the acquired basis" and "the source to produce qi and blood". The physiological relation between the spleen and stomach includes three aspects as follows.

2.3.1 Coordinative acceptance and transportation

The spleen dominates transportation and transformation, while the stomach dominates acceptance and decomposition. The two organs are closely cooperated in the digestive function, called the coordinative acceptance and transportation. The food

2.2 肺合大肠

肺气主肃降,大肠主传导。肺气肃降正常,津液下输大肠,肠腑濡润,可促进大肠传导下行;而大肠传导正常,腑气通利,也有利于肺气的肃降。所以肺之肃降与大肠的传导功能之间是互相协助的。在病理上,肺失肃降与大肠传导失司的病变往往相互影响,出现胸闷、咳喘、大便干结或便秘等肺与大肠同病的现象。

2.3 脾合胃

脾与胃同居中焦,二者的生理联系主要表现在人体的消化吸收功能方面,脾与胃共为"后天之本""气血生化之源"。脾与胃的生理关系可以概括为以下三个方面。

2.3.1 纳运协调

脾主运化,胃主受纳、腐熟,两者在消化功能上的密切配合,称为纳运协调。食物入胃,先由胃受纳和腐熟,这就为脾的运化奠定了基

enters into the stomach, which accepts and decomposes it. This process establishes the foundation for the spleen in transportation and transformation. The spleen dominates transportation and transformation, further digesting the food to absorb and transport the food essence. This process is to meet the need of stomach in continuously accepting food. The coordinative acceptance and transportation act to guarantee the normal digestive and absorptive function of human body.

2.3.2 Orderly up-flow and down-flow

The spleen qi acts to elevate the clear, while the stomach acts to subdue the turbid. The two organs are mutually assisted and retrained, with their qi up-flowing and down-flowing orderly. The spleen acts to elevate the clear, for the purpose to transfer the Qing (Clear) Qi of water and grain upwards to the heart and lung, while the stomach acts to subdue the turbid, for the purpose to transfer the Zhuo (Turbid) Qi of water and grain downwards. If the stomach fails to down-flow, the Zhuo (Turbid) Qi will be accumulated in the middle energizer and the Qing (Clear) Qi of water and grain cannot be transferred, so that the spleen qi cannot up-flow normally. If the spleen qi fails up-flow, the Qing (Clear) Qi of water and grain cannot be transferred upwards, but stays together with the Zhuo (Turbid) Qi in the abdomen, so that the stomach qi cannot down-flow normally. That is to say that none of the spleen's up-flow and stomach's down-flow is dispensable. Only with the orderly and harmonious up-flow and down-flow, can the whole digestive process be realized normally. Therefore, it is said in TCM that "the spleen is healthy when its qi up-

础;而脾主运化,进一步消化水谷,吸收并转输精微,又是适应胃继续受纳的需要。只有纳运协调配合,才能保证人体消化吸收功能的正常进行。

2.3.2 升降相因

脾气主升清,胃气主降浊,两者互助互制,称为升降相因。脾主升清,能将水谷精微向上输送至心肺;胃主降浊,能使水谷浊气通降下行。没有胃气之降,水谷浊气壅塞于中焦,精微之气不能转输,脾气就不能升;没有脾气之升,水谷之清不能上行,则与浊气相混于腹中,胃气就不能正常地降。也就是说,脾升与胃降缺一不可,只有升降相互协调,消化过程才能正常地进行,所以中医学有"脾宜升则健,胃宜降则和"的理论。

flows, while the stomach is harmonious when its qi down-flows".

2.3.3 Appropriate dryness and dampness

The spleen prefers dryness and dislikes dampness, while the stomach prefers moisture and dislikes dryness. The two organs are mutually complementary in their physiological features, called the appropriate dryness and dampness. The spleen and stomach are just opposite in preferring and disliking dryness and dampness. The spleen is a zang organ, pertaining to yin, so it is possible to maintain its functions in transporting and transforming and in elevating the clear when it gains the yang-dry featured qi. The dampness is a yin-type pathogen, often attacking the spleen to disturb its functions in transporting and transforming and in elevating the clear. Therefore, the spleen is featured in preferring dryness and disliking dampness. The stomach is a fu organ, pertaining to yang, so it is possible to maintain its functions in decomposing and subduing the turbid when it gains the yin-moist fluid. The dryness is a yang-type pathogen, often damaging the stomach's fluid and harmful for the stomach's functions in decomposing and subduing. Therefore, the stomach is featured in preferring dampness and disliking dryness. Physiologically, the spleen's yin-moist qi is beneficial to assist the stomach in decomposing and subduing, while the stomach's yang-dry qi is beneficial to assist the spleen in transporting and transforming and in elevating the clear. The appropriate dryness and dampness of the two organs play a very important role in their digestive and absorptive function.

The spleen and stomach are very closely related

2.3.3　燥湿相济

脾喜燥恶湿,胃喜润恶燥,两者生理特性上的相互济助,称为燥湿相济。脾胃两脏在喜恶燥湿方面的特性正好相反。脾为脏,属阴,得阳燥之气始能运化升清,而湿属阴邪,容易困脾,阻碍其运化升清的功能,所以脾的特性是喜燥恶湿;胃为腑,属阳,得阴液滋润则能腐熟润降,而燥属阳邪,易伤胃津,不利于胃的腐熟润降功能,因此胃的特性是喜润恶燥。在生理情况下,脾的阴润之气有利于胃的腐熟润降,胃的阳燥之气有利于脾的运化升清,两者燥湿相济,各得其利,在消化吸收功能中发挥着非常重要的作用。

由于脾胃生理关系十分

physiologically, so spleen disease and stomach disease are very easy to influence each other pathologically. Usually, the spleen disease may involve the stomach, while the stomach disease may involve the spleen, leading to the coincided disease of both the spleen and stomach, with the symptoms of poor appetite, epigastric and abdominal distension, vomiting, belching, diarrhea, etc.

2.4 Liver matching gallbladder

The physiological relation between the liver and gallbladder implies that the liver and gallbladder jointly dominate dredging and draining. The liver dominates dredging and draining, and secrets and discharges the bile, while the gallbladder is attached to the liver, and stores and discharges the bile. The bile originates from the liver, but is stored in the gallbladder. That the bile is discharged and infuses into the intestines to assist the digestion relies on the smooth qi activities, while the normal liver's function in dredging and draining is the prerequisite of the smooth qi activities. Simultaneously, whether the gallbladder is unblocked or not may also influence the liver's function in dredging and draining. The liver and gallbladder are mutually acted in the qi circulation, so it is said that the liver and gallbladder jointly dominate dredging and draining. If the liver fails to dominate dredging and draining, there can be gallbladder qi stagnation, leading to unsmooth discharge of the bile. On the contrary, if the bile is stagnant, the liver's function in dredging and draining is disturbed, leading to the liver qi stagnation. If the liver and gallbladder fail to dominate dredging and draining, the bile cannot be discharged smoothly, leading to the symptoms of hy-

密切,因此临床上脾病与胃病最易互相影响,往往脾病则胃亦病,胃病则脾亦病,出现食欲不振、脘腹胀满、呕吐、嗳气、腹泻等脾胃同病的症状。

2.4 肝合胆

肝与胆在生理上的关系,主要表现为肝胆同主疏泄。肝主疏泄,分泌和排泄胆汁;胆附于肝,贮存和排泄胆汁。胆汁来源于肝,贮藏于胆。胆汁排泄入肠以助消化,离不开气机的调畅,而肝气疏泄是保证气机调畅的前提;同时,胆腑通畅与否,也能影响肝气的疏泄。肝胆之间在气的运行方面的相互作用,称为肝胆同主疏泄。如肝失疏泄,可导致胆气不舒,胆汁排泄不畅;反之,胆汁瘀阻,也可影响肝之疏泄,使肝气郁结而不畅。肝胆失疏,胆汁排泄不畅,可出现胁痛、黄疸、食欲不振等症。

pochondriac pain, jaundice, poor appetite, etc.

2.5 Kidney matching bladder

The relation between the kidney and bladder embodies the mutual dependence and coordination in discharging the urine. Through the transforming function of the kidney qi, the turbid part of water inside the human body is transformed into urine, which is transferred downwards to the bladder and to be stored there temporarily, then discharged. The bladder's functions in storing urine and discharging urine are realized by the normal transforming function of the kidney qi. If the kidney qi is sufficient and its transforming function is normal, the bladder acts to open and close properly and the urine discharge is normal. If the transforming function of kidney qi is abnormal, the bladder's function is disturbed, leading to the symptoms of difficult urination, excessive urine, enuresis, etc. On the contrary, if there is the damp-heat in the bladder, disturbing the qi activities, the Xie (Pathogenic) Qi will flow reversely to the kidney to disturb the transforming function of the kidney qi. Therefore, besides the symptoms of poor transforming function of the bladder qi, as frequency of urination, urgency of urination, pain of urination, difficult urination, etc., there can be the symptoms of the kidney damage, as aching of low back, pain of low back, etc.

2.5　肾合膀胱

肾与膀胱的关系，主要表现为在排泄小便方面的相互依赖和协同作用。人体的水液通过肾的气化作用，其浊者形成尿液，下输膀胱以暂时贮留，然后排出体外。膀胱贮尿和排尿的功能，是在肾的气化功能正常的前提下完成的。肾气充足，气化正常，则膀胱开合有度，尿液排泄正常。如肾的气化失常，影响膀胱的功能，可出现小便不利或尿多、遗尿等症。反之，如膀胱湿热，气机不通，邪气逆行于肾，也会影响肾的气化功能，日久使肾脏受损，临床除有尿频、尿急、尿痛等膀胱气化不利、排尿不畅的表现外，还可出现腰酸、腰痛等肾脏受损的症状。

Chapter 4 Meridians and Collaterals

The meridians and collaterals are the important component part of the structural tissues of human body. Inside the human body, the circulation of qi, blood and body fluid, the functional activities of zang-fu organs and tissues, and their mutual links and coordination can be realized by the transferring, connecting and regulating functions of the meridian system, so as to form up an organic entirety.

The theory of meridians and collaterals is the doctrine to study the composite structure, physiological functions, pathological changes and relations to the zang-fu organs, the body constituents, sense organs, orifices, qi, blood and body fluid in the meridian system of human body, being the important component part of the theory system of TCM.

Section 1 Concept and System of Meridians and Collaterals

1 Concept of meridians and collaterals

The meridians and collaterals are the passage to circulate qi and blood, to connect the zang-fu organs, body constituents, sense organs and orifices and to communicate the upper with the lower and

第4章 经络

经络,是人体组织结构的重要组成部分。人体气血津液的运行,脏腑器官的功能活动,以及互相之间的联系和协调,均须通过经络系统的运输传导、联络调节的功能得以实现,并使之成为一个有机的整体。

经络学说,是研究人体经络系统的组成结构、生理功能、病理变化及其与脏腑形体官窍、气血津液等互相关系的学说,是中医理论体系的重要组成部分。

第1节 经络的概念与经络系统

1 经络的概念

经络是人体运行全身气血,联络脏腑形体官窍、沟通上下内外的通道。

the internals with the body surface inside the human body.

The meridians and collaterals are the important component part of the human structure. The meridians are the main trunks in the meridian system, while the collaterals are the branches in the meridian system. The collaterals branch out from the trunks of the meridians, and then they constantly branch repeatedly, becoming thinner and thinner, so as to form up a reticular framework all over the body. The major functions of the meridians and collaterals are to transport qi and blood, to connect the zang-fu organs and tissues, and to make the human body into an organic entirety.

2 System of meridians and collaterals

The system of meridians and collaterals is composed of five parts of the meridians, collaterals, muscle regions, cutaneous regions and zang-fu organs. In the system, the meridians and collaterals are the major part, acting to pertain and connect to the zang-fu organs internally and to link with the tendons, muscles and skins externally. The meridians and collaterals run through all the tissues including the zang-fu organs, body constituents, sense organs and orifices, spreading all over the system of meridians and collaterals of whole body.

2.1 Meridians and collaterals

The meridians are the most major component part in the system of meridians and collaterals, including the regular meridians, extraordinary meridians and divergent meridians.

The regular meridians include three yin meridians of hand, three yin meridians of foot,

经络是经脉和络脉的总称,是人体结构的重要组成部分。经脉是经络系统的主干部分,络脉是经络系统的分支部分。络脉从经脉主干上分出,并不断反复分支,越分越细,以至形成网状遍布全身。经络的作用主要是通行气血,沟通脏腑器官,把人体联系成一个有机的整体。

2 经络系统

人体经络系统,是有经脉、络脉、经筋、皮部和脏腑等五个部分组成。其中以经脉和络脉为主,在内连属于脏腑,在外连属于筋肉、皮肤。经脉和络脉贯串于脏腑器官、形体官窍等一切组织,并遍布全身各部的经络系统。

2.1 经脉与络脉

经脉是经络系统最为主要的组成部分,其有正经、奇经、经别之分。

正经有十二条,即手、足三阴经和手、足三阳经,合称

three yang meridians of hand and three yang meridians of foot, called "the twelve regular meridians".
The twelve regular meridians have their own start-
ing points and ending points respectively, the certain distributive areas and connecting orders, the
certain regulations in distribution and running directions on body and limbs, and the directly pertaining
and connecting relations to the zang-fu organs, as
the major passages of qi and blood circulation inside
the body.

　　The extraordinary meridians include the Governor Vessel, the Conception Vessel, the Thoroughfare Vessel, the Belt Vessel, the Yin Heel Vessel,
the Yang Heel Vessel, the Yin Link Vessel and the
Yang Link Vessel, called "the eight extraordinary
meridians". The eight extraordinary meridians
mainly function to dominate, connect and regulate
the twelve regular meridians.

　　The twelve divergent meridians derive from the
twelve regular meridians respectively, start from the
four limbs, run in the deep part of zang-fu organs in
the body cavity, and emerge from the neck. The divergent meridians of the yin meridians derive from
their regular meridians, run deep inside the body,
and join the yang meridians which are exterior-interior related to them, functioning to enhance the exterior-interior relations among the twelve regular
meridians and to supplement some regular meridians
through the body constituents and organs which the
regular meridians do not reach.

　　The collaterals are the branches of the meridians, and most of them have no certain fixed running
courses. The collaterals include the main collaterals, superficial collaterals and capillary collaterals.

为"十二经脉"。十二经脉有
一定的起止，一定的循行部
位和交接顺序，在肢体的分
布和走向有一定的规律，与
脏腑有直接的络属关系，是
人体气血循行的主要通道。

　　奇经有八条，即督脉、任
脉、冲脉、带脉、阴跷脉、阳跷
脉、阴维脉、阳维脉，合称为
"奇经八脉"。奇经主要具有
统率、联络和调节十二经脉
的作用。

　　十二经别，是从十二经
脉分出的较大的分支，分别
起于四肢，循行于体腔脏腑
深部，上出于颈项浅部。其
中，阴经之经别从本经别出
循行于体内，而与相为表里
的阳经相合，起到加强十二
经脉中相为表里两经之间的
关系，并能通过某些正经未
循行到的形体部位和器官，
以补正经之不足。

　　络脉是经脉的分支，多
数无一定的循行路径。络脉
有别络、浮络和孙络之分。

The main collaterals are the bigger branches. There are twelve main collaterals of the twelve regular meridians, the main collateral of the Governor Vessel, the main collateral of the Conception Vessel, and the great main collateral of the spleen, all together called "the fifteen main collaterals". The major function of the fifteen main collaterals is to enhance the superficial relation between the exterior-interior related meridians.

The superficial collaterals run at the superficial part (the skin) of the human body, often floating and being seen.

The capillary collaterals are the thinnest and smallest collaterals, functioning to "dispelling the pathogens" and to "communicate the Ying (Nutrient) Qi and Wei (Defensive) Qi" described in Huang Di Nei Jing.

2.2 Superficial connections with muscle regions and cutaneous regions

The muscle regions and cutaneous regions are the affiliated parts of the twelve regular meridians with the muscles and skin. It is believed in the theory of meridians and collaterals that the muscle tendons are the system in which qi of the twelve regular meridians "knots, accumulates, scatters and connects" at the muscles and joints. They are the affiliated parts of the twelve regular meridians, so called "the twelve muscle regions", functioning to connect four limbs and all bones, and to govern the joint movements. The skin of the whole body is the area where the functional activities of twelve regular meridians superficially reflect, and also the area where qi of meridians and collaterals spreads as well. "The twelve cutaneous regions" are the twelve parts divid-

别络也是较大的分支。十二经脉与督脉、任脉之别络,以及脾之大络,合为"十五别络"。别络的主要功能是加强相为表里的两条经脉之间在体表的联系。

浮络是循行于人体浅表部位(皮肤表面)而常浮现的络脉。

孙络是最细小的络脉,《黄帝内经》称之有"溢奇邪""通荣卫"的作用。

2.2　在外连属经筋皮部

经筋和皮部,是十二经脉与筋肉和皮肤的连属部分。经络学说认为,经筋是十二经脉之气"结、聚、散、络"于筋肉、关节的体系,是十二经脉的连属部分,故称之为"十二经筋",具有联缀四肢百骸,主司关节运动的作用。全身的皮肤,是十二经脉的功能活动反映于体表的部位,也是经络之气散布之所在。"十二皮部"就是把全身皮肤划分为十二个部分,分属于十二经脉。

ed in the skin of whole body, pertaining to the twelve regular meridians respectively.

2.3 Internally pertaining and connecting to six zang organs and six fu organs

The meridians and collaterals connect all tissues and organs of whole body, distribute to everywhere on body surface and enter deep in the body, so as to connect all the zang-fu organs. The regular meridians, the divergent meridians, the extraordinary meridians and the collaterals are all related to the zang-fu organs. The twelve regular meridians play a major and direct role in such a connection.

The twelve regular meridians link with the zang-fu organs directly, called "pertaining". The three yin meridians of hand link with the chest, pertaining to the lung, pericardium and heart respectively, while the three yin meridians of food link with the abdomen, pertaining to the spleen, liver and kidney respectively. The three yang meridians of foot pertain to the stomach, gallbladder and bladder respectively, while the three yang meridians of hand pertain to the large intestine, triple energizer and small intestine respectively.

The twelve regular meridians link with exterior-interior related zang-fu organs, called "connecting". All the yang meridians pertain to the fu organs and connect with the zang organs, while the yin meridians pertain to the zang organs and connect with the fu organs. For example, the Lung Meridian of Hand-Taiyin pertains to the lung and connects with the large intestine, while the Large Intestine Meridian of Hand-Yangming pertains to the large intestine and connects with the lung. The rest meridians can be deduced accordingly.

2.3 在内络属六脏六腑

经络联系全身的组织、器官,布散于体表各处,同时深入体内,连属各个脏腑。正经、经别、奇经、络脉都与脏腑有一定的联系。其中,十二经脉则起着主要和直接的连属作用。

十二经脉各与其本身脏腑直接相连,称之为"属"。手三阴经联系于胸部,内属肺、心包、心;足三阴经联系于腹部,内属于脾、肝、肾。足三阳经内属于胃、胆、膀胱;手三阳经内属于大肠、三焦、小肠。

十二经脉各与其相为表里的脏腑相联系,称之为"络"。阳经皆属腑而络脏,阴经皆属脏而络腑。如:手太阴肺经,属肺络大肠;手阳明大肠经,属大肠络肺。余皆依此类推。

The yin meridians and yang meridians of the twelve regular meridians pertain to and connect with the relevant zang-fu organs respectively, forming up the exterior-interior relation by yin and yang, meridians and zang-fu organs, as Yangming and Taiyin are exterior-interior related, Shaoyang and Jueyin are exterior-interior related, and Taiyang and Shaoyin are exterior-interior related. Furthermore, a kind of broad and complicated connection between the meridians and zang-fu organs is formed up through the running courses and crossing ways of meridians and collaterals, the branches of the divergent meridians and collaterals, and the other zang-fu organs.

The system of meridians and collaterals is as figure 4-1.

十二经脉中的阴经和阳经分别络属于相应的脏腑，构成了阴阳经脉与脏腑表里相合的关系。即阳明与太阴、少阳与厥阴，太阳与少阴均相为表里。此外，还通过经络的循行、交叉和经别、络脉等的分支，或与其它脏腑贯通联接等，从而构成了经络与脏腑之间广泛复杂的联系。

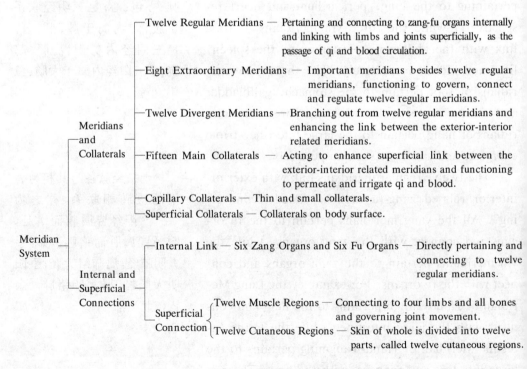

Figure 4-1   System of Meridians and Collaterals

经络系统简图如图4-1。

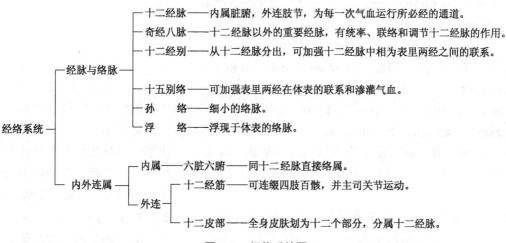

图4-1　经络系统图

Section 2　Twelve Regular Meridians

第 2 节 十二经脉

1　Nomenclature of twelve regular meridians

The concrete names of the twelve regular meridians are as follows.

The three yin meridians of hand: the Lung Meridian of Hand-Taiyin, the Pericardium Meridian of Hand-Jueyin and the Heart Meridian of Hand-Shaoyin.

The three yang meridians of hand: the Large Intestine Meridian of Hand-Yangming, the Triple Energizer Meridian of Hand-Shaoyang and the Small Intestine Meridian of Hand-Taiyang.

The three yin meridians of foot: the Spleen Meridian of Foot-Taiyin, the Liver Meridian of Foot-Jueyin and the Kidney Meridian of Foot-Shaoyin.

The three yang meridians of foot: the Stomach

1　具体名称

十二经脉的具体名称是：

手三阴经,包括手太阴肺经、手厥阴心包经、手少阴心经；

手三阳经,包括手阳明大肠经、手少阳三焦经、手太阳小肠经；

足三阴经,包括足太阴脾经、足厥阴肝经、足少阴肾经；

足三阳经,包括足阳明

Meridian of Foot-Yangming, the Gallbladder Meridian of Foot-Shaoyang and the Bladder Meridian of Foot-Taiyang.

The nomenclature of the twelve regular meridians is based upon: ① the running course of a meridian on the hand or foot, ② the yin-attribution or yang-attribution of a meridian, and ③ the zang or fu organ pertained by a meridian. For example, the Lung Meridian of Hand-Taiyin runs on the hand, attributes to Taiyin, and pertains to the lung.

2   Cyclical flow of qi in twelve regular meridians

One of the basic functions of the twelve regular meridians is to transport qi and blood. Qi and blood circulate in the twelve regular meridians in certain directions. For example, qi and blood circulate in the Lung Meridian of Hand-Taiyin, which starts from the lung, emerges to the body surface at the lateral aspect of the chest, and runs along the medial aspect and radial side of the upper limb, all the way downwards to the tip of the thumb. Qi and blood circulate inside one meridian to its end, and transfer and infuse into another meridian to circulate continuously. This kind of transferring and circulating phenomenon of qi and blood is called "the cyclical flow".

The cyclical flow of qi and blood in the twelve regular meridians has a certain order. After a circle of twelve regular meridians, qi and blood flow back to the original meridian. So that qi and blood go round and begin again, in a constant cycle.

The cyclical flow order of twelve regular meridians is as figure 4-2.

胃经、足少阳胆经、足太阳膀胱经。

十二经脉的名称含义有三：一是指出某一经脉在四肢循行的部位是手还是足。二是指出某一经脉的阴阳属性是阴经还是阳经。三是指出某一经脉所隶属的具体脏腑名称。如手太阴肺经循行于手，属太阴经，隶属于肺。

2   流注次序

十二经脉的基本功能之一是通行气血。气血在十二经脉中运行有一定的方向性，如手太阴肺经的气血是从肺发出，从胸部外侧出于体表，沿上肢内侧前缘向下运行至拇指端。气血沿某一经脉运行至其终端，就传注于另一经脉继续运行，这种气血在经脉之间相互传注的现象，称为"流注"。

十二经脉气血按一定次序流注，运行于十二经脉一周，又回到原来的经脉，这样周而复始，循环不息。

其流注次序如下图4-2。

Lung Meridian of Hand-Taiyin → Large Intestine Meridian of Hand-Yangming

Spleen Meridian of Foot-Taiyin ← Stomach Meridian of Foot-Yangming

Heart Meridian of Hand-Shaoyin → Small Intestine Meridian of Hand-Taiyang

Kidney Meridian of Foot-Shaoyin ← Bladder Meridian of Foot-Taiyang

Pericardium Meridian of Hand-Jueyin → Triple Energizer Meridian of Hand-Shaoyang

Liver Meridian of Foot-Jueyin ← Gallbladder Meridian of Foot-Shaoyang

Fig. 4-2   Cyclical Flow Order of Twelve Regular Meridians

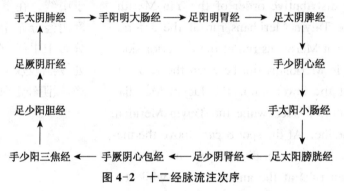

图 4-2   十二经脉流注次序

3   Distribution and Regulations of twelve regular meridians

The twelve regular meridians distribute on the body surface with certain regulations. According to the different distributive areas of the meridians, the regulations are as follows:

Head and face: The Hand-Yangming Meridian and Foot-Yangming Meridian run on the face and forehead, the Hand-Shaoyang Meridian and Foot-Shaoyang Meridian run on the temporal region of head on both sides, the Foot-Taiyang Meridian runs at the vertex of head and nape, while the Hand-Taiyang Meridian runs on the cheeks.

3   分布规律

十二经脉在体表的分布是有规律的。根据经脉所在部位的不同,其规律如下:

头面部:手阳明经、足阳明经行于面部、额部;手少阳经、足少阳经行于头部两侧;足太阳经行于头顶、后项;手太阳经行于面颊部。

Four limbs: The three Yin Meridians of Hand and three Yang Meridians of Hand run on the upper limb, while the three Yin Meridians of Food and three Yang Meridians of Foot run on the lower limb. The Yin Meridians run on the medial aspect of four limbs, while the Yang Meridians run on the lateral aspect of four limbs. The distributive order of the Yang Meridians is as: The Yangming Meridians run at the anterior side (radial side), the Taiyang Meridians run at the posterior side (the ulnar side), while the Shaoyang Meridians run between the two. The distributive order of the Yin Meridians is as: The Taiyin Meridians run at the anterior side, the Shaoyin Meridians run at the posterior side, while the Jueyin Meridians run between the two. At the lower part the lower limb, the Jueyin Meridian runs at the anterior side, while the Taiyin Meridian runs at the midline. At the spot 8 *cun* above the medial malleolus, the two meridians cross, and then the Taiyin Meridian runs at the anterior side, while the Jueyin Meridian runs at the midline.

Body trunk: The three Yang Meridians of Hand run at the scapular region, the Foot-Yangming Meridian runs at the anterior part (the chest and abdomen), the Foot-Taiyang Meridian runs at the posterior part (the back), and the Foot-Shaoyang Meridian runs at the lateral part. The three Yin Meridians of Hand emerge from the axilla, while the three Yin Meridians of Foot run at the chest and abdomen. On the chest and abdomen, the distributive order from the middle to the lateral is as the Foot-Shaoyin Meridian, the Foot-Yangming Meridian, the Foot-Taiyin Meridian and the Foot-Jueyin Meridian.

四肢部:手三阴经、手三阳经行于上肢,足三阴经、足三阳经行于下肢。其中阴经行于四肢内侧面,阳经行于四肢外侧面。阳经的排列顺序是,阳明经分布于前缘(拇指侧),太阳经分布于后缘(小指侧),少阳经分布于中线。阴经的排列顺序大致是,太阴经分布于前缘,少阴经分布于后缘,厥阴经分布于中线。在下肢的下半部,厥阴经分布于前缘,太阴经分布于中线,至内踝上八寸处,两经交叉,太阴经走向前缘,厥阴经走向中线。

躯干部:手三阳经行于肩胛部;足三阳经则阳明经分布于前(胸、腹面),太阳经分布于后(背面),少阳经分布于侧面;手三阴经均从腋下走出;足三阴经均行于胸、腹面。循行于胸、腹面的经脉自内向外的顺序为足少阴经、足阳明经、足太阴经、足厥阴经。

4 Exterior-interior relation of twelve regular meridians

The twelve regular meridians are divided into six couples, each couple of meridians are mutually exterior-interior related. In the coupled meridians, the Yin Meridian is termed as the interior, while the Yang Meridian is termed as the exterior. The coupled meridians connect at the terminals of four limbs. The pertaining zang-fu organs of the coupled meridians are also exterior-interior related. The coupled meridians and coupled zang-fu organs possess the mutual pertaining relation and mutual connecting relation. The Yin Meridian pertains to the zang organ and connects with the fu organ, while the Yang Meridian pertains to the fu organ and connects with the zang organ. The exterior-interior relation of the twelve regular meridians is as Table 4-1.

4 表里关系

十二经脉分为六对，每一对都是互为表里的。互为表里的经脉有阴阳之分，其阴经为里，阳经为表。表里两经在四肢末端相互交接。表里两经所隶属的脏腑也互为表里。表里两经与互为表里的脏腑形成相互属络关系，其阴经属脏而络腑，阳经属腑而络脏。

十二经脉的表里相合关系如表4-1。

Table 4-1   Exterior-Interior Relation of Twelve Regular Meridians

Interior	Exterior
Lung Meridian of Hand-Taiyin	Large Intestine Meridian of Hand-Yangming
Pericardium Meridian of Hand-Jueyin	Triple Energizer Meridian of Hand-Shaoyang
Heart Meridian of Hand-Shaoyin	Small Intestine Meridian of Hand-Taiyang
Spleen Meridian of Foot-Taiyin	Stomach Meridian of Foot-Yangming
Liver Meridian of Foot-Jueyin	Gallbladder Meridian of Foot-Shaoyang
Kidney Meridian of Foot-Shaoyin	Bladder Meridian of Foot-Taiyang

Note: For the concrete running courses of the twelve regular meridians, please refer to "*Chinese Acupuncture and Moxibustion*" of this Library.

表 4-1   十二经脉的表里相合关系

里	表
手太阴肺经	手阳明大肠经
手厥阴心包经	手少阳三焦经
手少阴心经	手太阳小肠经
足太阴脾经	足阳明胃经
足厥阴肝经	足少阳胆经
足少阴肾经	足太阳膀胱经

注：十二经脉的具体循行路线请参阅本文库《中国针灸》分册。

Section 3   Eight Extraordinary Meridians

第 3 节
奇经八脉

The eight extraordinary meridians, the Governor Vessel, the Conception Vessel, the Thoroughfare Vessel, the Belt Vessel, the Yin Heel Vessel, the Yang Heel Vessel, the Yin Link Vessel and the Yang Link Vessel, are the important component parts of the system of meridians and collaterals.

奇经八脉是督脉、任脉、冲脉、带脉、阴跷脉、阳跷脉、阴维脉、阳维脉的总称，是经络系统的重要组成部分。

Different from the twelve regular meridians which run all over the body, the eight extraordinary meridians do not distribute on the upper limb. Different from the twelve regular meridians which possess the yin-yang and exterior-interior relations of upward and downward distributions, internal and external connections and fair and counter flows of qi and blood, the eight extraordinary meridians, except the Belt Vessel which runs transversely surrounding the waist and abdomen, and Thoroughfare vessel which runs from the lower limb or lower abdomen upwards. The eight extraordinary meridians, except the Governor Vessel, do not pertain to or connect with the zang-fu organs directly, and do not possess the exterior-interior relation. Only some of the meridians link with the zang-fu organs, for example, the Governor Vessel enters the brain, connects with the kidney and infuses into the heart, the Thoroughfare Vessel, the Conception Vessel and the Governor Vessel link with the uterus. Due to the above-mentioned differences from the twelve regular meridians, they are called "the extraordinary meridians".

奇者，异也。奇经八脉不同于十二经脉遍布全身，如上肢无奇经分布；八脉之中，除带脉横绕腰腹，冲脉一分支下行之外，其余诸脉均从下肢或少腹部上行，不似十二经脉有上下、内外、顺逆的阴阳表里规律；奇经八脉（除督脉外）不与脏腑直接属络，无表里相配关系，只有部分经脉与脏腑连属，如督脉入属脑、络肾、贯心；冲、任、督三脉均与胞宫相联系。上述诸种有别于十二经脉，故称之为"奇经"。

The eight extraordinary meridians link with the twelve regular meridians in a crisscross network, and possess three functions as follows:

(1) Enhance the relations among the twelve regular meridians. In their running courses, the eight extraordinary meridians cross the other meridians, so as to enhance the mutual relations among all the meridians.

(2) Regulate qi and blood in the twelve regular meridians. The eight extraordinary meridians crisscross among the twelve regular meridians in the body. When qi and blood in the twelve regular meridians are sufficient and surplus, they infuse into the eight extraordinary meridians to be stored there for future possible use. When the body is in a motor state which needs qi and blood or when qi and blood in the twelve meridians are not sufficient, they flow out from the eight extraordinary meridians to irrigate and permeate in the tissues all over the body to support them.

(3) Be closely related to some organs. The eight extraordinary meridians are closely related to the zang organs of the liver and kidney and to the extraordinary fu organs of the uterus, brain and marrow. In terms of the uterus, brain and marrow, they are directly related to the extraordinary meridians. The Thoroughfare Vessel, the Conception Vessel and the Governor Vessel originate from the same source, while the Belt Vessel runs transversely surrounding the waist in a circle. All of them establish a complete system, which links with the Liver Meridians, so they are closely related to hernia, and menstruation, leucorrhea, pregnancy and delivery in female. Therefore, it can be seen

奇经八脉纵横交叉于十二经脉之间,主要具有三个方面的作用。

(1) 密切十二经脉的联系。奇经八脉在循行过程中,与其它各经交叉相接,加强了各条经脉之间的相互联系。

(2) 调节十二经脉的气血。奇经八脉错综分布、循行于十二经脉之间,当十二经脉气血旺盛有余时,则流注于奇经八脉,涵蓄备用;当人体活动需要或十二经脉气血不足时,可由奇经"溢出",渗灌于周身组织,予以补充。

(3) 与某些脏腑密切相关。奇经与肝、肾等脏及女子胞、脑、髓等奇恒之府的关系较为密切。如女子胞、脑髓主要与奇经直接联系;冲、任、督三脉一源而三岐,带脉环腰一周,共同构成一个完整的系统,且与肝经相通,故与疝气及女子的经、带、胎、产等密切相关。可见它们相互之间在生理和病理方面均有一定的影响。

that they are influenced each other physiologically and pathologically.

Note: For the concrete running courses of the eight extraordinary meridians, please refer to "*Chinese Acupuncture and Moxibustion*" of this Library.

注：奇经八脉的具体循行路线请参阅本文库《中国针灸》分册。

Section 4　Divergent Meridians, Muscle Regions, Cutaneous Regions and Main Collaterals

第4节 经别、经筋、皮部、别络

1　Twelve divergent meridians

The twelve divergent meridians are the braches of the regular meridians running in the deep part of the body cavity. They run deep and long, with the distributive features of "derive", "enter", "emerge" and "coincide". The twelve divergent meridians branch out from the regular meridians at the areas above the elbow and knee, pass the body trunk, and enter into the thoracic and abdominal cavities. The Yang Divergent Meridians, after entering into the thoracic and abdominal cavities, link with the zang-fu organs pertained and connected by their related regular meridians, and then emerge to the body surface from the vertex of head. The Yang Divergent Meridians coincide with their related regulated meridians, while the Yin Divergent Meridians coincide with the Yang Regular Meridians which are exterior-interior related to their related regular meridians.

The physiological functions of the twelve divergent meridians are as follows:

(1) Enhance the relationship between the exterior-interior related yin and yang meridians. The

1　十二经别

十二经别是正经别行深入体腔的支脉，其循行路线深而长，具有离、入、出、合的循行分布特点。它从肘膝以上的正经分出，经过躯干，深入胸腹腔。阳经经别在进入胸腹后均与其经脉所属络的脏腑联系，然后均在头项部出体表。阳经经别合于本经经脉，阴经经别合于相表里的阳经。

十二经别的生理作用主要有以下两点：

一是加强相为表里的阴阳两经的联系。十二经别进

twelve divergent meridians enter the body cavity, and the Yin and Yang Divergent Meridians run parallel to enhance the relationship between the exterior-interior related zang-fu organs. The Yin Divergent Meridians coincide with the Yang Regular Meridians which are exterior-interior related to their related regular meridians, so as to provide another reason why the exterior-interior relation among the twelve regular meridians are established.

(2) The twelve divergent meridians reach some organs and body constituents where the regular meridians do not reach, so they function to supplement the insufficient state of the regular meridians, so as to make the regular meridians closer to link the all parts of body and to enlarge the therapeutic scope of the meridian points. For example, the Bladder Meridian of Foot-Taiyang does not reach the anus, but the points as Chengshan（BL 57）of the meridian acts to treat hemorrhoids, it is because that the Divergent Meridian of Foot-Taiyang "runs deep to the buttock and enters the anus".

2 Twelve muscle regions

The twelve muscle regions are a system in which qi of the twelve regular meridians knots, converges, spreads and joins at the fascia, muscular tendons and muscles, distributing as three Yin Muscle Regions of Hand and Foot and three Yang Muscle Regions of Hand and Foot. The twelve muscle regions function to restrain the joints, govern the movement and protect the internals.

3 Twelve cutaneous regions

The twelve cutaneous regions are the division of skin on body surface according to the distribution of

入体腔后,阴阳两经并行,增强了表里相合脏腑间的联系。且阴经经别合于相表里的阳经,故十二经脉表里关系的确立也与经别的沟通有关。

二是由于其能通达某些正经未循行到的器官和形体部位,因而能补正经之不足,能使经脉对身体各部的联系更趋周密,从而扩大了经穴主治的范围。如足太阳膀胱经并不到肛门,但该经的承山等穴却可治疗痔疮,这正是足太阳经经别"深入尻下,别入于肛"的缘故。

2 十二经筋

十二经筋,是十二经脉之气结、聚、散、络于筋膜、肌腱和肌肉等的体系,按手足三阴三阳分布,称为十二经筋。十二经筋具有约束骨节、主持运动、保护内脏的作用。

3 十二皮部

十二皮部,是指体表的皮肤按十二正经分布部位的

the twelve regular meridians. They are closely related to the meridians, main collaterals and superficial collaterals, but different from them in some aspects. The meridians distribute in linear type, the collaterals distribute in reticular type, while the cutaneous regions distribute in zonal type. Therefore, their distributive scope is broader than that of the meridians and collaterals, but they are divided "according to the meridians".

4　Fifteen main collaterals

The fifteen main collaterals refer to those bigger collaterals, including the collaterals branching from the twelve regular meridians, the Governor Vessel and the Conception Vessel, and the great main collateral of the spleen.

Each of the main collaterals of the twelve regular meridians branches out from the Luo-Connecting Point of the meridian, and reaches its exterior-interior related meridian. The main collaterals locate more superficially, so they function to enhance the exterior-interior relation between the yin and yang meridians on the body surface.

The main collateral of the Governor Vessel branches from Changqiang (GV 1), the Luo-Connecting Point, spreads over the head, and joins leftwards and rightwards to the Foot-Taiyang Meridian. It functions to communicate the meridian qi at the back.

The main collateral of the Conception Vessel branches from Jiuwei (CV 15), the Luo-Connecting Point, and spreads over the abdomen. It functions to communicate the meridians qi at the abdomen.

The great main collateral of the spleen branches

分区。其不仅与经脉，而且与别络、浮络都有密切的关系，但各有侧重：经脉是呈线状分布；络脉是呈网状分布；而皮部则着重于"面"的划分。所以其分布范围比经络更为广泛一些，但总"以经脉为纪"。

4　十五别络

十五别络是主要的、较大的络脉，由十二经脉、督脉、任脉各分出一支络脉，再加上脾之大络组成。

十二经脉的别络，在四肢肘膝关节以下本经的络穴分出后，均走向其相表里的经脉。因别络分布较浅表，故十二别络可加强相为表里的阴阳两经在体表的联系。

督脉的别络，从长强穴分出后，散布于头部，左右别走足太阳经。它的作用主要是沟通背部经气。

任脉的别络，从鸠尾穴分出后，散布于腹部。其作用主要是沟通腹部经气。

脾之大络，从大包穴分

from Dabao（SP 21）, the great Luo-Connecting Point, and spreads over the chest and hypochondriac region. It functions to communicate the meridian qi at the lateral aspect of the body trunk.

Section 5   Basic Functions of Meridians and Collaterals

The meridians and collaterals possess two basic functions: first to communicate the exterior and the interior, the upper and the lower so as to connect zang-fu organs and tissues-organs, and second, to transport qi and blood and regulate yin and yang so as to nourish zang-fu organs, body and limbs.

1   Communicate the exterior and the interior, the upper and the lower so as to connect zang-fu organs and tissues-organs

The human body is an organic entirety, in which the zang-fu organs, body constituents, five sense organs and nine orifices are connected by the meridians and collaterals. The meridians and collaterals pertain to the zang-fu organs internally, connect with the limbs and joints externally, and act to link the surface with the internals and the upper with the lower, so as to connect everything broadly. The meridians and collaterals branch repeatedly, so they extend in all directions and reach everywhere. The connecting and communicating functions of the meridians and collaterals possess the following three ways.

(1) Enhance the relation of the zang-fu organs to the body constituents, sense organs and orifices.

出,散布于胸胁。它的作用主要是沟通躯干侧面的经气。

第 5 节
经络的基本功能

经络的基本功能有二,一是沟通表里上下,联络脏腑器官,二是通行气血阴阳,濡养脏腑形体。

1　沟通表里上下,联络脏腑器官

人体是一个有机的整体,而在脏腑、形体、五官九窍之间起联络作用的正是经络。经络内属于脏腑,外络于肢节,出入上下,联系极其广泛。由于经络可以反复分支,网络全身,所以经络四通八达,无所不至。经络的联络与沟通作用有以下三种基本方式。

一是加强脏腑与形体官窍之间的联系。经络联系脏

The meridians and collaterals act to connect the zang-fu organs with the body constituents, sense organs and orifices through the twelve regular meridians. The twelve regular meridians act to reach the exterior and the interior through their own meridians and branches on one hand, and act to enhance such a connecting relation through the twelve divergent meridians, the twelve muscle regions and the twelve cutaneous regions.

(2) Enhance the relation among the zang-fu organs. The twelve regular meridians possess the exterior-interior relation of six couples, so as to make the pertaining and connecting relations between the meridians and zang-fu organs. Furthermore, the meridian originates from the zang or fu organ also links with many other zang-fu organs in its process of the internal running course, and every zang or fu organ is linked by several meridians.

(3) Enhance the relation among the meridians and collaterals. The twelve regular meridians, due to their exterior-interior relation of yin and yang and the certain cyclic flow order, form up a major circulatory system. The twelve regular meridians and eight extraordinary meridians crisscross each other, while the eight extraordinary meridians are also related each other. The broad connection among the meridians and collaterals links the upper with the lower, the internals with the surface of the human body, form up an interwoven organic entirety.

2 Transport qi and blood and regulate yin and yang so as to nourish zang-fu organs, body and limbs

All the zang-fu organs and body constituents

腑与形体官窍,主要通过十二经脉来进行。十二经脉一方面通过其本经及其分支出入于表里,另一方面又通过十二经别、十二经筋、十二皮部来加强这种联系。

二是加强脏腑之间的联系。十二经脉构成六对表里相合关系,使相表里的脏腑之间具有相互属络关系。发源于脏腑的经脉在体内循行过程中还联系于多个其他脏腑,每一脏或腑都有数条经脉与之相联系。

三是加强经络之间的联系。十二经脉的阴阳表里相接,有一定的流注次序,并形成一个大的循环系统。十二经脉与奇经八脉之间纵横交错,奇经八脉之间又彼此相互联系。经络之间的广泛联系,使人体上下内外完全沟通起来,形成一个密不可分的有机整体。

2 通行气血阴阳,濡养脏腑形体

人体所有脏腑形体,都

need to be nourished by qi, blood, yin and yang, so as to maintain their normal physiological functions. Why qi, blood, yin and yang can reach everywhere of body, it relies on the transporting function of the meridians and collaterals. The meridians and collaterals are actually the passages of qi, blood, yin and yang, so the purpose of the meridians and collaterals to link the zang-fu organs with the body constituents is to transport qi and blood and regulate yin and yang. Through the broad distribution of the meridians and collaterals, qi, blood, yin and yang of human body may flow and infuse into the upper, the lower, the internals and the surface, so as to maintain the coordination and equilibrium of the whole body.

需要气血阴阳的濡养,才能维持正常的生理功能。气血阴阳之所以能通达全身,有赖于经络的传注输送。经络实质上是气血阴阳的通道,经络在脏腑与形体之间联络与沟通的目的就在于通行气血阴阳。通过经络的广泛分布,人体气血阴阳上下内外相互交通贯注,维持着整体的协调与平衡。

Section 6   Clinical Application of Theory of Meridians and Collaterals

第 6 节 经络学说的临床应用

1   Illustrate the mechanism of occurrence and progress of diseases

The theory of meridians and collaterals in traditional Chinese medicine is applied to illustrate the mechanism of occurrence and progress of diseases.

1   阐述疾病发生与传变的机理

无论是疾病的发生,还是病机的传变,中医学多用经络理论加以阐述。

1.1   Illustrate the mechanism of disease occurrence

The occurrence of the diseases due to external invasion is caused by the invasion of the exogenous pathogens. When the exogenous pathogens attack the human body, they first attack the skin, and then in succession the collaterals in which the Wei

1.1   阐述疾病的发生机理

外感病的发生,是由于邪气的侵袭。外邪最初侵入人体,是从肌表开始,首先侵入卫气空虚的络脉,然后逐步向里传变。内伤病的发生,或由于气血阴阳的不足,

(Defensive) Qi is deficient, and the internals. The occurrence of the diseases due to internal injury is caused by insufficiency of qi, blood, yin or yang, or by disharmony between qi and blood or between yin and yang. The insufficiency of qi, blood, yin or yang causes emptiness of meridians and collaterals, and the disharmony between qi and blood or between yin and yang leads to meridian qi stagnation or counter-flow, so as to result in the occurrence of diseases.

1.2 Illustrate the mechanism of disease progress

　　The meridians and collaterals are the ways to the progress of diseases. The exogenous pathogens attack the body from the exterior to the interior, from one meridian to another, then from meridians to the zang-fu organs. The diseases of zang-fu organs may transfer through the meridians. For example, the zang organ disease may transfer to the fu organ, and the fu organ disease may transfer to the zang organs, through the pertaining and connecting relations of the coupled meridians. Among the five zang organs, the diseases may transfer through various linking ways of the meridians and collaterals. For example, the liver disease may transfer to the lung or stomach, and the kidney disease may transfer to the heart or lung. The zang-fu organ diseases may transfer to the body surface through the meridians and collaterals, leading to the diseases of the body constituents, sense organs and orifices. For example, the disease of cardiac pain may lead to the painful sensation on the medial aspect of upper limb where the Heart Meridian of Hand-Shaoyin runs through. The disease of stomach fire may cause

或由于气血阴阳的失调。若气血阴阳不足,则经络空虚;若气血阴阳失调,则经气阻滞或逆乱,都能导致疾病发生。

1.2 阐述疾病的传变机理

　　疾病的传变常常以经络为途径。外邪由表入里,从络脉传入经脉,从经脉再传入脏腑。脏腑的病变,可以通过经络相互传变,如脏病可以传腑,腑病可以传脏,是通过表里经的相互属络关系进行传变。五脏之间也可以通过经络的多种相互联系而传变,如肝病传肺、胃,肾传心、肺等。内脏病变也可以通过经络传出体表,出现相关形体官窍的病变,如真心痛可在上肢内侧手少阴心经经过的部位有痛感,胃火病人可在阳明经所经过的牙龈出现肿痛,肝火上炎可见目赤等。

swelling and pain of the gum where the Stomach Meridian of Foot-Yangming goes through. The disease of liver fire flaring-up may result in redness of eyes.

2　Guide the diagnosis and treatment of diseases

The theory of meridians and collaterals in TCM is applied to guide the diagnosis and treatment of diseases.

2.1　Guide the diagnosis of diseases

The meridians and collaterals run through the areas of their given running courses and possess the pertaining zang-fu organs respectively, so that there are certain links between the various parts of body and the internal organs. According to the relation of the meridians and collaterals to the diseases or the diseased areas, it is possible to determine the pertaining meridians and zang-fu organs of the diseases, so as to make the diagnosis clinically. For example, the Liver Meridian distribute at the hypochondriac area, so hypochondriac pain is diagnosed as the liver disease. The Lung Meridian emerges from the sup-raclavicular fossa, so pain in the supraclavicular fossa is diagnosed as the lung disease. Headache may occur in different parts of the head. The frontal headache is related to the Yangming Meridians, the temporal headache is related to the Shaoyang Meridians, and the occipital headache is related to the Taiyang Meridians. Furthermore, some diseases may have the specific reaction spots on some specific meridian points on body surface. The tenderness of these reaction spots is the important basis in the diagnosis. For example, the tender-

2　指导疾病的诊断和治疗

无论是疾病的诊断,还是疾病的治疗,中医学每以经络学说为指导。

2.1　指导疾病的诊断

由于经络有一定的循行部位和所属脏腑,因此人体各部与内脏之间存在着特定的联系。临床上可以根据病变或证候所在的部位与经络的关系,判断疾病所属的经络与脏腑,从而作出诊断,如肝经布于胁,胁痛可以诊断为肝病;肺经出于缺盆,缺盆中痛可以诊断为肺病。又如头痛往往出现在不同部位,若前额痛则与阳明经有关,两侧头痛多与少阳经有关,后项头痛则与太阳经有关。此外,某些疾病在体表特定经穴有特殊反应点,该反应点出现压痛时往往是诊断的重要依据,如肠痈在足阳明经的阑尾穴有压痛,胆病在足少阳经的阳陵泉有压痛等。

ness may occur at the Lanweixue (EX-LE 7) on the Foot-Yangming Meridian in appendicitis, and the tenderness may occur at Yanglingquan (GB 34) on the Foot-Shaoyang Meridian in the gallbladder diseases.

2.2 Guide the treatment of diseases

The theory of meridians and collaterals is broadly applied in the treatment of diseases of various departments, possessing the important guiding significance in acupuncture-moxibustion, massage and herbal medicine. In the therapies of acupuncture-moxibustion and massage, it is advisable to select points near the disease or at distant area where the involved meridian runs through and to apply acupuncture-moxibustion or massage in the treatment of the disease of a certain meridian or a certain organ, for the purpose to regulat the functional activities of qi and blood of the meridians and collaterals. In the selection of point, it is necessary to make diagnosis first according to the theory of meridians and collaterals to determine which meridian is involved in the disease, and then it is possible to select the points according to running course, distributive area and related actions of the meridian. This is the so-called "selection of points along meridian".

The meridians and collaterals are also the ways to the therapy of herbal medicine. The efficacy of herbs can reach the diseased sites to realize the therapeutic function through the transportation of meridians and collaterals. According to the summary of the long-term clinical practice and experience, the theory of "meridian tropism of herbs" is established in TCM. It is believed in the theory of "meridian tropism of herbs" that the different herbal ef-

2.2 指导疾病的治疗

经络学说被广泛用于临床各科的治疗,特别是对针灸、按摩和药物治疗,具有重要指导意义。针灸疗法与按摩疗法,主要是对于某一经或某一脏腑的病变,在其病变的邻近部位或经络循行的远隔部位上取穴,通过针灸或按摩,以调整经络气血的功能活动,从而达到治疗的目的。而穴位的选取,首先必须按经络学说来进行辨证,断定疾病属于何经后,再根据经络的循行分布路线和联系范围来选定,这就是"循经取穴"。

药物治疗也是以经络为渠道,通过经络的传导转输,才能使药到病所,发挥其治疗作用。中医学通过长期的临床实践经验的总结,创立了"药物归经"的理论。"药物归经"理论认为,不同的药物将以不同的经络为通路,到达不同的脏腑器官。每一

ficacies may reach different zang-fu organs through the passages of the different meridians. Each herb may pertain to one meridian or to several meridians. In such a way, it is advisable on the basis of pattern identification to purposely choose the herbs which efficacies may reach the diseased area, so as to increase the therapeutic effect. For example, in the treatment of headache, it is advisable to choose *Notopterygii Rhizoma seu Radix* (Qiang Huo) for Taiyang Meridian type, *Angelicae Radix Dahuricae* (Bai zhi) for Yangming Meridian type, and *Bupleuri Radix* (Chai Hu) for Shaoyang Meridian type, because these herbs pertain to the related meridians respectively. Furthermore, a couple of herbs which pertain to the involved meridian may be added to the prescription in which most herbs do not pertain to the meridian, so as to guide the rest herbs to reach the diseased area. Those herbs which function to guide the other herbs are called "the meridian-guiding herbs".

种药物可以归入一经或数经。这样,临床治疗时就可以在辨证的基础上,有目的地选择能直达病所的药物,从而提高治疗效果,如治头痛,属太阳经的可用羌活,属阳明经的可用白芷,属少阳经的可用柴胡,这是因为这些药物能归入相应的经络。此外,处方时也可以在众多不具有直达病所作用的一般药物中加入一两味能归入某一经络的药物,以引导其他药物到达病所,这些起引导作用的药物被称为"引经药"。

Chapter 5　Etiology

The etiology, the pathogenic factors, refers to various causes of the occurrence of diseases in human body. The etiology is divided into four categories: ① the exogenous factors, including the six pathogenic pathogens and the Li (Epidemic) Qi; ② the endogenous factors, including the seven emotional factors, improper diet, overstrain and idleness; ③ the secondary pathogens, including the phlegm-rheum and stagnant blood; ④ the other pathogenic factors, including various traumatic injuries, physical-chemical factors, insect bites and animal damage. It is stressed on the six pathogenic pathogens, seven emotional factors, improper diet, overstrain and idleness, phlegm-rheum and stagnant blood in this book.

Section 1　Exogenous factors

1　Six Pathogenic pathogens

The six pathogenic pathogens refer to the wind, cold, summer heat, damp, dryness and heat (fire).

The wind, cold, summer heat, damp, dryness and heat (fire) are the six climatic changes found in the nature, called "the six types of qi". The human beings living in the natural environment are inevitable to be influenced by the various climatic changes in the nature. Under the normal conditions, the

第 5 章
病因

病因,即致病因素,指各种能使人发生疾病的原因。病因大体可分为四类:一是外感病因,包括六淫、疫疠等。二是内伤病因,包括七情、饮食失宜、劳逸过度等。三是继发病因,包括痰饮、瘀血等。四是其他病因,包括各种外伤、理化因素致伤、虫兽所伤等。本书重点介绍外感六淫、内伤七情、饮食失宜、劳逸过度、痰饮、瘀血等内容。

第 1 节　外感病因

1　六淫

六淫,即风、寒、暑、湿、燥、热(火)六种外感病邪的总称。

风、寒、暑、湿、燥、热(火),本是六种正常的自然气候因素,合称为"六气"。人生存在自然环境中,不可避免自然界各种气候变化的影响。正常情况下,人体对

human body is capable to adapt itself to the various climatic changes in the nature, while the orderly climatic changes in the nature are the necessary conditions of the human existence. If the coordinative relation between the human being and natural environment is broken, the human body cannot adopt itself to the climatic changes in the nature, so that the diseases occur. In such a situation, the six types of qi become the six pathogenic pathogens.

The diseases caused by the six pathogenic pathogens possess the pathogenic characteristics as follows:

Firstly, the invasion of the six exogenous pathogens are related to the seasonal climates and living environment. Since the occurrence of wind, cold, summer heat, damp, dryness or heat (fire) is related to the seasonal changes of the weather, i.e. the wind pattern mostly occurs in spring, the heat pattern or summer heat pattern mostly occurs in summer, the damp pattern mostly occurs in late summer, the dryness pattern mostly occurs in autumn, and the cold pattern mostly occurs in winter. The living environment is taken as the minor environment with the relevant minor climates. For example, if one lives in the humid place for long time, he is mostly attacked by the pathogenic damp. If one works in the high temperature environment, he is mostly attacked by the pathogenic dryness and heat.

Secondly, each of the exogenous pathogens may affect the body singly or in combination with others. For example, the pathogenic wind may affect the body in combination with the cold, damp, dryness, heat, etc. to cause the wind-cold pattern,

各种自然气候的变化具有充分的适应能力,自然气候有序的变化也是人类生存不可缺少的条件。如果人与自然环境相适应的协调关系被打破,不能适应自然气候的变化,就会导致疾病。此时,六气便成为致病因素六淫。

六淫致病,一般具有以下几个特点。

一是多与季节气候、居住环境有关。因为风、寒、暑、湿、燥、热(火)的出现与季节有某种特殊联系,所以春季易感受风邪,夏季易感受暑、热(火),长夏易感受湿邪,秋季易感受燥邪,冬季易感受寒邪。居住环境可视为小环境,也有相应的小气候。如久居湿地容易感受湿邪,在高温环境下工作容易感受燥热邪气等。

二是既可单独侵袭人体,也可相互兼挟侵入人体。如风邪可兼寒、湿、燥、热等邪,而形成风寒、风湿、风燥、风热等证。

wind-damp pattern, wind-dryness pattern, wind-heat pattern, etc.

　　Thirdly, the property of the disease caused by the six exogenous pathogens may change due to the individual constitutional factors. For example, the pathogenic cold affects the body, entering into the interior to transform into heat, or the pathogenic damp which accumulates in the body for long time may transform into heat. Due to different body constitutions, the diseases of different properties may occur when various exogenous pathogens affect the body. This phenomenon is called "the favorable transformation" in TCM. For example, when the person with the body constitution of yang excess or yin deficiency is affected by the exogenous pathogens, it is possible to transform the disease into the heat pattern. When the person with the body constitution of yin excess or yang deficiency is affected by the exogenous pathogens, it is possible to transform the disease into the cold pattern. When the person with the body constitution of damp excess or spleen deficiency is affected by the exogenous pathogens, it is possible to transform the disease into the damp pattern.

　　Fourthly, the exogenous pathogens may enter from the exterior (the body surface) to the interior to cause the disease, or may enter from the upper (the mouth and nose) to the lower to cause the disease. Therefore, the disease caused by the six exogenous pathogens is the exterior pattern in the early phase, and gradually transforms into the interior pattern during the progress when they transfer to the interior.

　　In addition to the diseases caused by six

　　三是六淫所致疾病的性质可因个体体质因素的差异而发生变化。如感受寒邪，可以入里化热，湿邪蕴积日久也可以化热。感受各种邪气，还可以因其体质不同而表现为不同性质的疾病，中医学把这种现象叫做"从化"。如素体阳盛或阴虚者，感受外邪后易从热化；素体阴盛或阳虚者，感受外邪后易从寒化；素体湿盛或脾虚者，感受外邪后易从湿化等。

　　四是既可从外（如肌表）感受，由表入里而发病，也可自上（如口鼻）而下，由上焦下传而发病。因此，外感六淫早期多先出现表证，然后逐步向里传变。

　　此外，临床上还有某些

exogenous pathogens occurring in the nature, there are many diseases caused by the functional disturbances of the zang-fu organs which nevertheless share the similar clinical manifestations. They are so called "the five endogenous pathogens" in TCM, i. e. the endogenous wind, the endogenous cold, the endogenous damp, the endogenous dryness and the endogenous heat (fire). The five endogenous pathogens are not caused by the six exogenous pathogens, but they are often induced by the six exogenous pathogens. For example, the exogenous pathogenic wind may induce the endogenous wind, while the exogenous pathogenic damp may induce the endogenous damp.

1. 1 Pathogenic wind

The wind is the predominant qi of spring, so the diseases caused by the pathogenic wind often occur in spring. The pathogenic wind is the mostly commonly-seen pathogen among the six exogenous pathogens. The exogenous pathogen, characterized by moving, opening, ascending, dispersing, outward and upward movement, most easily affecting human body, is the pathogenic wind. The properties and pathogenic characteristics of the pathogenic wind are as follows.

1. 1. 1 The wind is a yang pathogen, characterized by opening and dispersing and easily attacking the yang part of the body

The wind is characterized by moving without residence, ascending, dispersing, outward and upward movement, so it is termed as the yang pathogen. Opening and dispersing property implies that the pathogenic wind makes the sweating pores open, leading to the symptoms of sweating and a-

并非感受六淫外邪,而是由脏腑功能失调所致的类似于风、寒、湿、燥、热(火)的病理变化,中医学称为"内生五邪",如内风、内寒、内湿、内燥、内热(火)之类。内生五邪虽然不是由外感六淫所致,但常可因外感六淫邪气而引发,如外感风邪可引动内风,外感湿邪可引动内湿等。

1. 1 风邪

风为春季主气,故风邪为病以春令居多。风邪是外感六淫中最常见的病邪。凡自然界中具有善动不居、开泄升发、向上向外等特性,最易使人体患病的外邪,称为风邪。风邪的性质及致病特点如下。

1. 1. 1 风为阳邪,其性开泄,易袭阳位

风性善动而不居,具有升发、向上、向外的特性,故为阳邪。其性开泄,是指风邪易使腠理疏泄而开张,出现汗出恶风之症。易袭阳位,是指风邪易袭人体的上

version to cold. Attacking the yang part of the body implies that the pathogenic wind often attacks the upper part of human body, as the head, the face and the clear aperture in the upper, and attacks the lung system locating in the highest position, leading to the symptoms of the respiratory tract, and attacks the body surface, causing the exterior pattern.

1.1.2 The wind is characterized by constant movement and rapid changes

The constant movement implies that the wind in the nature blows in gusts, therefore being marked by the diseases with the migratory and infixed features. For example, in the Bi (Obstructive) Pattern (a kind of diseases with the major symptoms of joint or muscle pain, swelling or weightiness) caused by the intermingling pathogenic wind, cold and damp. The migratory Bi (Obstructive) Pattern with the symptoms of wandering joint pain and rapid changes is caused by the pathogenic wind as the prior pathogen. It implies that first, "the wind does not follow the routine", as the primary pathogen to cause many diseases, and second, the diseases caused by the pathogenic wind are often marked by migratory symptoms, rapid changes and abrupt onset. For example, urticaria caused by the pathogenic wind is characterized by itching of the skin and wheals, small as sesames or big as broad beans, in flakes, appearing and disappearing from place to place.

1.1.3 The wind is the major pathogen of many diseases

It implies that the pathogenic wind is the easiest to attack the human body among the six exogenous pathogens, being the leading pathogen of the exogenous pathogens to guide the other pathogens to at-

部,如风邪容易侵犯上部头面清窍;容易侵犯居位最高肺系而出现呼吸道症状;容易侵犯肌表而多出现表证。

1.1.2 风性善行而数变

善行,是指风本为气之激烈流动,故其致病多见病位游移、行无定处的特性。例如风寒湿三气杂至而为痹证(以关节或肌肉疼痛、肿大或重着为主症的一类疾患),其风邪为主者为"行痹",症见游走性关节疼痛。数变,一是指"风无常方",为病众多;二是指风邪为病,多变幻迅速无常。如荨麻疹发无定处,搔痒不已,小如麻粒丘疹,大如豆瓣,甚则成片,此起彼伏,发作无常。

1.1.3 风为百病之长

是指风邪为六淫之中最常见最易中人之邪,且常为外邪致病的先导,其他病邪每依附于风而侵袭人体。如

tack the human body. For example, the pathogenic wind brings the pathogenic damp to cause the wind-damp disease, brings the pathogenic cold to cause the wind-cold disease, and brings the pathogenic heat to cause the wind-heat disease. Therefore, it is said that the pathogenic wind is the representative of all the exogenous pathogens by the ancient physicians.

1.1.4 The wind is characterized by constant movement

The movement here implies the features of the wind to make the objects of human body move, shake and unstable. When the pathogenic wind attacks the human body, the symptoms of dizziness, blurring of vision, up-turn of eyes, trismus, rigidity of nape, convulsion of four limbs and opisthotonos may occur. According to the clinical practice, the above-mentioned symptoms mostly pertain to the category of "the endogenous wind". Some conditions, as tetanus with the symptoms of rigidity of nape, up-turn of eyes and convulsion of four limbs, belong to the category of "the exogenous wind".

1.2 Pathogenic cold

The cold is the predominant qi in winter, so the diseases caused by the pathogenic cold often occur in winter. But in the other seasons, the pathogenic cold may also attack the body to cause diseases due to being caught in rain, wading in water, exposure to cold after sweating, over-seeking for cold or abrupt decrease of temperature. The so-called pathogenic cold refers to the exogenous pathogen, characterized by cold property, stagnation and contraction, and attacking the human body to cause diseases.

风邪可兼挟湿邪而为风湿，兼挟寒邪而为风寒，兼挟热邪而为风热。古代医家甚至把风邪作为外感病邪的代称或总称。

1.1.4 风胜则动

动，是指风有使物体及人体动摇不定的特点。感受风邪，人体可出现头晕、目眩、上视、口噤、项强、四肢抽搐、角弓反张等症状。就临床实际看，上述诸症多以"内风"为多见。但也有属于外风的，如破伤风之见项强上视、四肢抽搐等症。

1.2 寒邪

寒为冬季主气，故寒邪为病冬令居多。其他季节也可因淋雨涉水、汗出当风、贪凉太过或气温骤降等而感受寒邪。所谓寒邪，是指自然界中具有阴凉、凝滞、收引特性，而导致人体患病的外邪。

1.2.1 The cold is a yin pathogen, often consu-ming the yang qi

The cold pertains to yin. If the yin cold is excessive, the yang qi inside the human body is not strong enough to expel the yin-cold pathogen, but damaged by the yin cold. Therefore, it is said that "yin preponderance leads to sickness of yang". If the pathogenic cold attacks the body, yang is consumed, leading to yin-cold excess pattern. If the pathogenic cold attacks the body surface, the Wei (Defensive) Yang Qi is obstructed, causing the symptom of aversion to cold. If the pathogenic cold directly attacks the spleen and stomach, the spleen yang is damaged, leading to the symptoms of cold pain at epigastria and abdomen, vomiting and diarrhea. If the pathogenic cold directly attacks the Shaoyin Meridians, yang of the heart and kidney is declined, causing the symptoms and signs of fear of cold, sleepiness, severe chills in hands and feet, diarrhea with indigested food in feces, clear and excessive urine, feeble and thready pulse, etc.

1.2.2 The cold is characterized by stagnation, causing pain

Stagnation implies the blockage of meridians. When the pathogenic cold attacks the human body, the yin cold is excessive and the yang qi is consumed, so that the meridians are blocked. Blockage causes pain. Therefore, if the pathogenic cold attacks the body to cause qi and blood stagnation, the various pains may occur. It is so called that "the excessive cold causes pain". For example, in the Bi (Obstructive) Pattern caused by the intermingling pathogenic wind, cold and damp, the painful Bi (Obstructive) Pattern with the symptom of cold

1.2.1 寒为阴邪,易伤阳气

寒性属阴,阴寒过盛,人体阳气不仅不足以驱除阴寒之邪,反而为阴寒所伤,即所谓"阴胜则阳病"。因此,感受寒邪,最易伤阳,而出现阴寒偏盛之证。若寒邪袭表,卫阳被遏,便见恶寒;寒邪直中脾胃,脾阳受损,则见脘腹冷痛、呕吐腹泻等症;寒邪直中少阴,心肾阳衰,则见畏寒倦卧、手足厥冷、下利清谷、小便清长、脉象微细等症。

1.2.2 寒性凝滞,其胜则痛

凝滞,即凝结、阻滞不通之意。寒邪入侵,阴寒偏盛,阳气受损,人体经脉易致凝涩不畅。不通则痛,故寒邪入侵,导致气血凝滞,最易出现各种痛证,即所谓"寒胜则痛"。如风寒湿三气杂至而为痹证,其寒邪为主者为"痛痹",临床以关节寒性疼痛为主。这种疼痛的特点是局部有寒冷感,遇寒加重,得热则

joint pain is caused by the pathogenic cold as the prior pathogen. This type pain is characterized by local cold pain which is worsened by cold and relieved by heat.

1.2.3　The cold is characterized by contraction

Contraction refers to contraction and dragging. When the pathogenic cold attacks the human body, it may cause the contraction or spasm of the skin, muscles, meridians and collaterals, blood vessels, limbs, joints, etc. If the skin and muscles are contracted, the symptoms of aversion to cold, fever and absence of sweating occur. If the meridians and blood vessels are contracted, the symptoms and signs of headache, aching of whole body, spasm, pale-white or purple-black skin, severe chills in four limbs and taut pulse occur. If the limbs and joints are contracted, the symptoms of curling-up body, spasm and pain of limbs and joints. The pathogenic cold may also restrain the qi activities of human body, to affect the internal organs. For example, if the pathogenic cold attacks the intestines and stomach, the symptom of spasmodic pain at abdomen may occur.

1.3　Pathogenic summer heat

The summer heat is the predominant qi of summer. Unlike other exogenous pathogens, the diseases caused by the summer heat are only seen in its own season, the summer. The summer heat is a pure exogenous pathogen, not endogenous. The so-called pathogenic summer heat is a kind of exogenous pathogen in summer characterized by scorching, burning, ascending and dispersing to cause sweating, damaging body fluid and consuming qi, and attacking the human body to cause diseases. The

减。

1.2.3　寒主收引,寒则气收

收引,即收缩牵引之意。寒邪入侵人体,可使皮毛肌腠、经络血脉、肢体关节等收缩挛急。皮毛肌腠收引,则见恶寒发热、无汗;经络血脉收引,则见头身疼痛、经脉拘急、皮肤苍白或青黑、四肢厥冷、脉紧;肢体关节牵引,则见形体蜷缩、肢节拘挛疼痛。因寒主收引可使人体气机收敛,故亦可影响内脏,如见肠胃受寒而出现痉挛性疼痛。

1.3　暑邪

暑为夏季主气,是夏季火热之气所化。暑邪伤人发病有明显的季节性,即独见于夏令。暑病只有外感,并无内生。所谓暑邪,是指暑季具有炎热燔灼、升散汗出、伤津耗气等特性,而导致人体患病的外邪。

暑邪的性质和致病特点如下。

properties and pathogenic characteristics of the pathogenic summer heat are as follows.

1.3.1 The summer heat is a yang pathogen, characterized by scorching and burning

The pathogenic summer heat is transformed from qi of heat and fire in midsummer, so it pertains to yang. When the pathogenic summer heat attacks the human body, there can be a series of symptoms and signs of excessive yang heat, such as high fever, red facial complexion, restlessness, surging pulse, etc. The summer heat is like the fire, with scorching and burning features, so the burning sensation is another symptom of the disease caused by the pathogenic summer heat.

1.3.2 The summer heat is characterized by ascending and dispersing

damaging body fluid and consuming qi. When the pathogenic summer heat attacks the human body, it make the sweating pores open, leading to profuse sweating. Qi is lost along with sweating, so both qi and body fluid are deficient, causing the symptoms of shortness of breath, lassitude, fatigue, dry lips and tongue, etc.

1.3.3 The summer heat disturbs the heart spirit and induces the liver wind

Both the summer heat and heart pertain to the fire in the five elements. It is believed that the pathogenic summer heat communicates with the heart fire by the ancients. So that the pathogenic summer heat disturbs the heart spirit, leading to restlessness, emotional turmoil, even sudden coma, loss of consciousness (in heat stroke), etc. Besides, the pathogenic summer heat induces the liver wind, leading to convulsion of four limbs, rigidity of neck

1.3.1 暑为阳邪,炎热燔灼

暑邪为盛夏火热之气所化,故暑性属阳。暑邪伤人多出现阳热亢盛的一系列临床症状,多见壮热、面赤、烦躁、脉洪大等症。暑性似火,腾炎燔灼,故感人发病,似有烧灼之感。

1.3.2 暑性升散,伤津耗气

暑性升散,暑邪侵入人体,使腠理开泄而多汗;汗多气随津泄,故多致气津两伤,气随汗泄,则致气虚,见气短、乏力、体倦、唇干舌燥等症。

1.3.3 暑扰心神,暑引肝风

暑在五行属火,心在五行亦属火,故古人认为暑邪内通心火,暑热之邪,易扰动心神,出现心中烦躁,闷乱不宁,甚则突然昏倒,不省人事(中暑)。暑热之邪,又易引动肝风,而见四肢抽搐,颈项强直,甚则角弓反张,古医籍称之为"暑风""暑痫"。

and nape, even opisthotonos. It is the so-called "wind due to summer heat" or "epilepsy due to summer heat" in the ancient classics.

1.3.4 The summer heat brings the damp to attack the body

In summer, it is not only hot and warm, but also humid due to frequent rain as well. The sunlight in the upper send out the powerful heat downwards, and the humid air from the earth steams upwards. The humid and hot air spreads all over the place where the human body stays, so the body is attacked by the heat and damp through respiration and skin contact. So the concurrent disease of both summer heat and damp occurs. Besides, when a person with the body constitution of excessive damp is attacked by the pathogenic summer heat, the concurrent disease of both summer heat and damp occurs. The major symptoms and signs are of the summer heat, as fever, thirst, etc. and also of the damp, as tiredness of four limbs, stuffy chest, nausea, loose feces, scanty and dark-colored urine, thick-sticky tongue coating, etc.

1.4 Pathogenic damp

The damp is the predominant qi of late summer, so the diseases caused by the pathogenic damp often occur in late summer. The so-called late summer refers to the period of time between the summer and autumn. The sunlight in the upper send out the powerful heat downwards, and the humid air from the earth steams upwards, so the body is the easiest to be attacked by the pathogenic damp. In the other seasons, the pathogenic damp may also attack the body to cause diseases due to being caught in rain, wading in water, working in water, living

1.3.4 暑多挟湿

夏季不仅气候炎热,且常多雨潮湿,所谓天暑下迫,地湿上蒸,湿热弥漫空间,人身之所及,呼吸之所受,均不离湿热之气。暑令湿盛必多兼感。又内湿素盛之人,容易感受暑邪,而成暑湿相合证。其临床特征,除发热、烦渴等暑热症状外,常兼见四肢困倦、胸闷泛恶、大便溏泄、小便短赤、舌苔厚腻等湿阻症状。

1.4 湿邪

湿为长夏主气,湿邪为病,长夏居多。所谓长夏,多指夏秋之交。所谓天之暑热下迫,地之湿气上蒸,人在其中,最易感受湿邪。其他季节,若涉水淋雨,水中作业,久居湿地,汗出衣里,亦易受湿浸渍,湿邪为病。所谓湿邪,即指自然界中具有重浊、粘滞、趋下等特性,而使人患病的外邪。

in humid place for long time, wearing wet shirt after sweating, etc. The so-called pathogenic damp
refers to the exogenous pathogen, characterized by
heaviness and turbidity, viscosity and stagnation,
and downward movement, and attacking the human
body to cause diseases.

1.4.1 The damp is a yin pathogen, easily blocking the qi activities and damaging the yang qi

The damp is characterized by heaviness and turbidity, similar to water, so it is termed as the yin
pathogen and a tangible pathogen as well. As a yin
pathogen, the pathogenic damp easily damages the
yang qi, especially damages the spleen yang (because both the spleen and damp pertain to the
earth), to make the spleen fail to transport and
transform food, leading to the symptoms of diarrhe-
a, edema, etc. As a tangible pathogenic factor, the
pathogenic damp easily blocks the qi activities to
make the unsmooth flow of qi in the zang-fu organs
and meridians, leading to the symptoms of stuffy
chest, epigastric distension, abdominal distension
and pain, scanty urine and difficult urination, unsmooth defecation, or tenesmus, etc.

1.4.2 The damp is characterized by heaviness and turbidity

It implies that when the pathogenic damp attacks the body, the symptoms of heavy sensation in
head, tiredness and heavy sensation in body, heavy
sensation in four limbs, etc occur. For example, in
the Bi (Obstructive) Pattern caused by the intermingling pathogenic wind, cold and damp, the fixed Bi
(Obstructive) Pattern with the symptoms of numbness of skin and muscle, pain and heavy sensation in

1.4.1 湿为阴邪,易阻气机,易伤阳气

湿性重浊,其性类水,故
为阴邪,又为有形之邪。因
其为阴邪,故易伤阳气,尤易
损伤脾阳(因脾为湿土之
脏),使脾失健运,而出现腹
泻、水肿等症。因其为有形
之邪,故易阻滞气机,使脏腑
经络气机壅滞不畅,而见胸
闷脘痞、腹胀腹痛、小便短
涩、大便不爽或里急后重等。

1.4.2 湿性重浊

重,即沉重、重着。是指
感受湿邪,常见头重如裹、周
身困重、四肢沉重等症。如
风寒湿三气杂至而为痹证,
其湿邪为主者称"着痹",临
床见肌肤不仁,关节疼痛沉
重。"浊"即秽浊、污浊。是
指分泌物及排泄物污秽混浊

joints is caused by the pathogenic cold as the prior pathogen. Turbidity refers to the turbid secretes and discharges.

1.4.3 The damp is characterized by viscosity and stagnation

The viscosity and stagnation of the pathogenic damp include two aspects. Firstly, it refers to the viscose and sticky secretes and discharges in the diseases caused by the pathogenic damp, as viscose and sticky feces which is difficult to discharge, difficult urination, thick and sticky leucorrhea, thick and sticky exudates in eczema, etc. Secondly, the diseases caused by the pathogenic damp tend to be prolonged and intractable, such as fixed Bi (Obstructive) Pattern, eczema and some damp-heat patterns.

1.4.4 The damp is characterized by downward movement

The damp, similar to water, tends to move downwards, leading to the diseases with the symptoms in the lower part, as edema in lower limbs, turbid urine, excessive and heavy leucorrhea, diarrhea, etc.

1.5 Pathogenic dryness

The dryness is the predominant qi of autumn, so the diseases caused by the pathogenic dryness often occur in autumn. The diseases caused by the pathogenic dryness are divided into the warm-dryness diseases and cool-dryness diseases. The former is caused by the pathogenic dryness and heat, while the latter is caused by the pathogenic dryness and cold. The pathogenic dryness refers to the exogenous pathogen characterized by dryness, unsmooth, damaging body fluid, loss of moisture, easily attac-

而言。

1.4.3 湿性黏滞

湿邪的黏腻停滞主要表现在两个方面,一是指湿病症状多有黏滞不爽的特点,如分泌物及排泄物黏腻滞涩,便溏粘滞不畅,小便滞涩难解,妇女带下粘滞,湿疹渗出黏滞等;二是指湿邪为病多缠绵难愈,病程较长或反复发作,如湿痹、湿疹及某些湿热病证即是如此。

1.4.4 湿性趋下

湿性类水,有就下之性,故为病多见下部症状,如下肢水肿、小便淋浊、赤白带下、大便泄痢等。

1.5 燥邪

燥为秋令主气,燥邪为病最常见于秋季。燥邪为病有温燥与凉燥之分。燥邪兼受寒气为病,发为凉燥;燥邪兼受热邪为病,发为温燥。所谓燥邪,是指自然界中具有干燥、干涩、伤津、失润、最易伤肺等特性,而导致人体患病的外邪。

king the lung, etc.

1.5.1 The dryness is characterized by dryness and unsmooth, easily damaging the body fluid

In the diseases caused by the pathogenic dryness, there are the symptoms of dryness, unsmooth and consumption of body fluid, as dry mouth and throat, thirst, dry skin, even chapped skin, lusterless hair, scanty urine, dry feces or constipation, etc.

1.5.2 The dryness easily damages the lung

Firstly, the lung is regarded as "the delicate organ", preferring moisture and disliking dryness. Secondly, the lung dominates the respiration, opens into the nose and is related to the skin and hair. When the pathogenic dryness attacks the body through the mouth, nose and skin, it damages and consumes the body fluid of the lung, which is disturbed and fail to disperse and descend, leading to the symptoms of dry cough without sputum, or dry cough with scanty and thick sputum which is difficult to spit out, dry mouth, nose and skin, even bloody sputum, chest pain, panting, etc.

1.6 Pathogenic heat (fire)

Both the pathogenic fire and pathogenic heat pertain to the yang pathogens. They are related but different. Firstly, they are different in degrees. The heat is the mild fire, while the fire is the extreme heat. Secondly, they are different in forms. The heat is intangible, while the fire is tangible. Thirdly, they are different in clinical manifestations. The diseases caused by the exogenous pathogenic heat are manifested by the heat and hyperactivity of the whole body, as fever, thirst, profuse

1.5.1 燥性干涩,易伤津液

"燥胜则干"。燥邪为病,易出现伤津干涩症状。如口咽干燥,口渴,皮肤干燥,甚则皮肤皲裂,毛发不荣,小便短少,大便干结等。

1.5.2 燥易伤肺

燥易伤肺:一是因肺为"娇脏",喜润而恶燥;二是因为肺司呼吸,开窍于鼻,外合皮毛,而燥邪本是指气候干燥,燥邪自口鼻、皮毛而入,劫伤肺的津液,影响肺的宣发和肃降,出现干咳少痰,或痰少而稠,难于咯出,口鼻、肌肤干燥,甚则痰中带血、胸痛喘逆等症。

1.6 热(火)邪

火邪与热邪,都属阳邪,故火热常并称,但又有差别:一是病邪程度有差别,热为火之渐,火为热之极。二是以形象言,热无形可见,而火有形可寻。三是临床表现不同,外感热邪多表现为全身性的阳热亢盛症状,如发热、口渴、大汗、脉洪大等,而火多表现为某一脏腑的功能亢

sweating, surging and big pulse, etc., while the diseases caused by the exogenous pathogenic fire are manifested by the hyperactivity of a certain zang or fu organ, as the heart fire, the liver fire, the stomach fire, etc. Fourthly, they are different in sources. The pathogenic fire is often endogenous, as the result of excess of yang qi inside the body, while the pathogenic heat is often exogenous.

进,如心火、肝火、胃火等。四是来源不同,火常由内生,是体内阳气过盛的表现,而热邪多属外感病邪。

1.6.1 The fire-heat, pertaining to yang, is characterized by scorching and flaming upwards

Yang dominates constant movement, while the fire-heat are scorching and burning, flaming upwards and rising, so it is called "flaming upwards" and pertains to yang. The fire is the extreme heat, so the excessive heat may transform into fire which is flaming upwards, with the symptoms of the yang heat hyperactivity pattern, as fever, aversion to heat, irritability, thirst, sweating, etc. If the excessive heat transforms into fire which is flaming upwards, there be the symptoms and signs of red complexion, red eyes, red tongue body, or ulcers in mouth and tongue, or swollen and painful gum, etc. If the fire-heat flames upwards to disturb the heart spirit, there can be the symptoms of irritability, insomnia, mania, or loss of consciousness, delirium, etc.

1.6.1 火热属阳,其性炎上

阳主躁动,火热燔灼,焚焰升腾,故称"炎上",并显属阳邪。火为热之极,故热盛易化火上炎。临床表现为发热、恶热、心烦、口渴、汗出等阳热亢盛的症状。若热盛化火,火性炎上,又可见面红目赤、舌质红,或口舌生疮,或牙龈肿痛等。若火热上扰心神,还可见心烦、失眠、狂躁妄动,或见神昏谵语等。

1.6.2 The fire-heat consumes qi and damages the body fluid

The excessive yang heat burns and consumes the body fluid, and forces the body fluid to spill out. In the diseases caused by the pathogenic heat, there are the symptoms and signs of body fluid consumption, as thirst with preference for drinking cold wa-

1.6.2 耗气伤津

阳热亢盛,消灼津液,且每迫津外泄,故热邪致病,津液耗伤之象多较明显,如见口渴喜冷饮、咽干舌燥唇裂、小便短赤、大便秘结等症。

ter, dry throat and tongue, cracked lips, scanty and dark-colored urine, constipation, etc. The pathogenic yang heat also consumes qi, so it is said that "the strong fire consumes qi". The excessive yang heat easily consumes the Zheng (Anti-Pathogenic) Qi and forces to sweat, causing loss of qi during sweating (because the body fluid functions to carry qi). As a result, the symptoms of qi and yin deficiency can be seen in the diseases caused by the pathogenic heat (fire), as fever, sweating, etc. of heat (fire), low spirit, lassitude, shortness of breath, etc. of qi deficiency.

1.6.3　The fire-heat stirs up the wind and disturbs the blood circulation

The excessive heat stirring up wind is also called that "the extreme heat producing wind". When the pathogenic heat is excessive and hyperactive to its utmost, it consumes and injures the yin blood and scorches and burns the tendons and vessels, so as to induce the liver wind, causing "the extreme heat producing wind" pattern, with the symptoms of high fever, convulsion of four limbs, rigidity of neck and nape, opisthotonos, up-turn of eyes, etc. Disturbing blood circulation implies that the pathogenic heat enters into the Ying (Nutrient) Phase and blood, to force the blood to circulate more rapidly and to burn and damage the vessels, so as to causing various bleeding symptoms, as spitting blood, nasal bleeding, bloody feces, bloody urine, subcutaneous bleeding, etc.

1.6.4　The fire-heat brings the toxin to cause sores and boils

The pathogenic fire-heat often brings the toxin to attack the blood and accumulates at the local area to

阳热之邪还可耗气,即所谓"壮火食气"。阳热亢盛,易耗正气,加之热迫汗出,气随汗泄(津能载气之故),致使热病患者多见气阴两伤,故感受热(火)病邪,除发热、汗出外,又常见神疲乏力、少气等气虚症状。

1.6.3　生风动血

热盛化风,又称"热极生风"。邪热亢盛至极,每易耗伤阴血,燔灼筋脉,引动肝风,而致热极生风。临床表现为高热、四肢抽搐、颈项强直、角弓反张、两目上视等症。动血,是热入营血,使血流薄急,甚则灼伤脉络,迫血妄行,而致各种出血见症,如吐血、衄血、便血、尿血和皮肤发斑等。

1.6.4　火热挟毒,易致肿疡

火热之邪,均易挟毒,侵入血分,聚于局部,腐肉成

corrode the flesh which becomes the pus, further leading to sores and boils. In the clinical pattern identification, those sores and boils with the features of local redness, swelling, feverish sensation and pain are diagnosed as the heat-toxin accumulation pattern.

2 Li (Epidemic) Qi

The Li (Epidemic) Qi is a kind of pathogen which is extremely infectious noxious epidemic. Generally speaking, the property of the Li (Epidemic) Qi is similar to that of the pathogenic heat (fire) in the six exogenous pathogens, so its pathogenic characteristics are same as those of the pathogenic heat (fire). But the Li (Epidemic) Qi is more severely toxic and can result in the much more severe diseases. The Li (Epidemic) Qi is characterized by the sudden onset of severe and risky diseases with similar symptoms, high infection and strong epidemic. According to the historical records, the Li (Epidemic) Qi may cause the extensive epidemic of diseases and high lethality.

The commonly-encountered diseases caused by the Li (Epidemic) Qi are erysipelas, epidemic parotitis, toxipathic dysentery, diphtheria, scarlet fever, smallpox, cholera, plague, etc.

Appendix: Five Endogenous Pathogens

The five endogenous pathogens refer to the endogenous wind, endogenous cold, endogenous damp, endogenous dryness and endogenous heat (fire). The names of the five endogenous pathogens of the wind, cold, damp, dryness and heat (fire) are same as those of the exogenous pathogens, but they are

脓,可发为肿疡。临床辨证,凡疮疡局部红肿高突灼热者,多属热毒积聚所致。

2 疠气

疠气,是一类具有强烈传染性的病邪。一般来说,疠气的性质与六淫中的热(火)邪颇为相似,故也具有热(火)邪的性质和致病特征。但是疠气为病具有比一般热(火)邪毒性更强的特点,主要表现在感受疠气后的发病情形更为严重。疠气致病具有发病急骤、病情重笃、症状相似及传染性强、易于流行等特点。从以往的记载来看,疠气可导致疾病大规模流行,而且患病死亡率高。

常见的疫疠所致的疾病有大头瘟(面部丹毒)、虾蟆瘟(流行性腮腺炎)、疫痢(中毒性痢疾)、白喉、烂喉丹痧、天花、霍乱、鼠疫等。

附:内生五邪

内生五邪,即内风、内寒、内湿、内燥、内热(火)的总称。内生五邪虽有风、寒、湿、燥、热(火)等名称,但其均由脏腑功能失常所产生,故冠以"内生"之名。

caused by the functional disturbances of the zang-fu organs, so called "the endogenous pathogens".

1　Endogenous wind

The endogenous wind is often transformed from the liver yang. Since the endogenous wind is caused by the liver yang hyperactivity, it is also called "the liver wind". The causes and symptoms are as follows: ① The extreme heat produces the wind. The pathogenic heat is scorching and excessive to burn and damage the liver yin which fails to nourish the tendons and vessels, leading to the wind pattern with symptoms of convulsion and spasm. ② The liver yang transforms into the wind. The liver yang is hyperactive, moving upwards to disturb the clear aperture, so as to cause the symptoms of dizziness, convulsion. ③ The yin deficiency stirs the wind. Due to the deficiency and exhaustion of the liver yin which fails to restrain yang, the yin fluid cannot moisturize and nourish the tendons and yang hyperactivity transforms the wind, so as to cause the symptoms of convulsion, spasm, etc. ④ The blood deficiency stirs the wind. Due to the deficiency of the liver blood which fails to nourish the liver and tendons, the wind is stirred to cause the symptoms of twitching of muscles, tremor, etc.

2　Endogenous cold

The endogenous cold is caused by yang deficiency. The kidney yang deficiency, or the spleen yang deficiency or the heart yang deficiency may cause the cold pattern of deficiency type in the relevant organ. The yang deficiency of different organs may present the relevant manifestations of the endogenous cold. The kidney yang is the basis of the yang qi of the whole body, so that the kidney yang deficiency is the chief causative factor to form the endogenous cold.

1　内风

内风,多由肝阳化风所致。因阳亢内风皆生于肝,故也称"肝风"。其常见的形成原因:一是热极生风。因热邪炽盛,灼伤肝阴,筋脉失养,而致动风,出现以抽搐为特征的病变。二是肝阳化风。因阳亢化风,上扰清窍,出现眩晕、惊厥等症。三是阴虚风动。由肝阴虚竭,阳不潜藏,阴液不能滋养其筋,又被阳亢化风所扰,从而发生惊厥、抽搐等症。四是血虚风动。由肝血亏虚,血不养肝,筋失濡养,而致风动,表现为肌肉蠕动、震颤等。

2　内寒

内寒,生于阳虚。或肾阳虚,或脾阳虚,或心阳虚,都可引起相应的脏腑虚寒。不同的脏腑阳虚,可见相应的内寒表现。由于肾阳为一身阳气之根本,故肾阳虚是形成内寒的首要因素。

3　Endogenous damp

The endogenous damp is transformed from the spleen. If the spleen is weak and fails to transport and transform the water, the water is accumulated to form the damp, a kind of pathological product. When the pathogenic damp is formed, it blocks the spleen to further disturb the transporting and transforming function of the spleen. Therefore, the spleen deficiency and endogenous damp are in the reciprocal causation. Furthermore, the accumulated damp may transform into the phlegm, which may cause other diseases.

4　Endogenous dryness

The endogenous dryness is caused by the insufficiency of the body fluid, related to the yin deficiency. Since the body fluid and blood share a same source, the deficiency of blood may also cause the endogenous dryness. The endogenous dryness often affects the intestines, stomach, lung and relevant orifices, to cause the symptoms of lack or loss of moisture, as dry nostrils, dry throat, dry mouth, dry eyes, scanty urine, dry feces or constipation, etc.

5　Endogenous heat (fire)

There are many different causative factors of the endogenous heat. The exogenous wind, cold, damp or dryness may transform into heat the emotional depression may transform into fire or yang excess and yin deficiency may produce the endogenous fire due to the equilibrium disturbance of yin and yang.

Section 2　Endogenous Factors

1　Seven emotional factors

The seven emotional factors are joy, anger,

3　内湿

内湿生于脾。凡脾虚失于健运,水湿不化,即能生湿,成为病理产物。湿邪既生,又可困阻于脾,妨碍脾的运化功能,由此而使脾虚与内湿互为因果。也可聚湿成痰、酿湿成饮,进一步发展变化成其他病变。

4　内燥

内燥都由津液不足所致,与阴虚相互关联。由于津血同源互化,故血虚也能生燥。内燥主要表现在肠胃、肺及有关的孔窍,因失于滋润而致鼻腔干燥、咽干口燥、两目干涩、小便短少、大便干结等。

5　内热(火)

内热形成原因众多。如外感风、寒、湿、燥,均可从热而化;情志不遂,五志郁而化火;阴阳不调,阳盛及阴虚也可内生火热。

第 2 节　内伤病因

1　七情

七情,是喜、怒、忧、思、

melancholy, worry, grief, fear and fright. The seven emotions are the normal emotional responses of the body to the external stimuli, pertaining to the normal psychological activities, and do not normally cause diseases. The abrupt, severe or continuous occurring emotional stimuli, however, which surpass the regulative adaptability of the human body, will cause the disturbance of qi activities, the disharmony between yin and yang and between qi and blood of zang-fu organs, resulting in the occurrence of diseases. The seven emotional factors, different from the six exogenous pathogens, directly affect the zang-fu organs, qi and blood. For this reason, they are considered to be the main causative factors of the endogenous diseases, and so called "seven emotional factors of endogenous diseases".

In Huang Di Nei Jing, it is believed that the seven emotions match the five zang organs to establish the theory of the five zang organs governing the five emotions, i.e. the heart governing the joy, the liver governing the anger, the spleen governing the worry, the lung governing grief, and the kidney governing the fear. Besides, the fright and melancholy are also closely related to the qi activities of the five zang organs.

The seven emotions pertain to the five zang organs respectively, but these relations are not absolute. Firstly, in the different physiological or pathological states of a same zang organ, there may be different emotional responses. For example, the liver qi excess leads to anger, while the liver qi deficiency causes fear. The heart qi excess leads to joy, while the heart qi deficiency causes grief. Secondly, all the emotional activities are actually reflected by

悲、恐、惊七种情志变化的总称。七情是人体对外界事物的不同反应，属正常的心理活动方式，一般不会致病。只有突然、强烈或长期持久的情志刺激，超过了正常的生理活动范围，导致人体气机紊乱，脏腑阴阳气血失调，才会导致疾病的发生。因七情生于内，直接影响脏腑气血，是导致内伤病的主要因素之一，所以称为"内伤七情"。

《黄帝内经》把七情与五脏相配合，建立了五脏主五志的理论，即心主喜、肝主怒、脾主思、肺主悲、肾主恐。惊和忧也与五脏气机运动密切相关。

七情虽分属五脏，但也不是绝对的。其一，同一内脏的不同生理病理状态，可有不同的情绪反应。如肝气实则表现为怒，肝气虚则表现为恐；心气实则表现为喜，心气虚则表现为悲。其二，所有情志活动实际上都必须通过心才能体现出来，一切

the heart, and all the emotional responses are essentially the manifestations of the heart spirit, so that the seven emotions are finally dominated by the heart. The pathogenic characteristics of the seven emotional factors are as follows.

1.1 Directly injure the internal organs

The seven emotional factors are endogenous, so they directly injure the zang organs. For example, the joy injures the heart, the anger injures the liver, the worry injures the spleen, the grief injures the lung, and the fear injures the kidney. Due to the various and complicated relations among the zang organs, one of the seven emotional factors injure a certain zang organ, but its pathological reactions may involve other zang organs. For example, the anger injures the liver, to make the liver qi transversely-reverse flow to attack the spleen and stomach, leading to the patterns of liver and spleen disharmony, liver and stomach disharmony, etc. Simultaneously, the heart is the predominant governor of all spiritual activities, so the diseases due to the seven emotional factors are all closely related to the heart. According to the clinical practice, the heart, liver and spleen are most closely involved with the pathological changes resulting from the seven emotional factors.

1.2 Disturb the qi activities

The seven emotional factors injure the internal organs, to influence the qi activities of the zang-fu organs, so as to cause the disturbance of the qi activities.

1.2.1 The joy makes qi flow slow and slack.

The joy is the emotion of the heart, it normally makes qi and blood to flow moderately, and Ying

情绪反应实质上仍是心神的表现,因此七情最终要归心所主管。

七情致病有以下特点。

1.1 直接伤及内脏

七情生于内,故直接伤及内脏。如喜伤心,怒伤肝,思伤脾,悲伤肺,恐伤肾等。由于内脏之间存在着多种复杂的关系,所以七情损伤某一内脏时,其病理反应会波及多个脏腑。如郁怒伤肝,肝气横逆,又常犯脾胃,出现肝脾不调、肝胃不和等证。同时,由于心为精神活动的最高主宰,故七情所伤都与心有密切关系。从临床来看,七情所伤以心、肝、脾三脏为多见。

1.2 导致气机紊乱

七情损伤内脏,主要是影响脏腑气机,最易导致气机紊乱。

1.2.1 喜则气缓

缓,有"缓和"与"涣散"双重含义。喜为心之志,正

(Nutrient) Qi and Wei (Defensive) Qi to flow smoothly, so the ease of mind presents. The over joy may cause the slack flow of the heart qi, so the spirit cannot be stored, leading to absence of mind, even the symptoms of loss of spirit, such as mania.

1.2.2　The anger makes qi flow upwards.

The severe anger makes the liver qi to rush upwards to disturb the upper, leading to the symptoms of dizziness, headache, red facial complexion, red eyes, or hematemesis, even sudden coma. The severe anger makes the liver qi to transversely-reverse flow to attack the spleen and stomach, leading to restraint of the spleen and stomach, with the symptoms of poor appetite, epigastria distension, belching, or dirrrhea.

1.2.3　The worry makes qi accumulated.

The worry is the emotion of the spleen. The over worry causes the spleen qi accumulation, disturbing the transporting and transforming function, so as to cause the symptoms of epigastria and abdominal distension, poor appetite, loose feces, etc. The continuous worry for long time consumes the yin blood, which fails to nourish the heart, so as to cause the symptoms of palpitation, poor memory, insomnia, dream-disturbed sleep, etc.

1.2.4　The grief makes qi depleted.

The grief is the emotion of the lung. The melancholy is similar to the grief. The over grief or melancholy makes the lung qi depleted, so the lung qi is restrained and fails to dominate dispersing, and the Ying (Nutrient) Qi and Wei (Defensive) Qi fail to distribute normally, leading the depletion of the Zong (Pectoral) Qi, with the symptoms of dizziness, lassitude, low spirit, etc.

常情况下,喜能使气血和缓、营卫通利,心情舒畅;若大喜过度则导致心气涣散,神不守舍,出现精神不集中,甚则失神狂乱等症状。

1.2.2　怒则气上

怒为肝之志,大怒使肝气横逆上冲,血随气逆,并走于上,可出现头昏胀痛、面红目赤,或呕血等症,甚至突然昏厥。大怒而肝气横逆,犯脾乘胃,则令脾胃受制,使人不欲饮食、脘闷嗳气,或见大便泄泻。

1.2.3　思则气结

思为脾之志,思虑过度则导致脾气郁结,运化功能障碍,从而出现脘腹胀满、食欲不振、大便溏薄等症。久思不解,阴血暗耗,心神失养,则出现心悸、健忘、失眠、多梦等症。

1.2.4　悲则气消

悲为肺之志。忧与悲类同。过悲忧可使肺气消减。凡悲忧至极,肺气过于敛肃,宣发输布失职,营卫不能布散,胸中大气(宗气)于是耗损。故悲忧伤肺者,常见头昏、乏力、精神不振等症。

1.2.5　The fear makes qi flow downwards.

The severe fear makes the kidney qi flow downwards excessively, so the kidney qi fails to check normally, leading to incontinence of urination or defecation. Due to failing to check normally, the kidney cannot store the essence, leading to the symptoms of aching or flaccidity of bones, seminal emission, etc. The continuous fear for long time makes qi fail to up-flow and outflow, so the functions of the zang-fu organs are disturbed and the Zheng (Anti-Pathogenic) Qi fails to protect the body surface, leading to the occurrence of diseases due to invasion of various exogenous pathogens.

1.2.6　The fright makes qi disturbed.

Both the fear and fright can be caused by the same external stimuli, but they are obviously different in the qi activities of the zang-fu organs. The fear originates from the kidney, leading to qi flow downwards, while the fright originates from the kidney, leading to qi disturbed. Therefore, if someone is frightened, he is at a loss and manifested by the heart qi disturbance, the spirit failing to be dominated, and the thinking activity failing to be stored. If the qi activities are disturbed, qi and blood are disharmonized, and the Wei (Defensive) Qi fails to protect the body surface. In such a situation, the exogenous pathogens attack the body which is deficient, leading to the occurrence of diseases.

1.3　Induce or worsen some diseases

The emotional factors may induce some diseases. For example, if a person with the body constitution of liver yang hyperactivity is irritated by something, the symptoms of sudden dizziness, co-

1.2.5　恐则气下

恐为肾之志,大恐则令肾气过度下沉,固摄无权,气泄于下,导致二便失禁;或精失所藏,而致骨酸痿厥、遗精等症。恐惧日久不解,气机不能升发,脏腑功能减退,正气不能卫外,也易感受各种外邪而发病。

1.2.6　惊则气乱

惊与恐可由相似的外界刺激因素所引起,但二者在脏腑气机上的反应有明显区别。恐生于肾,导致气机下行;惊生于心,引起气机紊乱。因此,人受惊吓之时,主要反应为心气紊乱,神无所主,虑无所定,不知所措。由于气机紊乱,于是气血不调,卫外不固,邪气便能乘虚而入,导致疾病的发生。

1.3　引发或加重某些疾病

情志因素可引发某些疾病。如素体肝阳偏亢者,若遇事恼怒,肝阳暴张,可突发眩晕、昏厥,或昏仆不语、半

ma, loss of consciousness, hemiplegia, deviation of mouth, etc. may occur. In the process of some disease, the abnormal emotional changes may worsen the disease. For example, a patient of heart disease may suffer from the sudden attack of heart disease and worsened condition due to some emotional stimuli, as fear, fright, etc.

2　Improper diet

The food intake is the necessary condition for human existence, and the major mode of human body to gain the nutritional substances from the external. However, it will be beneficial for the health when the food intake is acted in accordance with the normal regulation food intake of on the needs of human body for the nutritional substances. If the food intake is improper, it will damage the human body and become a causative factor of diseases.

The improper diet includes three aspects: improper hungry and full states, intake of unclean food, and overindulgence in particular foods.

2.1　Improper hungry and full states

The improper hungry and full states include over-hungry state and over-full state.

The over-hungry state includes two situations of the continuous hungry state and prolonged lack of food intake. In the continuous hungry state, the body fails to obtain the sufficient nutrients from the food, so the qi and blood cannot be transformed and functions of zang-fu organs decrease abruptly, leading to symptoms of dizziness, blurring of vision, weakness of four limbs, etc., even imperiling the life. The prolonged lack of food intake causes poor nutrition, so qi and blood of human body are be-

身不遂、口眼歪斜等。某些疾病过程中,可因异常的情绪波动而使病情加重,或迅速恶化,如心脏病患者,可因突然受惊恐刺激而骤然发病,并迅速恶化。

2　饮食

饮食是人类生存的必要条件,是人体从外界获得营养物质的主要方式。然而,饮食的摄取,应当遵循满足人体对营养素需求的正常进食规律,才能有益于健康。如果饮食失宜,反而会对人体造成伤害,而成为一种致病因素。

饮食失宜包括饥饱失度、饮食不洁、饮食偏嗜三个方面的内容。

2.1　饥饱失度

饥饱失度包括过饥和过饱两个方面。

过饥,有连续饥饿和长期摄食不足两种情况。在连续饥饿状态下,由于无法从饮食中获取充足的营养,气血生化乏源,脏腑功能骤然减退,会出现头昏目眩、四肢无力等症状,严重时可危及生命。长期摄食不足,营养不良,人体气血得不到足够的补充而逐渐亏虚,不但身

coming gradually deficient due to lack of sufficient supplement. In such a situation, the body is weak and depleted day by day, and is easy to be attacked by other pathogens to cause various secondary diseases.

The over-full state includes two situations of voracious intake of food and prolonged over-intake of food. The voracious intake of food surpassed the enduring ability of the spleen and stomach, so the food cannot be normally decomposed, transported and transformed, but retains in the middle energizer to damage the spleen and stomach, leading to the symptoms of epigastria and abdominal distension, belching, acid regurgitation, dislike of eating, vomiting, diarrhea, etc., and to injure the vessels of the intestines and stomach, leading to the symptoms of abdominal pain, bleeding due to hemorrhoids, etc. The prolonged over-intake of food causes supernutrition, so that the spleen is not enough to transform food into qi and blood, but makes the water accumulate inside the body to form the phlegm or rheum, which further blocks the qi and blood circulation, leading to the symptoms of over-weight, dizziness, blurring of vision, palpitation, stuffy chest, etc., or which is transformed into heat to attack the blood vessels, leading to the symptoms of carbuncles, furuncles, boils, sores, etc.

2.2　Intake of unclean food

If the food is mixed with some unclean objects, the unclean food eaten may cause diseases, as the diseases of the stomach and intestines, with the symptoms of abdominal pain, vomiting, diarrhea. If the food is mixed with the parasites' eggs, the food eaten may cause various parasitic diseases. If

体日渐衰弱,还容易感受其他邪气而继发多种疾病。

过饱,有暴饮暴食和长期摄入过量两种情况。暴饮暴食,超过脾胃的承受能力,饮食不能正常地腐熟和运化,阻滞于中,反使脾胃受伤,出现脘腹胀满、嗳腐泛酸、厌食、吐泻等症,严重者可伤损肠胃脉络,引起腹痛或痔疮出血等症。长期摄入过量,营养过剩,气化不及,水谷精微不化气血,反变生痰饮而停聚于体内,阻碍气血运行,出现形体肥胖、头昏目眩、心悸胸闷等症;或酿湿蕴热,侵淫血脉,变生痈疽疔疮等。

2.2　饮食不洁

饮食中混有不洁之物,食之可使人致病。一般不洁之物主要引起腹痛、吐泻等胃肠道病症;若饮食中混有寄生虫卵,可引起各种寄生虫病;若食物已腐败变质,则

the food is rotten and deteriorated, it becomes toxic and causes poisoning symptoms, as severe abdominal pain, vomiting, diarrhea, etc.

Drinking of unclean water is another important factor of diseases. In the industrial society, the natural water is often polluted to be mixed with various toxins or harmful substances. Drinking the water may cause various acute or chronic poisoning diseases.

2.3　Overindulgence in particular foods

The overindulgence in particular foods includes two aspects of overindulgence in cold or hot food, and overindulgence in any of the five flavors.

Overindulgence in cold or hot food: The foods are different in cool-cold property and warm-hot property, and in raw-cold nature and burning-hot nature. The overindulgence of cool-cold property foods or the raw-cold nature foods may injure the yang qi of the spleen and stomach, so as to cause the endogenous cold-damp, with the symptoms of abdominal pain, diarrhea, etc. The overindulgence of warm-dry property foods or the burning-hot nature foods may cause the accumulated heat in stomach and intestines, with the symptoms of thirst, abdominal distension and pain, constipation, or even hemorrhoids, etc.

Overindulgence of five flavors: The five flavors match the five zang organs, i.e. the sour flavor enters the liver, the bitter flavor enters the heart, the sweet flavor enters the spleen, the pungent flavor enters the lung, and the salty flavor enters the kidney. So that the overindulgence of the sour flavor food injures the liver qi, the overindulgence of the salty flavor food injures the kidney qi, the overindulgence of the sweet flavor food injures the spleen

有毒,食之可发生中毒症状,出现剧烈腹痛、吐泻等。

饮水不洁,也是重要致病因素之一。工业社会中的自然水源往往因受污染而混有多种有毒或有害物质,饮用这种水也会导致多种急性或慢性中毒性疾病。

2.3　饮食偏嗜

饮食偏嗜表现在两个方面,一是寒热偏嗜,一是五味偏嗜。

寒热偏嗜:饮食物也有寒凉、温热之性,又有生冷、炙热之别,若偏好寒凉饮食,或过食生冷,可损伤脾胃阳气,导致寒湿内生,发生腹痛、泄泻等症;若偏喜温燥之物,或多食炙热,可使胃肠积热,出现口渴、腹满胀痛、便秘,或酿成痔疮等。

五味偏嗜:五味与五脏各有归属,即酸味入肝,苦味入心,甘味入脾,辛味入肺,咸味入肾。若偏食酸味,易伤肝气;偏食咸味,易伤肾气;偏食甘味,易伤脾气;偏食苦味,易伤心气;偏食辛味,易伤肺气。

qi, the overindulgence of the bitter flavor food injures the heart qi, and the overindulgence of the pungent flavor food injures the lung qi.

3   Overstrain and over-idleness

The strain includes various types of labors and sports. The idleness refers to rest and comfort. Both the strain and idleness are the necessities in the human life, none is dispensable. The normal labors and sports are helpful to promote qi and blood circulation and strengthen the body. The necessary rest and comfort are able to relieve fatigue and recover the physical power and spirit. But the overstrain or over-idleness may cause diseases.

3.1   Overstrain

Overstrain includes three aspects of the physical overstrain, spiritual overstrain and sexual overstrain.

The physical overstrain implies the prolonged overuse of physics, as over physical labor or over sports, which consume qi and blood too much, and the body has not enough time to supplement and recover, so as to break the health down from overwork to cause diseases. Besides, the injuries caused by prolonged standing, prolonged walking, prolonged speaking, etc. also belong to the physical overstrain.

The spiritual overstrain implies that over-thinking activity consumes the heart blood, so as to causes the diseases of deficiency pattern. The spiritual overstrain not only consumes the heart blood, but also damages the spleen as well. As a result, there can be the symptoms of the heart spirit failing to be nourished as palpitation, poor memory, insomnia,

3   劳逸

劳,包括各种劳作和运动。逸,指休息和静养。劳和逸都是人类生活的需要,两者不可缺一。正常的劳作和运动,有助于流通气血,增强体质;必要的休息和静养,可以消除疲劳,恢复体力和精神。如果过度劳累,或过度安逸,都会使人致病。

3.1   过劳

过劳,包括劳力过度、劳神过度和房劳过度三个方面。

劳力过度,指长时间过度用力,如体力劳动过度、运动过度等,气血消耗太过,得不到及时补充和恢复,从而积劳成疾。诸如久立、久行、言语过久等所致损伤,也属劳力过度。

劳神过度,指用心思虑太过,耗伤心血,导致虚损性疾病。凡劳神太过,不仅心血耗伤,而且思虑则伤脾,故一方面表现为心神失养的心悸、健忘、失眠、多梦,同时多兼有脾不健运的纳呆、腹胀、

dream-disturbed sleep, etc. on one hand, and also the symptoms of the spleen failing to transport and transform as poor appetite, abdominal distension, loose feces, etc. on the other hand.

The sexual overstrain refers to the excessive sexual activity. The normal sexual activity acts to promote qi and blood circulation and harmonize yin and yang. But the excessive sexual activity may consume the kidney essence and exhaust qi and blood, so that the five zang organs fail to be nourished and become premature senility, leading to the symptoms of aching and weakness at low back and knee, dizziness, blurring of vision, tinnitus, low spirit, or impotence, seminal emission, premature ejaculation, etc.

3.2   Over-idleness

The over-idleness implies lack of necessary labors or sports. The prolonged over-idleness without physical exercises may slow down qi and blood circulation and decrease the functions of zang-fu organs, so as to lead to poor appetite, fatigue, low spirit, weakness of limbs and body, or over-weight, fattiness, intolerance in laboring, and palpitation, shortness of breath and sweating on exertion. As a result, the stagnant blood is produced internally, and the exogenous pathogenic wind, cold or damp attacks from the external, so as to cause various secondary diseases.

Section 3   Pathological Products

The phlegm-rheum and stagnant blood are the

便溏等症。

房劳过度,即房事过度。正常的房事活动,可以通行气血,调和阴阳。但房事太多,肾精耗损过度,气血也随之衰弱,五脏失养,导致早衰,出现腰膝酸软、眩晕耳鸣、精神萎靡,或阳痿、遗精、早泄等肾亏之症。

3.2   过逸

过逸,主要指缺乏必要的劳动或运动。长期过度安逸,缺少锻炼,气血运行迟缓,脏腑功能减退,使人食少乏力,精神不振,肢体软弱,或发胖臃肿,不耐劳动,动则心悸、气喘及汗出等。瘀血生于内,风寒湿邪袭于外,可继发多种疾病。

第 3 节
病理产物

痰饮和瘀血是人体受某

pathological products inside the human body formed during the process of disease caused by some pathogenic factors. When these pathological products are formed, they affect the zang-fu organs and tissues of human body directly or indirectly, to cause the secondary diseases. Therefore, the phlegm-rheum and stagnant blood are the pathological products, and also the pathogenic factors as well.

1 Phlegm-rheum

1.1 Concept of phlegm-rheum

The phlegm-rheum is a kind of pathological product formed due to the disturbance of the body fluid metabolism in human body. The thick and turbid type is regarded as the phlegm, while the clear and thin type as the rheum.

The phlegm is divided into the tangible phlegm and the intangible phlegm. The tangible phlegm refers to the spitted sputum which is visible and audible. The intangible phlegm refers to the invisible and inaudible phlegm, which has the similar pathological manifestations to those of phlegm, such as scrofula and nodule between the skin and muscle. Besides, the patterns of phlegm misting the heart orifice, phlegm retaining in meridians and collaterals, pertain to the intangible phlegm.

The rheum is divided into four types in *Essential Prescriptions of the Golden Coffer* (Jin Kui Yao Lüe) as the phlegmatic rheum, the suspending rheum, the overflowing rheum and the branching rheum. These terms are given according to the different locations of the rheum. That locates in the abdomen is called "the phlegmatic rheum", that locates in the chest and diaphragm is called "the sus-

种致病因素作用后在疾病过程中所形成的病理产物。这些病理产物形成之后，又能直接或间接作用于人体脏腑或形体，导致继发性疾病。所以痰饮、瘀血既是病理产物，又是致病因素。

1 痰饮

1.1 痰饮的基本概念

痰饮是人体津液代谢障碍所形成的病理产物。一般以较稠浊的称为痰，较清稀的称为饮。

痰可分为有形之痰与无形之痰。有形之痰，是指视之可见、闻之有声的痰，指咯吐所出之痰液。无形之痰是指视之不见、闻之无声的痰，但其有因痰所致的病理表现，如皮肤肌肉间形成的瘰疬、痰核。另如痰迷心窍、痰留经络等，均属无形之痰。

《金匮要略》将饮分为四类，即痰饮、悬饮、溢饮、支饮。这是根据饮邪所在部位不同而规定的名称。如饮停于腹中名"痰饮"，饮悬于胸膈名"悬饮"，饮留于两胁名"支饮"，饮溢于肌肤名"溢饮"。

pending rheum", that locates in the hypochondria on both sides is called "the branching rheum", and that locates in the skin and muscles is called "the o-verflowing rheum".

There are four types of pathological products of phlegm, rheum, water and damp due to the disturbance of body fluid metabolism. There are some differences in them. That is diffusing and formless is termed as the damp, while the stopped and accumulated damp is termed as the rheum. The clear-thin type of rheum is called the water, while the rheum which is thickened and condensed be-comes the phlegm. That is to say that they all origi-nate from the disturbance of body fluid metabolism and act to mutually transform.

1.2 Formation of phlegm-rheum

Both the phlegm and rheum are produced by the disturbance of body fluid metabolism, and many zang-fu organs as the spleen, lung, kidney, liver, triple energizer, etc. are involved. Various patho-genic factors, such as the six exogenous pathogens, the seven emotional factors, the improper food in-take, the improper strain and idleness, etc., may injure the zang-fu organs and disturb their qi activi-ties, leading to the disturbance of body fluid metab-olism, so as to cause retention of water and further produce the water, damp, phlegm and rheum.

The spleen dominates the transportation and transformation of water, the lung dredges and regu-lates the water passage, the kidney dominates the water, the liver dominates dredging and draining so as to promote the body fluid metabolism, and the triple energizer acts as the water passage. There-fore, if the spleen fails to transport and transform

痰、饮、水、湿四者都是津液代谢障碍所形成的病理产物,但相互之间有一定区别。其弥漫无形者为湿,停聚有形者为饮;饮之清稀者为水,饮之煎炼而成者为痰。也就是说,四者皆源于津液代谢障碍,并可互相转化。

1.2 痰饮的形成

痰饮皆由津液代谢障碍所致,涉及到脾、肺、肾、肝、三焦等多个脏腑。各种致病因素,如外感六淫、内伤七情、饮食失宜、劳逸失当等,都可损伤脏腑,使其气化功能失常,津液代谢障碍,停聚而成水湿痰饮。

因脾主运化水湿,肺主通调水道,肾主水,肝主疏泄能促进津液代谢,三焦为水道,若脾失健运,或肺失通调,或肾不主水,或肝失疏泄,或三焦气化失常,使水湿不化,津液停聚,皆可聚湿而

the water, or if the lung fails to dredge and regulate the water passage, or if the kidney fails to dominate the water, or if the liver fails to dominate dredging and draining, or if the triple energizer's function is disturbed, the body fluid cannot be transpired and transformed, but retains and accumulates to become the phlegm-rheum. After the phlegm-rheum is formed, it affects the zang-fu organs to disturb the transforming function of zangu-fu organs, so as to cause the repeated formation of the phlegm-rheum. If the phlegm blocks the lung to cause cough and panting, the actual cause is the deficiency of the spleen. Therefore, it is said by the ancients that "the spleen is the source to produce the phlegm, while the lung is the container to store the phlegm" by the ancients.

Furthermore, the formation of phlegm-rheum is also related to the factors of cold and heat. The cold and heat can be the exogenous type, or are caused by the dysfunction of zang-fu organs. If the pathogenic cold attacks the zang-fu organs, their transforming function may decrease even stop, so that the body fluid cannot be transpired and trans- formed, becoming the phlegm-rheum. If the patho- genic heat attacks the zang-fu organs, the body fluid may be thickened and condensed into phlegm- rheum. For example, the pathogenic cold attacks the lung to make the rheum staying in the lung, leading to cough with clear, thin or foamy sputum. This condition is called "the cold-rheum hiding in lung". The pathogenic heat attacks the lung to cause cough with yellow, thick or pus-like sputum. This condition is called "the phlegm-heat blocking lung".

成痰饮。痰饮形成以后,又可在脏腑之间相互影响,进而使多个脏腑气化失常,导致痰饮的反复形成。如痰湿蕴肺而致咳嗽、气喘,临床多责之于脾虚,故古人有"脾为生痰之源,肺为贮痰之器"的说法。

痰饮的形成还与寒热因素有关。寒热可由外感而得,也可由脏腑阴阳失调所致。脏腑有寒,则气化迟滞,津液不化,形成痰饮。脏腑有热,则煎熬津液,也可形成痰饮。如肺寒可致饮停于肺,咳吐清稀泡沫痰液,称为"寒饮伏肺"。肺热可致痰阻于肺,咳吐黄稠脓痰,称为"痰热蕴肺"等。

1.3 Pathogenic characteristics of phlegm-rheum

1.3.1 Impede the qi and blood circulation in the meridians

The phlegm-rheum can reach everywhere along with qi circulation. If the phlegm-rheum infuses into the meridians and collaterals, it blocks the meridians and collaterals and disturbs the qi and blood circulation, leading to numbness and motor impairment of limbs and body, even hemiplegia, etc. If it accumulates in some local areas, there can be scrofula, nodules, yin-type subcutaneous ulcer, etc.

1.3.2 Obstruct the up-flow and down-flow of qi of the zang-fu organs

The phlegm-rheum, accumulated by the water and damp, retains in the zang-fu organs to obstruct the qi activities, so as to disturb the normal up-flow and down-flow of qi of the zang-fu organs. The lung qi tends to descend. If the phlegm-rheum retains in the lung, the lung fails to dominate dispersing and descending, leading to the symptoms of stuffy chest, cough, panting, etc. The stomach qi tends to descend. If the phlegm-rheum retains in the stomach, the stomach qi fails to descend, causing the symptoms of nausea, vomiting, etc.

1.3.3 Mist and afflict the spirit

The turbid phlegm disturbs the upper to mist and afflict the Qing (Clear) Yang, leading to the symptoms of dizziness, blurring of vision, etc. The phlegm mists the heart aperture, or the phlegm-fire disturbs the heart, the heart spirit is misted, causing the symptoms of stuffy chest, palpitation, loss of consciousness, delirium, even mental disorders as Dian (Depressive) Pattern, Kuang (Manic) Pat-

1.3 痰饮致病的特点

1.3.1 阻碍经脉气血运行

痰饮随气流行，无所不至。若痰饮流注于经络，易使经络阻滞，气血运行不畅，出现肢体麻木、屈伸不利，甚至半身不遂等。若结聚于局部，可形成瘰疬痰核、阴疽流注等。

1.3.2 阻滞脏腑气机升降

痰饮为水湿所聚，若停滞于脏腑，易于阻遏气机，使脏腑气机升降失常。如肺以肃降为顺，若痰饮停肺，肺失宣肃，可出现胸闷、咳嗽、喘促等症；胃以降为和，痰饮停胃，胃失和降，则出现恶心呕吐等症。

1.3.3 易于蒙蔽神明

痰浊上扰，蒙蔽清阳，可致头昏目眩；痰迷心窍，或痰火扰心，心神被蒙，可致胸闷心悸、神昏谵妄，或引起癫狂惊痫等。

tern, convulsion, epilepsy, etc.

1.3.4 Possess the complicated symptoms and multiple changes

The phlegm-rheum is formed by many causes and related to lots of areas, moves upwards and downwards along with the qi movement, and reaches everywhere in the upper, the lower, the internal and the external. So that the diseases caused by the phlegm-rheum cover a wide range, influencing many zang-fu organs and tissues and causing the complicated symptoms with multiple changes. According to the clinical manifestations, the five zang organs, six fu organs, all body constituents, sense organs, orifices, four limbs and all bones can be diseased due to the phlegm-rheum, with symptoms of stuffy chest, cough, panting, spitting sputum, nausea, vomiting, palpitation, dizziness, mental disorders, numbness of limbs and body, pain or swelling of joints, subcutaneous tumor or ulcer with pus, edema, ascites, diarrhea, etc. Furthermore, all types of difficult, complicated and miscellaneous diseases without confirmed causes are related to the phlegm-rheum. Therefore, it is said by the ancients that "the strange diseases are often related to the phlegm", and that "all diseases are evil influenced by the phlegm".

Since the phlegm-rheum moves upwards and downwards along with the qi circulation, the diseases caused by the phlegm-rheum possess the features of multiple changes and repeated attacks. For example, the disease of epilepsy has the repeated attacks, because the attack occurs if qi up-flows, and the attack stops if qi down-flows.

1.3.4 症状复杂,变化多端

由于痰饮形成的原因多,痰饮关联部位广,并且能随气升降,上下内外无所不至,故痰饮所致疾病种类多,影响脏腑组织也多,症状极为复杂,且变化多端。从临床表现来看,五脏六腑、形体官窍、四肢百骸,皆可因痰饮而致病,其症状表现如胸闷、咳嗽、气喘、咯痰、恶心、呕吐、心悸、眩晕、癫狂、肢体麻木、关节疼痛或肿胀、皮下肿块或溃破流脓,以及水肿、腹水、泄泻等。凡种种疑难杂病、不明原因疾病,都可能与痰饮有关,所以古人有"怪病多痰""百病多由痰作祟"的说法。

由于痰饮可以随气升降,故其病证往往容易变化,呈反复发作性。如癫痫病,痰随气升则病发,痰随气降则病止,反复多次。

2 Stagnant blood

2. 1 Concept of stagnant blood

The stagnant blood is a kind of pathological product formed due to the disturbance of the blood circulation.

The normal blood constantly circulates inside the vessels by the promoting function of the heart qi. The stop of blood flow, or the slow flow of blood due to various causes, may lead to blockage of meridians or zang-fu organs. The blood flows away from the vessels to be accumulated inside the body. These conditions are called the stagnant blood.

The stagnant blood differs from the blood stagnation in their concepts. The stagnant blood is a kind of pathological product, while the blood stagnation refers to a kind of pathological process. The stagnant blood is produced during the process of blood stagnation, while the stagnant blood is the necessary product during the pathological process of blood stagnation.

2. 2 Formation of stagnant blood

There are many causes in the formation of blood. The pathogenic cold of the six exogenous pathogens attacks the body to cause the obstruction of the blood vessels, while the worry and melancholy of the seven emotional factors make qi accumulated, so as to slow down the blood circulation. Besides, the deficiency, overstrain or injury are also the causative factors. In summary, the mechanism in the formation of stagnant blood is as follows.

2. 2. 1 Qi stagnation

The blood flows along with qi, so qi stagnation causes the blood stasis, further leading to the for-

2 瘀血

2. 1 瘀血的基本概念

瘀血,是由血液运行障碍所产生的一种病理产物。

正常血液由心气推动着在血脉中不停地运行,若因某种原因导致血液停滞,或血行迟缓,阻滞于经脉或脏腑,或离经之血存积体内,皆称为瘀血。

瘀血与血瘀的概念不同,瘀血是一种病理产物,而血瘀则是一个病理过程。血瘀的过程可以产生瘀血,瘀血必然是血瘀病理过程的产物。

2. 2 瘀血的形成

瘀血形成的原因很多。有外感六淫所致者,如寒性凝滞,可使血脉瘀滞;有内伤七情所致者,如忧思气结,可使血行迟缓;也有虚损、劳伤等因素所致者。归纳起来,瘀血的形成机理有以下几个方面。

2. 2. 1 气滞

血随气行,气滞则血瘀,可导致瘀血。外感寒、湿阴

mation of blood stasis. The exogenous pathogenic cold or damp, the yin pathogen, attacks the body to obstruct the qi activities. The worry or melancholy makes qi accumulated, so as to cause dysfunction of liver to maintain dredging and draining. The turbid phlegm accumulates internally, so as to disturb the smooth qi activities. All these factors may obstruct the blood circulation, so as to form up the stagnant blood. For example, the liver qi stagnation may cause the obstruction of the blood vessels, and then the abdominal masses occur, leading to the symptoms and signs of hypochondriac pain, palpable hard masses, etc.

2.2.2 Qi deficiency

Qi is the commander of the blood. If qi is deficiency, it fails to promote the blood circulation and the blood flow slows down, so as to cause the formation of stagnant blood. Therefore, the functional decrease of the zang-fu organs, or the deficiency, strain and injury, or the improper food intake, or the chronic disease, or the weak body after delivery, may cause qi deficiency, further leading to the formation of stagnant blood. For example, in the patient with chronic disease, his qi is deficient and his blood circulation is not smooth, so that the ordinary treatment is not very effective. It is necessary to reinforce qi so as to move the blood. When qi and blood are sufficient and vigorous, they may dispel the pathogens, so as to cure the disease.

2.2.3 Cold in blood

The blood can flow with gain of heat, while it stagnates with gain of cold. If there is the cold in the blood, the blood flow slows down to cause the formation of stagnant blood. The exogenous patho-

邪,阻碍气机运行;或忧思气结,肝气失疏;或痰浊内阻,气机不畅等,皆可使血行受阻而形成瘀血。如肝气郁滞,血脉瘀滞,日久则形成癥积,出现胁下疼痛,可触及坚硬肿块等。

2.2.2 气虚

气为血帅,气虚则推动无力,血行迟缓,而形成瘀血。凡脏腑功能减退,或虚损劳伤,或饮食失调,或久病,或产后,皆可导致气虚而易致瘀血。如久病之人,往往气虚,血行不畅,所以一般治疗不易收效,必须补气以行血,待气血畅旺,方能祛邪外出,促使疾病痊愈。

2.2.3 血寒

血液得温则行,得寒则凝。若血中有寒,则血行迟缓,从而形成瘀血。外感寒邪侵淫血脉,湿盛日久损伤

genic cold which attacks the blood vessels, or the prolonged damp which injures and consumes the yang qi, or the fire declining at the Vital Gate which causes the insufficiency of the Yuan (Primary) Yang, may lead to the cold in blood so as to cause the formation of stagnant blood. For example, in females, when the cold blocks the uterus, the blood vessels are obstructed, leading to the symptoms of lower abdominal pain, purple or black color of menstrual blood, clots in menstrual blood, or delayed menstruation, or amenorrhea, which are all related to the stagnant blood.

2.2.4　Heat in blood

The blood can flow with gain of heat. But the excessive heat may force the blood flow recklessly to cause bleeding, after which the blood away from the meridians retains in the body to lead to the formation of stagnant blood. When the heat attacks the blood, it injures and consumes the yin fluid in the blood to make the blood thickened, so as to cause the formation of blood.

2.2.5　Traumatic injury

The traumatic injury, besides damages the tendon, bone or muscle, also damages the blood vessels, so as to cause the formation of stagnant blood. Therefore, the local hematoma occurring in the patient of traumatic injury is a typical phenomenon of the stagnant blood. Besides, the traumatic injury causes bleeding, so the blood away from the meridians retains inside the body, to cause the formation of stagnant blood.

2.2.6　Bleeding

The blood away from the meridians cannot circulate along with qi. If the blood away from the

阳气,命门火衰元阳不足等,皆可使血寒而致瘀血。如女子寒阻胞宫,血脉瘀滞,可见经行少腹疼痛,经色紫黑或挟有瘀血块,或经期延后,或经闭不来等,都与瘀血有关。

2.2.4　血热

血液得温则行,但温热太过,则血热妄行,造成离经之血积存体内,而形成瘀血;或血与热结,阴津耗伤,血液凝结而成瘀血。

2.2.5　外伤

外伤除了能损伤筋骨肌肉外,也可损伤血脉,形成瘀血,故外伤患者一般都有局部血肿,是瘀血的特征表现。若外伤出血,血液离经而积存于体内,也形成瘀血。

2.2.6　出血

血液离经,便不能再随气运行。离经之血若未能排

meridians cannot be dispelled, it retains at the local area to cause the formation of stagnant blood. There are many causative factors of bleeding, such as bleeding due to qi deficiency, the spleen failing to control blood, the liver failing to store blood, reckless flow of blood due to heat, reckless flow of blood due heat transformed from the five emotional factors, bleeding due to traumatic injury, etc.

2.3　Pathogenic characteristics of stagnant blood

There are many manifestations of the diseases caused by the stagnant blood, but their common features are as follows.

2.3.1　Pain

It is a type of sharp-stabbing pain which is fixed, worsened by pressure and more severe at night. If the pain in the stagnant blood is caused by qi and blood deficiency in the chronic disease, it is a kind of continuous dull pain.

2.3.2　Masses

The prolonged stagnant blood which is not dissolved may gradually form up the masses. The masses caused by the stagnant blood are featured by hard property and fixed location. If the masses locate on the body surface, there can be blue or purple color on the skin. If the masses locate in the internals, there can be the abdominal masses which are as hard as stones.

2.3.3　Bleeding

If the stagnant blood obstructs the wounded vessels, the wounds cannot be cured, to causing bleeding repeatedly. In the treatment for bleeding caused by the stagnant blood, it is necessary to activate the blood so as to dissolve the stasis, for the

出体外,停积于局部,就成为瘀血。导致出血的原因很多,如气虚出血、脾不统血、肝不藏血、血热妄行、五志化火动血、外伤出血等。

2.3　瘀血致病的特点

瘀血致病的表现很多,归纳起来主要有以下共同特点。

2.3.1　易致疼痛

主要表现为刺痛,痛处固定不移,拒按,夜间痛甚。若因久病、气血虚衰而致瘀血疼痛,可表现为隐痛绵绵。

2.3.2　易成肿块

瘀血日久,凝结不化,逐渐形成肿块。瘀血所致肿块,质地坚硬,固定不移。肿块在体表,可见皮色青紫;肿块在内脏,则形成癥积,坚硬如石。

2.3.3　易致出血

瘀血阻于损伤的血络,则其损伤不能愈合,可导致反复出血。此时瘀血成了出血的原因,必须活血化瘀,使损伤的血络得到修复,出血

purpose to cure the wounded blood vessels so as to stop bleeding. The blood in bleeding due to stagnant blood is purple or dark in color with blood clots.

2.3.4 Purple color

In the patient of stagnant blood, the purple color can be seen, such as purple-colored complexion, skin, lips and nails. The tongue body is purple or dark in color, or the purple spots or patches can be seen on the tongue.

Besides, the pulse can be thready, choppy, deep, wiry, knotted or intermittent.

Section 4 Other Pathogenic Factors

1 Traumatic injury

The traumatic injury includes the bullet wound, injuries from falls, fractures, contusions and strains, sprain due to carrying heavy objects, burn and scald, frostbite, drowning, insect and animal bites, lightning wound, etc.

1.1 Bullet wound, injuries from fall, factures, contusions and strains, and sprain due to carrying heavy objects

This type of traumatic injuries all directly damage the skin, muscles, tendons, vessels, bones and internals of human body, causing local swelling and pain, bleeding, fracture, or joint dislocation in mild conditions, and causing injury of internals, excessive bleeding, coma, convulsion, or collapse of yang in severe conditions.

1.2 Burn and scald

The burn and scald are mostly caused by the

才可治愈。瘀血所致出血，其血色紫暗，常伴有血块。

2.3.4 易现紫色

瘀血患者可见面色、肤色、口唇、爪甲呈青紫色。舌质可呈紫暗色，或出现瘀点、瘀斑。

此外，脉象多见细、涩、沉、弦，或出现结、代脉。

第 4 节 其他病因

1 外伤

外伤包括枪弹、金刃伤、跌打损伤、持重努伤、烧烫伤、冻伤、溺水、虫兽伤和雷击伤的等。

1.1 枪弹、金刃伤、跌打损伤、持重努伤

这些外伤，均能直接损伤人体的皮肤、肌肉、筋脉、骨骼以及内脏，轻则可引起皮肤肌肉瘀血肿痛，出血或筋伤骨折、脱臼；重则损伤内脏，或出血过多，导致昏迷、抽搐、亡阳等严重病变。

1.2 烧烫伤

烧烫伤多由沸水、沸油、

boiling water, boiling oil, high temperature objects, raging fire, high voltage electroshock, etc. which attack the human body. The burn and scald pertain to the diseases caused by the fire-toxin. If the body is attacked by the pathogenic fire-toxin, various symptoms may occur at the injured areas. In mild conditions, the skin is injured, causing local redness, swelling, hotness, pain or blisters. In severe conditions, the muscle, tendons and bones are injured, causing local leather-like changes, as wax-white, burnt-yellow, or carbonization, disappearance of painful sensation. In the most severe conditions, the pathogenic fire-toxin attacks the zang-fu organs internally, leading to the symptoms of restlessness, fever, thirst, scanty urine, retention of urine, etc., even death due to collapse of yin or yang.

1.3 Frostbite

The frostbite refers to the general or local injury due to attack of low temperature to the human body, as working or walking in snowy storm, or being thinly clad in low temperature environment, or poor winter protection, or absence of movement for long time, etc. Therefore, the frostbite is quietly commonly seen in the northern areas in China. Generally speaking, the lower the temperature is, or the longer time being frostbitten, the more severe injury occurs in frostbite. The frostbite is divided into the general frostbite and local frostbite.

1.4 Drowning

Due to incapability to swim or other factors, one sinks in water to drown, leading to suffocation, even death. When the body is sinking in the water, the water enters the lung and stomach to block the

高温物品、烈火、高压电流等作用于人体所引起。烧伤属于火毒为患,机体受到火毒侵害,受伤的部位一般立即可以出现各种症状。轻者,损伤肌肤,创面红、肿、热、痛或起水泡。重者,损伤肌肉筋骨,出现创面呈皮革样,或蜡白,或焦黄,或炭化,痛觉反而消失。更甚者,火毒内侵脏腑,可出现烦躁不安,发热,口渴,尿少尿闭等症,有的可亡阴亡阳而死亡。

1.3 冻伤

冻伤是指人体遭受低温侵袭引起的全身性或局部性损伤。如在暴风雪中作业,行走,或在低温环境中衣着单薄,防寒设备不良,长时间不活动均能发生冻伤。因此,冻伤在我国北方冬季最为常见。一般来说,温度越低,受冻时间越长,则冻伤程度越重。冻伤可分为全身性冻伤和局部性冻伤。

1.4 溺水

因不会游泳等原因沉溺水中可导致人体窒息,甚则死亡。人体沉溺水中,水入肺胃,气道窒塞,呼吸不通。

respiratory tract, leading to respiratory difficulty. In mild conditions, one comes back to life after rescue. In severe conditions, drowning causes death.

1.5 Insect and animal bites

1.5.1 Insect sting

Some insects may sting the human body with their poisonous spines, bristles or mouthparts to sting and suck, so as to cause diseases. The commonly seen insect sting includes the bee sting, centipede bite, scorpion sting, bristle worm sting, etc. There are the symptoms of local redness, swelling and pain in mild conditions, while the symptoms of high fever, shiver, etc. in severe conditions.

1.5.2 Animal bite

There are descriptions of the tiger bite, lion bite, wolf bite, etc. in the ancient classics, but they are rarely seen currently. Herein only the rabid dog bite is introduced. The disease caused by the rabid dog bite is called "the rabies" in modern medicine. The pathogenic toxin in the saliva of a rabid dog may enter the human body after its bite, stay in the body for a certain long period of time, and then the disease comes on. In the early stage of the rabid dog bite, there can be local redness, swelling, pain and bleeding, and the wound is healed after treatment. When the disease comes on, there are the symptoms of headache, restlessness, hydrophobia, wind phobia, sound phobia, trismus, convulsion, etc., even death.

1.5.3 Poisonous snake bite

When a poisonous snake bites the human body, its venom enters the human body through its poison fangs. The different poisonous snakes have different venoms, which cause different injuries to the

轻者,可经抢救复苏;重者,每致溺死。

1.5 虫兽伤

1.5.1 虫蛰伤

某些虫类可通过它们的毒刺及毒毛刺蛰或口器刺吮损伤人体而导致发病,常见的虫蛰伤有蜂蛰伤,蜈蚣咬伤,蝎蛰伤以及毛虫伤人等。这些虫蛰伤,轻者局部红肿疼痛,重者可引起高热、寒战等全身中毒症状。

1.5.2 兽咬伤

兽咬伤中医书籍载有虎、狮、狼咬伤等,这些现在均已罕见。这里仅介绍疯狗咬伤。疯狗咬伤致病现代医学称为"狂犬病"。这是由于狂犬的唾涎中含有毒邪,人被狂犬咬伤时邪毒随之进入人体,潜伏体内,经过相当时日,而后发病。狂犬咬伤之初仅见局部红肿疼痛,出血,经治疗后伤口愈合。发病时可见头痛、烦躁不安、恐水、恐风、恐声、牙关紧闭、抽搐等症,甚则导致死亡。

1.5.3 毒蛇咬伤

毒蛇咬伤人体,其毒汁可通过毒牙侵入人体而致人发病。不同的毒蛇含有不同的毒汁,对人体损害也不同,

human body with different symptoms. Due to the different clinical manifestations, the poisonous snake bite is divided into three types of wind-toxin, fire-toxin and wind-fire-toxin.

1.6   Lightning wound

The lightning wound refers to the damage of human body by the lightning. The lightning wound includes the lightning wound and electroshock. In mild conditions, there are symptoms of local burn of skin, or numbness of skin and muscles. In severe conditions, the zang-fu organs, tissues and organs may be damaged, leading to loss of consciousness, coma, convulsion, severe burn of body, even death.

2   Drug poisoning

2.1   Formation of drug poisoning

2.1.1   Overdose

If the herbs, especially those poison-containing herbs, are applied in overdose, it may cause poisoning condition. The herbs of raw *Aconiti Radix* (Chuan Wu), raw *Aconiti Kusenzoffii Radix* (Cao Wu), *Strychni Semen* (Ma Qian Zi), *Asari Radix et Rhizoma* (Xi Xin), *Crotonis Fructus* (Ba Dou), raw *Pinelliae Rhizoma* (Ban Xia), *Realgar* (Xiong Huang), etc. are poison-containing. Therefore, the routine doses of these herbs are determined strictly in clinical practice, the overdose may cause poisoning.

2.1.2   Improper processing method

The toxicity of some poison-containing herbs may be decreased through proper processing methods. For example, Chuan wu can be processed by fire-burning or honey-preserving, Ban xia can be

因而其临床表现也不一样。根据毒蛇咬伤后临床表现，一般可分为风毒、火毒和风火毒三类。

1.6   雷击伤

雷击伤是指雷电对人体造成的损害。雷击伤包括雷击伤和电灼伤，其实皆为电流击伤。轻者，仅有肌肤灼伤或肢节肌肤不仁，重者可以引起机体脏腑及组织器官的损害，出现神志不清、昏迷抽搐、肢体焦灼，甚则死亡。

2   药邪

2.1   药邪的形成

2.1.1   用药过量

特别是一些含有毒性的药物，过量则易中毒。例如生川乌、生草乌、马钱子、细辛、巴豆、生半夏、雄黄等均含有毒性，临床使用时有常用量的规定，用量过大则易引起中毒。

2.1.2   炮制不当

有些含有毒性的药物经过适当的炮制可减轻毒性。例如，乌头火炮或蜜制，半夏姜制，附子浸漂、水煮等就能

processed by baking with ginger, *Aconiti Lateralis Radix Praeparata* (Fu Zi) can be processed by soaking and rinsing or water-boiling. These processing methods may decrease the toxicity. If the processing methods do not conform to the standards, there can be poisoning.

2.1.3　Improper compatibility

　　The joint application of some herbs may increase their toxicity, as the joint application of *Radix* et *Veratri Nigri Rhizoma et Radix* (Li Lu) and *Ginseng Radix* (Ren Shen), the joint application of *Hydrargyrum* (Shui Yin) and *Arsenicum Album* (Pi Shuang), etc. As the regulation, "the eighteen incompatibilities" and "the nineteen antagonisms" are summarized by the ancients. Therefore, the improper compatibility of herbs may also cause poisoning.

2.1.4　Incorrect application

　　If the prohibited herbs are applied during pregnancy, it is possible to cause some other diseases and to injure the fetus. Some poison-containing herbs should be decocted first so as to decrease their toxicity, if they are not decocted first, they may cause poisoning of human body.

2.2　Pathogenic characteristics of drug poisoning

2.2.1　Symptoms of poisoning

　　The misapplication or overdose of poison-containing herbs may cause poisoning symptoms, which are related to the composition and dosage of the poison-containing herbs. In mild conditions, there are symptoms of dizziness, palpitation, nausea, vomiting, abdominal pain, diarrhea, numbness of tongue, etc. In severe conditions, there are symp-

減輕毒性。若对这些药物炮制不规范,则易致中毒。

2.1.3　配伍不当

　　还有某些药物相互合用则会使毒性增加。例如藜芦和人参、水银与砒霜等,古人分别概括成"十八反""十九畏"。因而,配伍不当,也会引起中毒。

2.1.4　用法不当

　　如妇女妊娠时使用了应该禁忌的药物也会变生他疾,并伤及胎儿。此外,有些药物先煎可减低毒性,应先煎而未先煎也会导致人体中毒。诸如此类,均为药物炮制、配伍、用法不当而致病。

2.2　药邪致病特点

2.2.1　多表现为中毒症状

　　误服或过服有毒性的药物,临床上多表现为中毒症状,并且其中毒症状与毒性药物的成分、剂量有关。轻者表现为头晕心悸、恶心呕吐、腹痛腹泻、舌麻等症状,重者可出现全身肌肉颤

toms of twitching of muscles of whole body, restlessness, jaundice, cyanosis, bleeding, coma, even death.

2.2.2 Abrupt onset of disease and worsening condition

After taking overdose of poison-containing herbs, the acute poisoning may occur with an abrupt of onset. If the correct toxin-relieved methods are not applied promptly, the condition will be worsened rapidly, so as to cause severe damages to the zang-fu organs of human body, even cause death.

2.2.3 Worsening of disease to induce other diseases

If the herbs are not applied properly, it is possible to assist the Xie (Pathogenic) Qi and injure the Zheng (Anti-Pathogenic) Qi, so as to worsen the primary disease on one hand, and to induce some other disease on the other hand. For example, if the herbs are not applied properly during pregnancy, it is possible to cause miscarriage, teratism or stillbirth.

3 Mala praxis

The mala praxis refers to the doctors' fault. The doctors' fault may worsen the disease or induce some other disease, so that the mala praxis is one of the causative factors of diseases.

3.1 Formation of *mala praxis*

3.1.1 Improper words

As a doctor, he should talk to the patients with nice words, which is beneficial to increase the patients' confidence in curing the diseases and to function as the supplementary treatment. On the contrary, if a doctor talks to the patients with re-

动、烦躁、黄疸、紫绀、出血，昏迷乃至死亡。

2.2.2 发病急,病势易趋危重状态

服了毒性大的药物往往会引起急性中毒,发病急骤。若不及时采取正确的解毒等治法,往往病情会迅速恶化,对机体脏器造成严重的损害,甚至死亡。

2.2.3 加重病情,变生他疾

药物使用不当,会助邪伤正,一方面使原有的病情加重,另一方面还会引起新的疾病,如妇女妊娠期用药不当会引起流产、畸胎或死胎等。

3 医过

所谓医过是指医生的过失。医生的过失可造成病情加重或滋生他疾,故医过也属于引起疾病的原因之一。

3.1 医过的形成

3.1.1 语言不妥

医生使用美好的语言有利于增强病人战胜疾病的信心,能起到辅助治疗作用。反之讲话不注意场合、分寸或语言粗鲁,均会增加患者

gardless words in some circumstance and propriety or even rude words, it is possible to increase a load on patients' mind, to worsen the condition, even to induce some other diseases. Besides, the undignified or unease manner of the doctor may bring the patients with the harmful stimuli, even make the patients to refuse treatment or worsen the condition.

3.1.2　Inconformity to standard in writing

When a doctor prescribes the drugs, he should write the common names of drugs, with a clear and legible handwriting. On the contrary, if some alternative names or rarely used names of drugs are written intentionally, it is possible to cause misunderstanding, and the pharmacists fail to make the prescription promptly, so as to bungle the chance of curing the disease.

3.1.3　Mistreatment

It is the mistakes made by a doctor in therapeutic methods and drug prescription due to the incorrect identification of pattern. For example, the reinforcing herbs are misused in the excess pattern which is misdiagnosed as the deficiency pattern, or the reducing herbs are misused in the deficiency pattern which is misdiagnosed as the excess pattern.

3.1.4　Improper operation

It is necessary in the treatment of patients to be serious and careful, and to be scrupulous about every detail. On the contrary, any carelessness or rude movement in the diagnosis and treatment may cause a medical mistake or accident.

3.2　Pathogenic characteristics of *mala praxis*

The different modes of mala praxis lead to different diseases and patterns. The improper words are similar to seven emotional factors. The damage

的思想负担,加重病情,甚至产生新生病症。此外医生的举止鲁莽、不端,同样会给患者带来不良刺激,有的会因此拒绝治疗或加重病情。

3.1.2　文字不规范

医生开处方,药名要通俗易懂,字迹要工整清晰。反之,故意开些别名、僻名,则易使配药人员难以理解,因而在危急之际,就会贻误病情。

3.1.3　误治

由于医生临床辨证不正确导致治法、用药的错误。如明为实证而判为虚证,误用补药;实为虚证而断为实证,误用泻药,不仅旧病难以治愈,反又添新疾。

3.1.4　操作不当

诊治病人必须认真细致,一丝不苟。反之,诊治病人过程中粗心大意,动作粗鲁,往往会造成医疗差错或事故。

3.2　医过的致病特点

不同的医过方式可造成不同的病证。语言不妥与七情致病特点相近。文字不规

of the patient caused by inconformity to standard in writing or by mistreatment is similar to the drug poisoning. The pathogenic characteristics of improper operation are similar to those of traumatic injury. These are the general conditions, but the specific conditions should be dealt with in different ways.

4   Innate factors

The innate factors imply the causative factors of diseases formed before birth, due to the parents' body constitutions or the fetus development, the so-called congenital pathogens. For example, if the parents are old in age, or weak in body, or sick, or lack of essence and blood, their born child is weak in body and easy to die young. If the mother, during her pregnancy, has an abnormal daily life, or drinks alcohol, or is angry or frightened, her fetus' development will be influenced.

范、误治对患者造成的损害则类同于药邪。操作不当与外伤的致病特点较为相似，这些一般仅是情况，特殊的又当别论。

4   先天因素

先天因素是指人未出生前因父母体质或胎儿发育过程中形成的病因，即先天性致病因素。例如由于父母年老、体衰、多病、精血亏虚，则所生之子体弱易于夭折。假使母妊之时，调摄失常，醉酒嗜饮，忿怒惊扑，则势必会影响胎儿的发育。

Chapter 6 Pathogenesis

第6章 病机

The pathogenesis refers to the mechanism of the occurrence, development and mutation of diseases. The pathogenesis is divided into the pathogenic mechanism and pathological mechanism.

病机,指疾病发生、发展与变化的机理。病机,可分为发病机理与病变机理。

Section 1 Pathogenic Mechanism

第1节 发病机理

It is believed in TCM that the harmony between yin and yang of the human body is the healthy state, reflected in the harmony and integration among the zang-fu organs, meridians and collaterals, qi, blood and body fluid of the human body, and between the human body and environment. If this state of harmony and integration is disturbed due to various pathogenic factors, a disease occurs. The occurrence of the disease is actually related to two basic aspects of the Xie (Pathogenic) Qi and the Zheng (Anti-Pathogenic) Qi. Besides, the various body constitutions also possess the important influence on the occurrence of the disease.

中医发病学认为,人体阴阳平和,即是健康状态,表现为人体各脏腑、经络、气血津液之间,以及人体与环境之间的协调与统一。如果在各种致病因素的作用下,这种平衡协调与统一状态被破坏,就会发生疾病。疾病的发生,实际上关系到邪气与正气两个基本方面,不同的体质对发病也有重要影响。

1 Xie (Pathogenic) Qi and Zheng (Anti-Pathogenic) Qi related to disease occurrence

1 邪正与发病

The occurrence of the disease is a very complicated process, but its essential is the mutual

疾病的发生是一个极其复杂的过程,但其本质在于

conflict between the Xie (Pathogenic) Qi and Zheng (Anti-Pathogenic) qi, and such a mutual conflict runs through the whole process of the disease.

邪气与正气的相互抗争，邪正相争贯穿于疾病过程的始终。

1.1 The deficiency of the Zheng (Anti-Pathogenic) Qi and the attack of the Xie (Pathogenic) Qi are the important factors to cause diseases

The occurrence of the disease should possess two conditions: the first is the insufficiency of the Zheng (Anti-Pathogenic) Qi, and the second is the attack of the Xie (Pathogenic) Qi. Opposite to the Xie (Pathogenic) Qi, the Zheng (Anti-Pathogenic) Qi is the fundamental substance to form up the human body and to maintain the vital activities of the human body, functioning to realize the normal actions of the zang-fu organs, meridians and collaterals. When the Xie (Pathogenic) Qi attacks the human body, this type of substance functions to resist the Xie (Pathogenic) Qi and preserve the human body.

The Zheng (Anti-Pathogenic) Qi should be kept sufficient and vigorous, and then it is capable to resist the invasion of the Xie (Pathogenic) Qi. The sufficiency of the Zheng (Anti-Pathogenic) Qi is based upon the substances of essence, qi, blood and body fluid and their normal functions, while the sufficiency and vigorousness of these substances directly influence the sufficiency of the Zheng (Anti-Pathogenic) Qi. If the Zheng (Anti-Pathogenic) Qi is not sufficient, the ability of human body in resisting the Xie (Pathogenic) Qi decreases, and the Xie (Pathogenic) Qi is easy to attack the human body to cause diseases.

1.1 正虚、邪侵是发病的重要因素

疾病的发生必须具备两个条件，一是正气不足，二是邪气侵袭。正气，是相对于邪气而言的，是构成人体和维持人体生命活动的基本物质，一般情况下发挥着维持脏腑经络正常功能的作用。当邪气侵袭人体时，这种物质又担负着抗御邪气、维护人体的作用。

正气必须保持充盛，才能抗御邪气的侵袭。正气的充盛与否，取决于精、气血、津液等物质及其所发挥的功能是否正常，这些物质的充足与否直接影响着正气的盛衰。如果正气不足，人体抵抗邪气的能力下降，邪气即易于侵袭人体而导致发病。

The Xie (Pathogenic) Qi is the factor to directly disturb the normal physiological functions of human body, including the six exogenous pathogens,
the Li (Epidemic) Qi, the seven emotional factors,
the improper food intake, the improper strain and
idleness, the phlegm-rheum, the stagnant blood,
etc. The occurrence of the disease is the result of
the mutual conflict between the Zheng (Anti-Pathogenic) Qi and Xie (Pathogenic) Qi after the invasion of the Xie (Pathogenic) Qi into the human
body. Why the Xie (Pathogenic) Qi can attack the
human body, it is because that the Zheng (Anti-
Pathogenic) Qi is not sufficient inside the human
body. Only when the Zheng (Anti-Pathogenic) Qi
is deficient, can the Xie (Pathogenic) Qi attack the
human body. This type of Xie (Pathogenic) Qi is
called "the Xie (Pathogenic) Qi due to deficiency"
in TCM. The Xie (Pathogenic) Qi due to deficiency
is combined with the deficiency of the Zheng (Anti-
Pathogenic) Qi inside the human body, as the two
necessary conditions in the occurrence of the disease. There is such a theory of "the mutual conflict
between two deficiencies" in Huang Di Nei Jing.

1.2　The actions of the Zheng (Anti-Pathogenic) Qi are different from those of the Xie (Pathogenic) Qi during the process of the disease occurrence

The insufficiency of the Zheng (Anti-Pathogenic) Qi and the attack of the Xie (Pathogenic) Qi
are the two important factors to cause diseases, but
the actions of the Zheng (Anti-Pathogenic) Qi are
different from those of the Xie (Pathogenic) Qi
during the process of the disease occurrence.

邪气是直接干扰人体正
常生理功能的因素,包括六
淫、疫疠、七情致病、饮食所
伤、劳逸失当、痰饮、瘀血等。
疾病的发生,是邪气侵入人
体,与正气相互抗争的结果。
邪气之所以能侵入人体,与
人体正气的不足有密切关
系。由于邪气只有在正气虚
弱时才能侵袭人体,故中医
学把这种邪气称为"虚邪"。
虚邪与人体正气之虚相合,
是疾病产生的两个必要条
件,所以《黄帝内经》有"两虚
相搏"而致病的理论。

1.2　正气与邪气在发病过程中的不同作用

虽然正气不足与邪气侵
袭是发病的两个重要因素,
但正气与邪气在发病过程中
所起的作用有所不同。

1.2.1 The insufficiency of the Zheng (Anti-Pathogenic) Qi is the intrinsic basis of the disease occurrence

It is believed in TCM that the functions of the Zheng (Anti-Pathogenic) Qi inside the human body are very important. If the zang-fu organs function normally, the Zheng (Anti-Pathogenic) Qi will be vigorous, qi and blood will be sufficient, and the defending function is normal, and the pathogens cannot attack to cause the diseases. Therefore, it is said in Huang Di Nei Jing that "when the Zheng (Anti-Pathogenic) Qi stays normally inside, the Xie (Pathogenic) Qi has no way to attack". When the Zheng (Anti-Pathogenic) Qi of human body is weak and its defending function is abnormal and unable to resist the Xie (Pathogenic) Qi, the Xie (Pathogenic) Qi is capable to get a chance to attack the body, to cause the disharmony of yin and yang and the disturbance of zang-fu organs of human body, so as to lead to the occurrence of disease. Therefore, it is also said in Huang Di Nei Jing that "why the Xie (Pathogenic) Qi attacks, it is because that the Zheng (Anti-Pathogenic) Qi is deficient". It is stressed in TCM that the Zheng (Anti-Pathogenic) Qi plays an leading role in the process of disease occurrence.

There are different conditions that the insufficiency of the Zheng (Anti-Pathogenic) Qi causes the attack of the Xie (Pathogenic) Qi. There is the condition of the general Zheng (Anti-Pathogenic) Qi insufficiency, and also the condition of the local Zheng (Anti-Pathogenic) Qi insufficiency as well. There is the condition of the persistent insufficiency of the Zheng (Anti-Pathogenic) Qi, and also the

1.2.1 正气不足是发病的内在根据

中医发病学非常重视人体正气的作用,认为若内脏功能正常,正气旺盛,气血充盈,卫外固密,病邪难以侵入,疾病就无从发生。所以,《黄帝内经》有"正气存内,邪不可干"的论述。只有在人体正气相对虚弱,卫外不固,抗邪无力的情况下,邪气方能乘虚而入,使人体阴阳失调,脏腑功能紊乱,从而导致发病。故《黄帝内经》又说:"邪之所凑,其气必虚。"由此而论,中医学强调正气在发病中的主导地位。

正气不足导致邪气侵袭有不同情况,既有整体正气不足的,也有局部正气虚弱的;既有一贯正气不足的,也有一时正气虚弱的。整体正气不足的,感邪后易导致全身性疾病,或邪气先侵犯局部,然后向其他部位传变,病

condition of the temporary insufficiency of the Zheng (Anti-Pathogenic) Qi. In the condition of the general Zheng (Anti-Pathogenic) Qi insufficiency, the Xie (Pathogenic) Qi attacks the body to cause the general disease, or to cause the local disease which transfers to other parts of the body and broadens the sick scope. In the condition of the local Zheng (Anti-Pathogenic) Qi insufficiency, the Xie (Pathogenic) Qi attacks the weak area to cause the local disease, which usually does not transfer to other parts of the body. In the condition of the persistent insufficiency of the Zheng (Anti-Pathogenic) Qi, the body constitution is weak, so the Xie (Pathogenic) Qi has more chances to attack the body to cause diseases. In the condition of the temporary insufficiency of the Zheng (Anti-Pathogenic) Qi, the body constitution is not very poor. The factors as fatigue, hunger, mental scar, sexual activity, menstruation, or delivery, etc. may cause the temporary insufficiency of the Zheng (Anti-Pathogenic) Qi. In such a situation, it is advisable to nourish and protect the body properly, so as to avoid the invasion of the Xie (Pathogenic) Qi. Any carelessness may cause the invasion of the Xie (Pathogenic) Qi.

The different degrees of the Zheng (Anti-Pathogenic) Qi insufficiency may cause the different seriousness of the Xie (Pathogenic) Qi attacking, and also the different degrees of the pathological reactions induced by the Xie (Pathogenic) Qi as well. Generally speaking, in the condition in which the Zheng (Anti-Pathogenic) Qi insufficiency is more severe, the Xie (Pathogenic) Qi attacking the body is also more severe. In the condition in which the Zheng (Anti-Pathogenic) Qi insufficiency is not se-

变范围容易扩展。局部正气虚弱的,邪气主要侵犯虚弱之处而形成局部性病变,一般不易向别处传变。一贯正气不足的,体质较弱,邪气侵入机会多,发病机会也多。一时正气虚弱的,平时体质尚好,若遇疲劳、饥饿、精神创伤、房事后、妇女经期、分娩等情形,即可出现一时性正气虚弱。此时若养护得法,可免受邪气侵袭。稍有不慎,邪气就会乘虚而入。

正气不足程度不同,所感邪气轻重不同,感邪后引起的病理反应强弱也不一样。一般地说,正气虚弱较甚者,感邪较重;正气虚弱不甚者,感邪也较轻。感邪引起的病理反应强弱,与邪正斗争的激烈程度有关。凡正气不足较严重者,抗邪无力,其病理反应往往较弱,多形

vere, the Xie (Pathogenic) Qi attacking the body is also less severe. The degrees of the pathological reactions induced by the Xie (Pathogenic) Qi are related to the degrees of the conflict between the Xie (Pathogenic) Qi and Zheng (Anti-Pathogenic) Qi. In the condition in which the Zheng (Anti-Pathogenic) Qi insufficiency is rather severe, the Zheng (Anti-Pathogenic) Qi is unable to resist the Xie (Pathogenic) Qi, leading to the lighter pathological reactions and forming the deficiency patterns or the intermingling patterns of both deficiency and excess. In the condition in which the Zheng (Anti-Pathogenic) Qi insufficiency is not severe, the Zheng (Anti-Pathogenic) Qi is strong enough to fight against the Xie (Pathogenic) Qi, to cause a fierce conflict between the Xie (Pathogenic) Qi and Zheng (Anti-Pathogenic) Qi and the strong pathological reactions, leading to the excess patterns.

1.2.2 The attack of the Xie (Pathogenic) Qi is the important condition of the disease occurrence

In TCM, it is believed that the Zheng (Anti-Pathogenic) Qi plays the major leading role in the occurrence of disease, but the important action of the Xie (Pathogenic) Qi is also stressed. In the person with the insufficiency of the Zheng (Anti-Pathogenic) Qi, there are no any manifestations of diseases if the body is not attacked by the Xie (Pathogenic) Qi. Only when the Xie (Pathogenic) Qi attacks the body to fight against the Zheng (Anti-Pathogenic) Qi, can the obvious manifestations of diseases occur. That is to say that the attack of the Xie (Pathogenic) Qi is the important condition of the disease occurrence. In some specific conditions,

成虚证或虚实错杂证;正气不足不甚严重者,由于正气尚能奋起抗邪,邪正相争激烈,其病理反应也较强,多形成实证。

1.2.2 邪气侵袭是发病的重要条件

中医学虽重视正气,强调正气在发病中的主导地位,但并不排斥邪气在发病中的重要作用。一般正气不足之人,在未感受邪气之时,可无疾病表现,只有当邪气侵袭之后,邪气与正气相争,才会表现出明显的疾病症状。也就是说,邪气侵袭是疾病发生的一个重要条件。在某些特殊情况下,邪气也可以在发病中起主导作用,如高温、高压电流、化学毒

as high temperature, high-voltage electroshock, chemical or toxic agent, bullet wound, poisonous snake bite, etc., the Xie (Pathogenic) Qi plays the major leading role in the occurrence of disease, even when the Zheng (Anti-Pathogenic) Qi is sufficient. Besides, the Li (Epidemic) Qi is often the decisive factor of the disease occurrence, leading to the severe epidemic diseases. Therefore, it is advanced by the ancients the preventive thought of "avoiding the poisonous Xie (Pathogenic) Qi" in the life preservation, at the same time when one has to protect and strengthen the Zheng (Anti-Pathogenic) Qi.

As the important condition of the disease occurrence, the Xie (Pathogenic) Qi is also related to the pathological changes after the disease occurrence, the property of the Xie (Pathogenic) Qi, the seriousness of the Xie (Pathogenic) Qi and the location where the Xie (Pathogenic) Qi attacks.

Influence of property of the Xie (Pathogenic) Qi on the disease occurrence: The Xie (Pathogenic) Qi of different properties cause the diseases of different properties. In the diseases caused by the six exogenous pathogens, the manifestations of the diseases are different, as the wind pattern occurs if the pathogenic wind attacks the body, the cold pattern occurs if the pathogenic wind attacks the body, the damp pattern occurs if the pathogenic damp attacks the body, and the heat pattern occurs if the pathogenic heat attacks the body. The Li (Epidemic) Qi is more poisonous that the six exogenous pathogens, therefore the diseases caused by the Li (Epidemic) Qi is featured of strong infection, tendency to spread, abrupt onset and serious and critical condi-

剂、枪弹杀伤、毒蛇咬伤等，即使是正气强盛之人，也不免被伤害而致病。又如疫疠病邪，常常成为疾病发生的决定因素，因而导致疾病的大流行。因此，在注意保护和增强正气的同时，古代中医养生学也提出了"避其毒气"的预防思想。

邪气作为发病的重要条件，还表现为感邪后所导致的病理变化与邪气的性质、感邪轻重以及邪气作用的部位有关。

邪气性质对发病的影响：不同性质的邪气，可导致不同性质的疾病。如感受六淫邪气，各有不同的病证表现，感受风邪则形成风证，感受寒邪则形成寒证，感受湿邪则形成湿证，感受热邪则形成热证等等。疫疠之邪比一般六淫邪气毒性更强，所以疫疠致病往往传染性强，容易流行，且发病急骤，病情重笃。

tions.

Influence of the seriousness of the Xie (Pathogenic) Qi on the disease occurrence: The seriousness of the diseases due to the attack of the Xie (Pathogenic) Qi is related to the strength of the Zheng (Anti-Pathogenic) Qi, and also to the seriousness of the Xie (Pathogenic) Qi as well. Generally speaking, if the attacked Xie (Pathogenic) Qi is less serious, the conflict between the Xie (Pathogenic) Qi and Zheng (Anti-Pathogenic) Qi is more moderate, so the disease caused is milder. If the attacked Xie (Pathogenic) Qi is more serious, the conflict between the Xie (Pathogenic) Qi and Zheng (Anti-Pathogenic) Qi is fiercer, so the disease caused is more severe.

感邪轻重对发病的影响:感邪后发病的轻重,既与正气的强弱有关,也与感邪的轻重有关。一般来说,感邪轻者,其邪正相争较缓和,故发病较轻;感邪重者,其邪正相争也激烈,故发病较重。

Influence of the location where the Xie (Pathogenic) Qi attacks on the disease occurrence: Due to the different locations of human body where the Xie (Pathogenic) Qi attacks, the reactions of diseases are different. For example, if the pathogenic cold attacks the body surface and meridians, there are the symptoms of headache, aching of four limbs and body. If the pathogenic cold attacks the lung, there are the symptoms of cough and panting. If the pathogenic cold attacks the stomach, there are the symptoms of epigastric pain, vomiting, etc.

邪气作用部位对发病的影响:邪气侵入人体的部位不同,所形成的病证反应也不同。如寒邪客于肌表经脉,则头身四肢疼痛;寒邪袭肺,则咳嗽、气喘;寒邪犯胃,则脘痛、呕吐等。

2　Body constitution related to disease occurrence

The body constitution is closely related to the occurrence of disease. Therefore, the body constitution factors are highly stressed in TCM.

2.1　Concept of body constitution

The body constitution refers to some characteristic property of human body in the aspect of the or-

2　体质与发病

体质与发病的关系非常密切,所以中医学历来重视人的体质因素。

2.1　体质的概念

体质,是指人体在形态结构、生理功能、心理状态等

ganic structures, physiological functions and psychological states. The body constitution is formed from the congenital, and nourished by the acquired.

It is believed in TCM that the body constitution is the manifestation of the functional states of the zang-fu organs, meridians and collaterals, tissues and organs in human body, reflecting the volume states of qi, blood, yin and yang of human body. The strength of the anti-pathogenic ability is the manifestation of the body constitution in the occurrence of disease.

2.2　Formation of body constitution

The formation of the body constitution is based upon the congenital Jing (Essence) Qi from the parents, the so-called "natural endowment". If a person has a highly natural endowment, his body constitution is strong. If a person has a low natural endowment, his body constitution is weak. Due to the difference in body constitutions, the susceptibility to the diseases is different. Many genetic or familial diseases are related to the body constitutions and diseases of the parents. Simultaneously, the nourishment and nursing during pregnancy are also important to the formation of the fetus body constitution, so it is why it is stressed on the nourishment of fetus in TCM.

After birth, the congenital body constitution is formed and usually not changeable. From this sense, the congenital body constitution may determine the whole life of a person. But the acquired life state, as the factors of food intake, life habit, sports and diseases may influence on the basically formed body constitution. It is believed in TCM that various kinds methods of life preservation

方面综合的相对稳定的某种特质。体质形成于先天，得养于后天。

中医学理论认为，体质的本质是人体脏腑经络等组织器官功能状态的表现，它反映了人体气血阴阳的盛衰状况。抗邪能力的强弱，是体质因素在发病中的表现。

2.2　体质的形成

体质形成的基础秉承于父母的先天精气，中医将此称之为"禀赋"。凡禀赋强者体质也强壮，禀赋弱者体质也虚弱。体质强弱不等，对邪气的易感性差异就很大。许多遗传性或家族性疾病都与父母的身体素质及其患病情况有关。同时，母体怀孕期间的养护对胎儿体质的形成也有重要影响，所以中医学历来重视养胎。

婴儿出生后，其先天的体质基础已经形成，一般是不易改变的。从这个意义上讲，先天的体质基础可以影响人的一生。但是，后天的生活状况，如饮食、起居、运动、疾病等因素也会影响到已经基本形成的体质。中医

function "to collect the essence and to supplement the spirit", so as to give full play to the congenital advantages of body constitution or to make up for the congenital deficiency of body constitution, for the purpose to strengthen the body constitution. Thus, the strong body constitution will be stronger, and the weak body constitution will be strengthened. On the contrary, if a person is careless in life preservation, his strong congenital body constitution will be weaken or even premature, or his weak congenital body constitution will be weaker, so he will be severely sick and even die young. Certainly, the change of the body constitution is a gradually slow and long process.

Due to affection of some pathogens or inoculations make the body to gain some specific immunity to some diseases. This is an important mode to form up some specific body constitution through the acquired ways.

2.3 Classification of body constitution

It is believed in the theory of body constitution in TCM that the human body constitutions are different. The study on this type of differences forms up the classified theory of the body constitution. The classification of body constitution is importantly significant for further illustration on the pathogenesis.

Generally, the body constitution is often divided into two types of the strong and weak body constitutions. In order to illustrate the mechanism of the diseases of different properties in details, it is put forward more concrete classification of body constitution in TCM.

According to the records in ancient classics,

学认为,后天的诸多养生方法可以"积精全神",更充分地发挥先天的体质优势,或弥补先天的体质不足,从而达到增强体质的目的。这样,先天体质强者可以更强,先天体质弱者可以由弱转强。反之,若不注意养生,先天体质强者会由强变弱或过早衰竭,先天体质弱者则更促其多病甚或夭折。当然,体质的改变是一个缓慢渐进的过程。

因感受某种病邪或经预防接种后可获得对某种疾病的特异免疫力,这是后天通过获得性方式形成某种特异体质的重要形式。

2.3 体质的分类

中医体质学说认为,人类体质是有差异性的。对这种差异性进行研究,就形成了关于体质的分类理论。体质的分类对进一步阐明发病学原理具有重要意义。

一般情况下,人们常把体质划分为强、弱两类。为了更详细地阐述各种不同性质的疾病发生的原理,中医体质学提出了更具体的体质分类法。

从文献记载看,体质的

there are many methods to classify the body constitutions, such as: ① the classified method according
to yin and yang; ② the classified method according
to five elements; ③ the classified method according
to zang-fu organs; ④ the classified method according to qi, blood and body fluid; ⑤ the comprehen-
sively classified method. All these classified methods are complicated and overlapped, so some commonly-seen body constitutions in clinic are
introduced here as follows.

2.3.1　Body constitution of qi deficiency

The body constitution of qi deficiency refers to
the body constitution in which the Yuan (Primary)
Qi is deficient. The person with the body constitution of qi deficiency is manifested in several aspects. If qi is deficient and fails to protect the body
surface, there are the manifestations of susceptibility to catch cold and profuse sweating. If qi is deficient and fail to promote, there are the manifestations of fatigue, lassitude and weak pulse. If qi is
deficient and fails to elevate the clear yang to nourish the clear aperture, there are the manifestations
of dizziness and blurring of vision. If qi is deficient
and fails to transport and transform the water and
disturbs the body fluid metabolism, the phlegm and
rheum may be produced.

2.3.2　Body constitution of blood deficiency

The body constitution of blood deficiency refers
to the body constitution in which the blood is
deficient. If the blood is deficient, it fails to moisturize and nourish the zang-fu organs, leading to the
manifestations of lusterless complexion, dizziness,
blurring of vision, numbness of limbs and body,
weakness in four limbs, poor sleep, dream-disturbed

分类方法很多，归纳起来大
致有以下几种：①阴阳分类
法；②五行分类法；③脏腑分
类法；④气血津液分类法；
⑤综合分类法。由于各种分
类方法内容繁杂，且相互交
叉重叠，这里选择临床常见
的几种体质类型加以介绍。

2.3.1　气虚质

气虚质，指元气偏虚体
质。气虚体质的人，其表现
涉及多个方面。如气偏虚则
卫外无力，肌表不固，容易感
冒，容易汗出；气偏虚则推动
无力，易致倦怠乏力、脉欠有
力；气偏虚则清阳不升，清窍
不充，易致头晕目眩；气偏虚
则运化无力，水液不化，输布
障碍，易致内生痰湿。

2.3.2　血虚质

血虚质，指血液偏虚体
质。血偏虚则濡养脏腑功能
不足，可有面色少华，容易出
现头昏眼花、肢体发麻、四肢
无力、少寐多梦等表现。妇
女容易出现月经量少、色淡、
舌质偏淡、脉搏偏于虚弱。

sleep, scanty volume and light color of blood in menstruation, pale tongue body and weak pulse.

2.3.3 Body constitution of yang deficiency

The body constitution of yang deficiency refers to the body constitution in which the yang qi is deficient. If yang is deficient and its warming function is weak, there may be the manifestations of fear of cold and chills in four limbs. If yang is deficient and its exciting function is weak, there may be the manifestations of low spirit and sleepiness. If yang is deficient and its transpiring function is weak, or if the yang qi of spleen and stomach is deficient, there may be the manifestations of unformed feces, pale tongue body and weak pulse. Yang deficiency also leads to yin excess and susceptible to incur the pathogenic cold or damp to cause diseases, or to cause the cold-transforming diseases after attack of other pathogens.

2.3.4 Body constitution of yin deficiency

The body constitution of yin deficiency refers to the body constitution in which the yin essence is deficient. The body constitution of yin deficiency has two features. Firstly, the body fluid, i. e. the normal water is deficient and fails to moisturize, leading to the manifestations of dryness, as dry throat, dry mouth, dry skin, dry feces, red and dry tongue body, etc. Secondly, if yin is deficiency, it fails to restrain yang, leading to the manifestations of internal heat or internal fire, as afternoon tidal fever, feverish sensation in palms and soles, vexation, poor sleep, thready and rapid pulse, etc.

2.3.5 Body constitution of phlegm-damp

The body constitution of phlegm-damp refers to the body constitution in which the metabolic function is weak and the phlegm and damp is then

2.3.3 阳虚质

阳虚质,指阳气偏虚的体质。阳虚体质之人,温煦功能偏弱,平素较为怕冷,四肢欠温;兴奋功能偏低,以致精神欠佳、睡眠偏多;阳虚蒸腾无力,脾胃阳气偏虚,易致大便欠实、舌淡脉弱。阳虚则阴盛,容易招致寒湿之邪入侵为病,或感受其他病邪而容易寒化。

2.3.4 阴虚质

阴虚质,指阴精偏虚的体质。阴虚体质的人,有两方面特点:一是体内津液,即正常水液偏少,失于滋润,容易出现干燥诸象,如咽干口燥、皮肤干燥、大便偏干、舌红欠润等。二是阴虚不能制约阳热,容易出现内热、内火,如午后潮热、手足心热、心烦少寐、脉细偏数等。

2.3.5 痰湿质

痰湿质,指津液代谢功能偏弱而痰湿偏重的体质。痰湿体质的人,形体多见肥

formed. In the body constitution of phlegm-damp, there are the manifestations of fat body, fatty and greasy skin on face, profuse sticky sweating, swollen tongue body, stickiness in mouth, unformed feces or pasty feces, etc. The damp is featured of heaviness and turbidity, leading to the manifestations of muddleheaded sensation, weighty sensation in body, excessive volume of leucorrhea, sticky tongue coating, wiry or rolling pulse.

2.3.6 Body constitution of damp-heat

The body constitution of damp-heat refers to the body constitution in which the damp and heat are heavy. In the body constitution of damp-heat, there are the manifestations of fatigue, lassitude, weighty sensation in head and body, fatty and greasy skin on face, frequent occurrence of acnes, bitter taste in mouth, foul breath, heavy body odor, pasty and stinking feces, dark-yellow color and heavy odor of urine, red tongue body, yellow-sticky tongue coating, yellow color of leucorrhea, pruritus vulvae, scrotum eczema, etc.

2.3.7 Body constitution of qi stagnation

The body constitution of qi stagnation refers to the body constitution in which the liver qi is susceptible to be stagnant and the qi activities are not smooth. In the body constitution of qi stagnation, there are the manifestations of severely emotional changes, emotional depression, low spirit, nervousness, anxiety, sentimentality, susceptibility to be frightened, sleep disturbance, frequent sighing, and distension and pain in breasts, irregular menstruation in fenales, etc.

2.3.8 Body constitution of blood stasis

The body constitution of blood stasis refers to

胖,面部皮肤油脂较多,多汗且黏,舌体胖大,口中黏腻,大便不成形或黏滞不爽。湿性重浊,故多见头脑昏沉、身重不爽、妇女带下量多、舌苔偏腻、脉多弦滑。

2.3.6 湿热质

湿热质,指湿热偏重的体质。湿热体质的人,常见倦怠乏力,头身沉重,面部油脂分泌偏多,易生痤疮,常感口苦、口臭,体味偏重,大便多粘滞不爽、臭秽难闻,小便偏黄且异味重,舌质偏红,舌苔可见黄腻。女性可见带下色黄,外阴瘙痒;男性可见阴囊湿疹等。

2.3.7 气郁质

气郁质,指容易肝气郁滞、气机不畅的体质。气郁体质的人,情绪波动较大,常感到闷闷不乐,情绪低沉,容易紧张,焦虑不安,多愁善感,容易惊吓,容易睡眠障碍,经常叹气。女性又多变现为乳房胀痛、月经不调等。

2.3.8 血瘀质

血瘀质,指血液运行失

the body constitution in which the blood circulation is not smooth. In the body constitution of blood stasis, there are the manifestations of dark complexion, pains occurring in head, body and limbs, irregular menstruation, dysmenorrhea, black-colored blood or blood clots in menstruation, dark tongue body with purple spots or purple patches, thready or choppy pulse.

The above-mentioned body constitutions may be concurrent, as the concurrent body constitution of yang deficiency and qi deficiency, the concurrent body constitution of phlegm-damp and blood stasis, etc.

2.4　Influence of body constitution on disease occurrence

Generally speaking, if the body constitution is strong, the Zheng (Anti-Pathogenic) Qi is sufficient, so the Xie (Pathogenic) Qi is not easy to attack the body to cause diseases. If the body constitution is weak, the Zheng (Anti-Pathogenic) Qi is deficient, so the Xie (Pathogenic) Qi is easy to attack the body to cause diseases. Furthermore, the different body constitutions possess some specific influences on the occurrence of diseases.

2.4.1　The different body constitutions possess the different susceptibilities to the different types of Xie (Pathogenic) Qi

The different body constitutions possess the different susceptibilities to the Xie (Pathogenic) Qi. The person with the body constitution of yin deficiency is susceptible to be attacked by the yang pathogens, as the pathogenic wind, heat, etc. The person with the body constitution of yang deficiency is susceptible to be attacked by the yin pathogens, as

畅的体质。可表现为面色晦暗、头身肢体容易出现疼痛；妇女易见月经不调，或痛经、或经色紫黑有瘀血块，舌质多偏暗，或有瘀点瘀斑，脉多细涩。

以上各型体质可以相兼，如阳虚质可兼气虚质，痰湿质可兼瘀血质等。

2.4　体质对发病的影响

一般说来，体质强者，正气充盛，邪气不易侵入，故较少发病；体质弱者，正气不足，易被邪气侵袭，故容易发病。除此而外，不同的体质类型对疾病的发生还有一些特殊的影响。

2.4.1　不同体质类型对不同邪气的易感性不同

体质类型不同，对邪气的易感性也不同。如阴虚体质的人，易感受风、热等阳邪；阳虚体质的人，易感受寒、湿等阴邪；津血偏虚体质的人，易感受燥邪等。

the pathogenic cold, damp, etc. The person with the body constitution of body fluid and blood deficiency is susceptible to be attacked by the pathogenic dryness.

2.4.2 In different body constitutions, the regulations of disease occurrence are different

The location and property of the disease due to invasion of the Xie (Pathogenic) Qi are determinedly influenced by the body constitution. In terms of the disease location, the pathogen is susceptible to attack the weak area of the body so as to cause some specific disease. In the person with the spleen qi deficiency, the Xie (Pathogenic) Qi is susceptible to attack or transfer to the spleen to cause the spleen disease. In the person with the lung qi deficiency, the Xie (Pathogenic) Qi is susceptible to attack or transfer to the lung to caused the lung disease. In the person with the heart qi deficiency, the Xie (Pathogenic) Qi is susceptible to attack and transfer to the heart to cause the heart disease. In the person with the Wei (Defensive) Qi deficiency, the Xie (Pathogenic) Qi is susceptible to attack the body surface to cause the exterior pattern.

The different body constitutions also act to decide the different properties of the diseases after the attack of the Xie (Pathogenic) Qi. In the body constitution of yang excess, the exogenous pathogens attack the body and are susceptible to be transformed into heat or dryness. In the body constitution of yin excess, the exogenous pathogens attack the body and are susceptible to be transformed into cold or damp. Therefore, in the different body constitutions, which attacked by the same type of

2.4.2　不同体质类型感邪后的发病规律不同

邪气侵入人体后的发病部位及形成何种性质的疾病,受其体质类型的决定性影响。从发病部位来看,素体有虚弱之处,感邪后即易传向体虚部位而形成某种特殊病变。如脾气偏虚者,邪气易传向脾而形成脾病;肺气偏虚者,邪气易传向肺而形成肺病;心气偏虚者,邪气易传向心而形成心病;卫气偏虚者,邪气易逗留于外而形成表证。

体质类型还能决定感邪后形成病证的性质。如阳盛体质,感受外邪后容易热化、燥化,阴盛体质感受邪气后容易寒化、湿化。因此,在同一环境中感受相同的邪气,不同体质者将形成不同性质的疾病。中医体质学把这种现象称为"从化"。

Xie (Pathogenic) Qi in the same environment, the diseases of different properties will be caused. This type of phenomenon is called "the sequential transformation" in the theory of body constitution of TCM.

Section 2   Pathological Mechanism

The pathological mechanism refers to the mechanism of the development and mutation after the occurrence of the disease, including the basic property and developing regulation after the formation of the disease.

The occurrence of the disease is the result of the conflict of the Xie (Pathogenic) Qi and Zheng (Anti-Pathogenic) Qi, and such a conflict runs all over the whole process of the disease. During the process of the disease, if the Zheng (Anti-Pathogenic) Qi is injured, the equilibrium and harmony between yin and yang are disturbed, or the functions of the zang-fu organs and meridians-collaterals are disturbed, or the circulations of qi, blood and body fluid are disturbed, so as to cause various pathological changes in the whole body or local areas. Therefore, the diseases are various in types and their clinical manifestations are complicated, but each disease or symptom possesses its own pathological mechanism, which is nothing but the regulations of the pathological changes, as the conflict between Xie (Pathogenic) Qi and Zheng (Anti-Pathogenic) Qi, the disharmony of yin and yang and the abnormalities of qi, blood and body fluid.

第 2 节

病变机理

病变机理,是疾病发生以后发展变化的机理,包括疾病形成后的基本属性及其传变的规律。

疾病的发生,是邪正相争的结果,整个疾病过程,始终贯穿着邪正相争。在疾病过程中,如果正气受到损伤,阴阳平和被破坏,并使脏腑、经络的功能失调,或使气血津液运行紊乱,就会产生全身或局部的多种多样的病理变化。因此,尽管疾病的种类繁多,临床表现错综复杂,每种疾病或症状都有各自的病变机理,但从总体来说,都离不开邪正盛衰、阴阳失调、气血津液失常等病机变化的一般规律。

1 Conflict between Xie (Pathogenic) Qi and Zheng (Anti-Pathogenic) Qi

The conflict between the Xie (Pathogenic) Qi and Zheng (Anti-Pathogenic) Qi refers to the strength ratio of both sides during the disease process when the Zheng (Anti-Pathogenic) Qi of human body fights against the Xie (Pathogenic) Qi. The result of the conflict between the Xie (Pathogenic) Qi and Zheng (Anti-Pathogenic) Qi, influences the change of deficiency and excess in the property of the disease on one hand, and directly influences the development, improvement and prognosis of the disease on the other hand.

1.1 Conflict between Xie (Pathogenic) Qi and Zheng (Anti-Pathogenic) Qi related to the mutations of deficiency and excess

In terms of the concepts of the deficiency and excess, it is said in Huang Di Nei Jing that "the preponderance of the Xie (Pathogenic) Qi is the excess, while the loss of the Jing (Essence) Qi is the deficiency". That is to say that "the excess" refers to the attacked Xie (Pathogenic) Qi, while "the deficiency" refers to the insufficient Zheng (Anti-Pathogenic) Qi.

1.1.1 Excess pattern

The excess pattern is a kind of pathological reflection in which the preponderance of the Xie (Pathogenic) Qi is the predominant cause. In this condition, the Zheng (Anti-Pathogenic) Qi is not deficient, or is generally healthy even it is damages in some degree, so it is strong enough to fight against the Xie (Pathogenic) Qi. The conflict between the Xie (Pathogenic) Qi and Zheng (Anti-

1 邪正盛衰

邪正盛衰,是指在疾病过程中,人体正气和致病邪气之间由于相互抗争所发生的双方力量对比的盛衰变化。邪正盛衰变化的结果,一方面影响着病证性质的虚实变化,另一方面直接影响着疾病的转归预后。

1.1 邪正盛衰与虚实变化

《黄帝内经》对虚和实有明确的定义,即"邪气盛则实,精气夺则虚"。也就是说,"实"是针对邪气入侵而言的,"虚"是针对正气不足而言的。

1.1.1 实证

实证,是以邪气偏盛为主要特点的一种病机反映。此时正气未虚,或虽有某种程度的耗损,但整体正气尚属较盛,足以与邪气抗争。由于邪正相争剧烈,故疾病的反应多较明显,出现一派有余的症状,所以称为实证。

Pathogenic) Qi is rather fierce, and the symptoms of the disease are more obvious and surplus, so it is called the excess pattern. The excess pattern is often seen in the early and middle stages of the diseases caused by the attack of the six exogenous pathogens, or the diseases caused by the phlegm-rheum, stagnant blood, food retention, or water-damp which retains inside the body. The clinical manifestations, as accumulation of phlegm and rheum, internal obstruction of stagnant blood, food retention due to poor digestion, overflow of water and dampness, high fever, mania, loud and heavy voice in speaking, abdominal pain which is worsened by pressure, retention of urine, constipation, forceful pulse, etc., are of the excess pattern.

1.1.2 Deficiency pattern

The deficiency pattern is a kind of pathological reflection in which the deficiency of the Zheng (Anti-Pathogenic) Qi is the predominant cause. In this condition, the Xie (Pathogenic) Qi has gone, or its remnants exist but are not strong enough to cause more harms on the Zheng (Anti-Pathogenic) Qi, so the conflict between the Xie (Pathogenic) Qi and Zheng (Anti-Pathogenic) Qi is rather moderate. The conflict between the Xie (Pathogenic) Qi and Zheng (Anti-Pathogenic) Qi is not fierce, and a series of symptoms of the disease are of the functional decrease of zang-fu organs due to insufficiency of the Zheng (Anti-Pathogenic) Qi, so it is called the deficiency pattern. The deficiency pattern is often seen in the late stage of the diseases caused by the attack of the exogenous pathogens, when the weakened Zheng (Anti-Pathogenic) Qi is not recovered, or in the conditions due to severe

实证常见于外感六淫致病的初期和中期,或由于痰饮、瘀血、食积、水湿等滞留于体内而引起的病证。如临床上可见到痰涎壅盛、瘀血内阻、食积不化、水湿泛滥等病变,以及壮热、狂躁、声高气粗、腹痛拒按、大小便不通、脉实有力等症,都属于实证的表现。

1.1.2 虚证

虚证,是以正气虚损为主要特点的一种病机反映。此时邪气已去,或虽然余邪未尽,但不会对正气造成大的伤害,邪正相争趋于缓和。由于邪正相争不甚激烈,主要表现为一系列正气不足及脏腑功能减退的症状,所以称为虚证。虚证多见于外感病的后期,正气虚损未复,或素体虚弱,或由于大病、久病、慢性病等消耗精气,或因大汗、剧烈呕吐下利、大出血等耗伤人体气血津液所导致。凡临床见到神疲体倦、面色憔悴、心悸气短、自汗、盗汗,或五心烦热,或畏寒肢冷,脉虚无力等,都属于虚证

diseases, or chronic diseases which exhaust the Jing
(Essence) Qi, or in the conditions due to profuse
sweating, severe vomiting, severe diarrhea, or severe bleeding which consumes qi, blood and body
fluid of human body. The clinical manifestations, as
low spirit, fatigue, haggard face, palpitation,
shortness of breath, spontaneous sweating, nocturnal sweats, feverish sensation in palms and soles, or
fear of cold and chills in limbs, weak pulse, etc.,
are of the deficiency pattern.

1.1.3 Mutual complication of deficiency pattern and excess pattern

During the process of the disease, the volume
changes of the Xie (Pathogenic) Qi and Zheng (Anti-Pathogenic) Qi not only cause the simple excess
pattern and deficiency pattern, but also lead to the
pathological changes of the complication of deficiency and excess, the so-called the complicated
pattern of deficiency and excess. If the excess pattern is not treated promptly or properly, the pathogens may retain to damage the Zheng (Anti-Pathogenic) Qi of human body. If the Zheng (Anti-Pathogenic) Qi is deficient already, it fails to dispel the
pathogens, so the pathological products as the water-damp, phlegm-rheum, stagnant blood, etc. occur. Both the conditions may cause the pathological
change of the complication of deficiency and excess.

There are two types of the complicated pattern
of deficiency and excess. The first one is the deficiency pattern complicated with excess, implying
that the pathological change of the disease pertains
to the deficiency pattern, but some excess-type
pathogens are also involved. For example, the

的表现。

1.1.3 虚证和实证的相互错杂

在疾病过程中,邪正的消长盛衰,不仅可以导致较为单纯的实证和虚证,也可以出现虚实相兼的病机变化,即虚实错杂证。若实证失治,或治疗不当,以致病邪久留,损伤人体的正气;或因正气本虚,无力驱邪外出,而致水湿、痰饮、瘀血等病理产物凝结阻滞,都可以形成虚实错杂的病机变化。

虚实错杂有两种情形,一是虚中夹实,是指疾病的病机变化以虚证为主,又兼实邪。如脾阳不振遂见水肿,多属虚中夹实。二是实中夹虚,是指疾病的病机变

spleen yang deficiency pattern, in which edema can be seen, pertains to the deficiency pattern complicated with excess. Another one is the excess pattern complicated with deficiency, implying that the pathological change of the disease pertains to the excess pattern, but some manifestations of the Zheng (Anti-Pathogenic) Qi deficiency are also involved. For example, in the severe stage of the febrile disease due to attack of the exogenous pathogens, the heat of excess type injures and consumes the yin fluid, pertaining to the excess pattern complicated with deficiency.

1.1.4 Mutual transformation of deficiency pattern and excess pattern

After the formation of the deficiency pattern or excess pattern, it is not immutable. Due to the constant change of the strength ratio of both sides in the conflict of the Xie (Pathogenic) Qi and Zheng (Anti-Pathogenic) Qi, the deficiency pattern and excess pattern are often transformed mutually.

There are two types of mutual transformation of the deficiency pattern and excess pattern. The first one is the excess pattern transforming into the deficiency pattern. Due to mistreatment or wrong treatment, the disease may lasts for long time. Although the Xie (Pathogenic) Qi is being dispelled gradually, the Zheng (Anti-Pathogenic) Qi and physiological functions of zang-fu organs of human body are damaged, in the end the property of the disease is transformed from the excess pattern to the deficiency pattern gradually. Another one is the deficiency pattern transforming into the excess pattern. In the original deficiency pattern without Xie (Pathogenic) Qi, the gradual decrease of the zang-

化以实证为主,又夹正虚。如外感热病的热盛期,常见实热耗伤阴津,多属实中夹虚。

1.1.4　虚证和实证的相互转化

虚证和实证形成之后,并不是一成不变的。由于邪正斗争中双方力量对比经常发生变化,因而虚证和实证之间也常发生相互转化。

虚证和实证相互转化有两种形式。一是由实转虚:实证正气本不虚,若由于误治、失治,使病情迁延日久,虽然邪气渐去,但人体的正气、脏腑的生理功能也受到损伤,其疾病的性质也就逐渐由实转虚。二是因虚致实:原属虚证,并无邪气,若因正虚而脏腑功能减退,导致气、血、水等不能正常运行而出现了气滞、瘀滞征象,就形成了夹实的病机。此时虽有实邪,但正气仍然不足,所

fu organs functions due to the Zheng (Anti-Pathogenic) Qi deficiency, may lead to abnormality of qi, blood or body fluid circulation, so as to cause the manifestations of qi stagnation, blood stasis or water retention, the so-called excess pattern. In such a condition, there is the excess-type Xie (Pathogenic) Qi, while the Zheng (Anti-Pathogenic) Qi is not sufficient, so it is called "the excess pattern caused by deficiency", and also becoming the complicated pattern of deficiency and excess.

1.2 Conflict between Xie (Pathogenic) Qi and Zheng (Anti-Pathogenic) Qi related to the development and improvement of diseases

During the process of the conflict between the Xie (Pathogenic) Qi and Zheng (Anti-Pathogenic) Qi, the Zheng (Anti-Pathogenic) Qi is capable to dispel the Xie (Pathogenic) Qi, while the Xie (Pathogenic) Qi also acts to damage the Zheng (Anti-Pathogenic) Qi. Therefore, in the process of the conflict between the Xie (Pathogenic) Qi and Zheng (Anti-Pathogenic) Qi, it is accompanied by the constant change of the strength ratio of both sides, and such a change finally determines the development and improvement of the disease.

The results of the disease change are the improvement and the development, the two different results of the conflict between the Xie (Pathogenic) Qi and Zheng (Anti-Pathogenic) Qi. If the Zheng (Anti-Pathogenic) Qi wins and the Xie (Pathogenic) Qi withdraws, the disease is improving and recovered. If the Xie (Pathogenic) Qi wins and the Zheng (Anti-Pathogenic) Qi declines, the disease is worsened or even developing to death.

以称其为"因虚致实"。因虚致实也可导致虚实错杂证。

1.2 邪正盛衰与疾病转归

在邪正斗争过程中，正气有祛除邪气的能力，邪气也有损伤正气的作用。因此，邪正相争的过程必然伴随着正气与邪气双方力量对比的不断变化，这种变化最终将决定疾病的转归。

疾病的转归有两种基本形式，一是向愈，一是恶化。这两种转归实际上是邪正相争的不同结果。若正胜邪退，则疾病趋于好转或痊愈；若邪胜正衰，则疾病趋于恶化或死亡。

1. 2. 1 Zheng (Anti-Pathogenic) Qi wins and Xie (Pathogenic) Qi withdraws

It is the necessary condition of the improvement and recovery of the disease that the Zheng (Anti-Pathogenic) Qi wins and the Xie (Pathogenic) Qi withdraws. The Zheng (Anti-Pathogenic) Qi is sufficient and vigorous, and its anti-pathogen ability is increasing constantly, so the Xie (Pathogenic) Qi will be dispelled gradually. Due to the prompt and proper treatment, the Xie (Pathogenic) Qi is dispelled or weakened, the Zheng (Anti-Pathogenic) Qi which has be consumed will be recovered gradually, and finally, the functions of zang-fu organs are completely recovered and the Xie (Pathogenic) Qi is completely dispelled, and then the disease declares cured.

The process in which the Zheng (Anti-Pathogenic) Qi wins and the Xie (Pathogenic) Qi withdraws can be long or short, different according to individuals. In the diseases due to attack of exogenous pathogens, the excess pattern and the diseases with short course, the Xie (Pathogenic) Qi is not that deep and the Zheng (Anti-Pathogenic) Qi is not severely damaged, its improvement and recovery are fast. In the diseases due to internal injury, deficiency pattern and the disease with long course, the Xie (Pathogenic) Qi enters the body deeply and the Zheng (Anti-Pathogenic) Qi is damaged severely, its improvement and recovery are slow. Generally, if the treatment is prompt and proper, the process in which the Zheng (Anti-Pathogenic) Qi wins and the Xie (Pathogenic) Qi withdraws will be shortened, otherwise it is prolonged.

1. 2. 1 正胜邪退

正胜邪退,是疾病趋于好转和痊愈的必要条件。由于正气充盛,抗御病邪的能力不断增强,邪气将逐渐被清除;或因得到及时正确的治疗,邪气被祛除或削弱,正气的耗伤逐渐得到修复;最终脏腑功能完全恢复正常,邪气被完全祛除,疾病即告痊愈。

正胜邪退的过程长短不一,因人而异。一般外感疾病、实证、病程短者,邪气侵入不深,正气损伤不重,则好转快,痊愈也快。若属内伤疾病、虚证、病程长者,邪气侵入深,正气损伤重,则好转慢,痊愈也慢。如果治疗及时而恰当,正胜邪退的过程就会缩短,反之则会延长。

1.2.2　Xie (Pathogenic) Qi wins and Zheng (Anti-Pathogenic) Qi declines

It is the basic cause of the development of disease or death that the Xie (Pathogenic) Qi wins and the Zheng (Anti-Pathogenic) Qi declines. If the Zheng (Anti-Pathogenic) Qi in human body is not sufficient, so it fails to stop the development of the Xie (Pathogenic) Qi. If the Xie (Pathogenic) Qi is too preponderant, it overpasses the resisting ability of the body. If the mistreatment or wrong treatment damages the Zheng (Anti-Pathogenic) Qi, the Xie (Pathogenic) Qi becomes stronger. In these conditions, the Zheng (Anti-Pathogenic) Qi ability is decreasing, and the pathological damage of body is being severe, so as to cause the functional failure of zang-fu organs, the separation of yin and yang, and even the death.

Besides, in the process of the conflict between the Xie (Pathogenic) Qi and Zheng (Anti-Pathogenic) Qi, if the Zheng (Anti-Pathogenic) Qi is deficient and fails to dispel the Xie (Pathogenic) Qi, and the Xie (Pathogenic) Qi does not develop further, the condition in which the Xie (Pathogenic) Qi and Zheng (Anti-Pathogenic) Qi are locked in stalemate, or the condition in which the Zheng (Anti-Pathogenic) Qi is deficient and the Xie (Pathogenic) Qi keeps retaining to block the complete recovery of the Zheng (Anti-Pathogenic) Qi occurs. As a result, the disease transform from the acute type to the chronic type, or the disease is left with some sequelae, or the disease becomes durable and incurable.

1.2.2　邪胜正衰

邪胜正衰,是疾病趋于恶化或死亡的根本原因。由于人体正气本来不足,无力制止邪气的发展;或因邪气过于亢盛,超过了机体的抵御能力;或因失治、误治损伤正气,助长邪气,使正气抗邪能力日益低下,机体的病理损害日趋严重,脏腑功能衰竭,阴阳离决而死亡。

此外,在邪正消长盛衰的过程中,若正气不足以祛除邪气,邪气也不能进一步发展,出现邪正相持或正虚邪恋,正气难以完全恢复等情况,常可导致许多疾病由急性过程转入慢性阶段,或留下某些后遗症,或经久不愈。

2   Disharmony of yin and yang

The disharmony of yin and yang refers to the pathological changes occurring in the loss of the normal equilibrium and harmony relation between yin and yang. The disharmony of yin and yang is the most basic pathogenesis, and also the highest summary of all pathogenesis changes. The zang-fu organs dysfunction, meridians and collaterals disturbance, qi and blood disharmony, etc., are the concrete manifestations of the disharmony of yin and yang.

In normal situation, yin and yang of human body maintain a kind of dynamic equilibrium and harmony relation. If the factors, as the six exogenous pathogens, the seven emotional factors, the improper food intake, the improper strain and idleness, etc., destroy such a relation, it may cause the disharmony of yin and yang. If yin and yang are disharmonious, there can be various complicated pathogenesis mutations.

The disharmony of yin and yang includes the pathogenesis mutations of the preponderance and weakness of yin and yang, the mutual damage of yin and yang, the mutual refusal of yin and yang, the mutual transformation of yin and yang, the collapse of yin and yang, etc.

2.1   Preponderance and weakness of yin and yang

The preponderance and weakness of yin and yang refer to the pathogenesis mutations of preponderance or weakness of yin or yang due to various causes, leading to the excess or deficiency pattern and the cold or heat pattern. The preponderance of

2   阴阳失调

阴阳失调,是指阴阳之间失去正常的协调平和关系从而出现的病机变化。阴阳失调是最基本的病机,是一切病机变化的最高概括。凡脏腑失常、经络失调、气血失和等,都是阴阳失调的表现形式。

正常情况下,人体的阴阳之间维持着一种动态的协调平和关系。若因外感六淫、内伤七情、饮食失宜、劳逸失当等因素,破坏了这种关系,就会导致阴阳失调。阴阳一旦失调,便会出现错综复杂的病机变化。

阴阳失调主要表现为阴阳盛衰、阴阳互损、阴阳格拒、阴阳转化、阴阳亡失等病机变化。

2.1   阴阳盛衰

阴阳盛衰,是由各种原因导致的阴或阳的偏盛和偏衰的病机变化。阴阳盛衰直接导致实证和虚证,阴阳偏盛则形成实证,阴阳偏衰则

yin or yang causes the excess pattern, while the weakness of yin or yang leads to the deficiency pattern. The preponderance of yang or the weakness of yin causes the heat pattern, while the preponderance of yin or weakness of yang leads to the cold pattern.

2.1.1 Preponderance of yin and yang

"The preponderance of the Xie (Pathogenic) Qi is the excess", so the preponderance of yin or yang causes the excess pattern. The preponderance of yang causes the heat pattern of excess, while the preponderance of yin leads to the cold pattern of excess.

Preponderance of yang: The preponderance of yang refers to a kind of pathological state of the yang qi excess and functional excitement due to disharmony of yin and yang, featured by the heat pattern of excess in which yang is excessive while yin is not deficient. Its major causative factors are the attack of the pathogens of yang-heat type, the attack of the pathogens of yin-cold type which transform into yang-heat type, the fire transformed from the emotional depression, and the fire transformed from the phlegm-rheum or food retention. The preponderance of yang leads to heat, so fever is a major symptom, with other manifestations of profuse sweating, thirst, red complexion, red tongue body with yellow tongue coating, surging or rapid pulse, or the manifestations caused by the internal disturbance of pathogenic fire, such as vexation, insomnia, mania, constipation, scanty and dark-colored urine, etc.

Since the preponderance of yang damages yin, there are also the manifestations of consumption of

形成虚证。阴阳盛衰还决定了疾病性质的寒和热,阳盛、阴虚则形成热证,阴盛、阳虚则形成寒证。

2.1.1 阴阳偏盛

"邪气盛则实",阴偏盛或阳偏盛都会形成实证。阳偏盛则形成实热证,阴偏盛则形成实寒证。

阳偏盛:阳偏盛是由于人体阴阳平和失调,表现为阳气偏盛、功能亢奋的一种病理状态,其病机特点多表现为阳盛而阴未虚的实热证。形成的主要原因,常见于感受阳热之邪,或感受阴邪从阳化热,或情志内郁化火,或痰浊、食积等郁而化火。阳盛则热,故临床表现以发热为主症,兼见多汗、口渴、面红、舌红苔黄、脉洪大或数;或火邪内扰,出现心烦、失眠、狂躁、大便干结、小便短赤等症。

由于阳盛则伤阴,所以阳偏盛者往往有耗伤阴津、

the yin fluid or the Yuan (Primary) Qi in the condition of the yang preponderance, leading to the excess pattern with deficiency. For example, during the process of the febrile disease due to attack of exogenous pathogens, there can be the symptoms of low spirit, lassitude, thirst, preference for drinking lots of water, etc.

Preponderance of yin: The preponderance of yin refers to a kind of pathological state of the yin qi excess, functional inhibition and pathological product retention due to disharmony of yin and yang, featured by the cold pattern of excess in which yin is excessive while yang is not deficient. Its major causative factors are the attack of the pathogens of yin-cold type, and the over-intake of raw and cold food. The preponderance of yin leads to cold, and the yang qi loses its warming function due to blockage, so feeling of cold is the major symptom, with other manifestations of aversion to cold, shiver, low spirit, pale complexion, absence of sweating, preference for drinking warm water, chills in four limbs, thin feces, clear urine, white tongue coating, deep and slow pulse, etc.

Since the preponderance of yin damages yang, there are also the manifestations of the yang qi blockage or damage in the condition of the yin preponderance, leading to the excess pattern with deficiency, with the manifestations of low spirit, pale-puffy face, pale and swollen tongue body, thready and weak pulse, etc.

2.1.2　Weakness of yin and yang

"The loss of the Jing (Essence) Qi is the deficiency", so the weakness of yin or yang causes the deficiency pattern. The weakness of yang causes the

元气的表现,便会形成实中夹虚证,如外感热病过程中,容易出现精神疲乏、口渴多饮等症。

阴偏盛:阴偏盛是由于人体阴阳平和失调,表现为阴气偏盛、功能衰减及其病理性代谢产物滞留的一种病理状态,其病机特点多表现为阴盛而阳未虚的实寒证。其形成原因多为感受寒湿阴邪,或过食生冷,致使人体阴气偏盛而形成。阴盛则寒,阳气被遏而不得舒展,也失去其温煦作用,故临床表现以发寒为主症,常见恶寒战栗、精神不振、面色苍白、无汗、喜热饮、四肢逆冷、大便稀、小便清、舌苔白、脉沉迟等症。

由于阴盛则阳病,所以阴偏盛往往有阳气受遏或损伤的表现。阴偏盛的疾病过程中,便会形成实中夹虚证,如出现精神萎靡、面色㿠白、舌质淡胖、脉搏细弱等症。

2.1.2　阴阳偏衰

"精气夺则虚",阴偏衰和阳偏衰都会形成虚证。阳偏衰则形成虚寒证,阴偏衰

cold pattern of deficiency, while the weakness of yin leads to the heat pattern of deficiency.

Weakness of yang: The weakness of yang is often caused by the disharmony of yin and yang in which the yang qi is over-consumed, or by the congenital deficiency which leads to the fire decline of the vital gate, or by the acquired malnutrition which damages the yang qi, or by the insufficiency of the yang qi due to some diseases. The weakness of yang causes cold, as the cold pattern of deficiency, and the functional decrease or weakness of zang-fu organs, with the manifestations of fear of cold, chills in four limbs, low spirit, lassitude, poor appetite, loose feces, clear and excessive urine, deep, slow and weak pulse, etc.

The yang deficiency pattern often involves the spleen and kidney, especially causing the kidney yang deficiency pattern. Since the kidney yang is the basis of the yang qi of all zang-fu organs, the yang qi of all zang-fu organs will become insufficient if the kidney yang is deficient.

Due to the deficiency of yang which fails to restrain yin, there can be the internal accumulation of the yin cold, or retention of water-damp, or internal blockage of stagnation blood, further obstructing the qi activities and causing severe disturbance of znag-fu functions, so as to form the deficiency pattern complicated with excess.

Weakness of yin: The weakness of yin is often caused by the disharmony of yin and yang in which the yin essence is over-consumed, or by the congenital deficiency which leads to the yin fluid depletion and deficiency, or by the acquired malnutrition which consumes the yin fluid, or by the insufficien-

则形成虚热证。

阳偏衰：阳偏衰多由人体阴阳平和失调，阳气消耗过度；或先天禀赋薄弱，命门火衰；或后天调养失当，损伤阳气；或因病阳气受损，使机体阳气不足而形成。阳虚则寒，故临床主要表现为虚寒证，脏腑功能减退或衰弱，出现畏寒怕冷、四肢不温、精神疲乏、食欲不振、大便溏泄、小便清长、脉沉迟无力等症。

阳虚证主要表现在脾、肾二脏，尤以肾阳虚为重点。因为肾阳为各脏腑阳气的根本，所以肾阳一虚，诸脏阳气均可因此而不足。

由于阳虚则不能制阴，可导致阴寒内盛，或水湿停聚，或瘀血内阻，进一步阻滞气机，可致脏腑功能严重障碍，从而形成虚中夹实之证。

阴偏衰：阴偏衰多由人体阴阳平和失调，阴精消耗过度；或先天禀赋薄弱，阴液亏虚；或后天调养失当，阴液耗竭；或因病阴液受损，使机体阴液不足而形成。阴虚则

cy of the yin fluid due to some diseases. The weakness of yin causes heat, as the heat pattern of deficiency, and the relatively functional excitement, with the manifestations of emaciation, low-grade fever, feverish sensation in palms and soles, vexation, nocturnal sweats, dry mouth, dry feces, scanty urine, red tongue body with scanty or with no tongue coating, thready and rapid pulse, etc.

The yin deficiency pattern often involves the liver and kidney, especially causing the kidney yin deficiency pattern. Since the kidney yin is the basis of the yin of all zang-fu organs, yin of all zang-fu organs will become insufficient if the kidney yin is deficient.

Due to the deficiency of yin which fails to restrain yang, there can be the internal production of fire or heat, or liver yang hyperactivity, leading to red facial complexion, red eyes, headache, distension in head, restlessness, anger, etc., so as to form the deficiency pattern complicated with excess.

2.2 Mutual damage of yin and yang

Since yin and yang are mutually rooted on, the insufficiency of yin or yang may influence the opposite. The prolonged yin deficiency may involve the yang qi, leading to the yang qi deficiency as well. The prolonged yang deficiency may involve the yin essence, causing the yin essence deficiency as well. Such a pathogenesis process in which yin and yang influenced each other is called the mutual damage of yin and yang. The result of the mutual damage of yin and yang is the deficiency pattern of both yin and yang.

热,故临床主要表现为虚热证,脏腑功能相对亢奋,出现形体消瘦、低热、五心烦热、盗汗、口干、大便干结、小便短少、舌红苔少或无苔、脉细数等症。

阴虚证主要表现在肝、肾二脏,尤以肾阴虚为重点。因为肾阴为各脏腑之阴的根本,所以肾阴一虚,诸脏之阴均可不足。

由于阴虚则不能制阳,可导致火热内生、肝阳亢盛而出现面红目赤、头胀头痛、急躁易怒等虚中夹实之证。

2.2 阴阳互损

由于阴阳是互根的,所以阴或阳的任何一方不足,都可影响另一方。阴虚日久,则累及阳气,导致阳气也虚;阳虚日久则累及阴分,导致阴精虚亏。这种阴阳之间虚损相互影响的病机过程,称为阴阳互损。阴阳互损的结果,最终导致阴阳两虚证。

2.2.1　Damage of yin involving yang

The damage of yin involving yang implies that the deficiency of the yin fluid involves the yang qi, to make the yang qi fail to be produced enough or make it scatter and be consumed due to absence of residence, so as to lead to yang deficiency on the basis of yin deficiency, forming the pathological state in which both yin and yang are deficient but the yin deficiency as the predominant. For example, in the liver yang hyperactivity pattern, the pathogenesis is the insufficiency of kidney yin, failing to restrain the liver yang. The Jing (Essence) Qi in the kidney is the substantial foundation of the kidney yin and kidney yang. If the kidney yin is further deficient, the Jing (Essence) Qi in the kidney will be consumed, and then to involve the kidney yang, leading to the manifestations of yang deficiency, as fear of cold, chills in limbs, clear and excessive urine at night, pale or grey-black complexion, further developing into the deficiency pattern of both yin and yang.

2.2.2　Damage of yang involving yin

The damage of yang involving yin implies that the deficiency of the yang qi involves the yin fluid, to make the yin fluid fail to be produced enough, so as to lead to yin deficiency on the basis of yang deficiency, forming the pathological state in which both yin and yang are deficient but the yang deficiency as the predominant. For example, in the kidney yang insufficiency pattern, the transforming function of the kidney qi is disturbed, to cause retention of body fluid and overflow of water and damp, leading to edema. If the kidney yang is further deficient, it consumes and damages the Jing (Essence) Qi in the

2.2.1　阴损及阳

阴损及阳,是指由于阴液亏损,累及阳气,使阳气生化不足或无所依附而耗散,从而在阴虚的基础上又导致了阳虚,形成了以阴虚为主的阴阳两虚的病理状态。例如肝阳上亢,其病机根本在于肾阴不足,不能制约肝阳所致。肾中精气是肾阴、肾阳的物质基础,若肾阴进一步亏损,则肾中精气耗伤,继而损及肾阳,出现畏寒、肢冷、夜尿清长、面色白而晦黯等阳虚症状,就发展成阴阳两虚证。

2.2.2　阳损及阴

阳损及阴,是指由于阳气虚损,累及阴液,使阴液生化不足,从而在阳虚的基础上又导致了阴虚,形成了以阳虚为主的阴阳两虚的病理状态。例如肾阳不足,气化失司,津液停聚,水湿泛滥而浮肿。若肾阳进一步亏损,必耗伤肾中精气,使肾阴亦伤而出现烦躁升火,甚至阳升风动、抽搐等阴虚症状,形成阴阳两虚证。

kidney, and then to involve the kidney yin, leading the manifestations of yin deficiency, as vexation, restlessness, feverish sensation, even convulsion due to the hyperactive yang stirring the wind, further developing into the deficiency pattern of both yin and yang.

2.3 Mutual refusal of yin and yang

The mutual refusal of yin and yang is a specific pathogenesis in the disharmony of yin and yang, including two types of preponderance of yin refusing yang and preponderance of yang refusing yin. The mechanism of the mutual refusal of yin and yang is that due to some causative factors, yin or yang is preponderant and accumulated inside, to refuse the opposite's entering, so as to lead to the complicated pathological phenomena in which the property of the disease is different from the manifestations of the disease.

2.3.1 Preponderance of yin refusing yang

The preponderance of yin refusing yang implies that the yin cold inside the body is excessive to refuse the yang qi's entering, leading to a kind pathological change of the true cold and false heat. The property of the disease is the cold pattern, but the refused yang qi possesses the false appearances of heat. For example, when the disease of the yang deficiency causing the internal cold develops to the critical stage, the yin cold becomes severely excessive, and yang is floating at the body surface, so as to form the pathological change of the preponderance of yin refusing yang, leading to the manifestations of excess of yin cold, as chills in four limbs, diarrhea with indigested food in feces, extremely weak pulse, etc., and also the manifestations of

2.3 阴阳格拒

阴阳格拒，是阴阳失调中比较特殊的一种病机，包括阴盛格阳和阳盛格阴两方面。形成阴阳格拒的机理，主要是由于某些原因引起阴或阳的一方偏盛至极而壅遏于内，将另一方排斥格拒于外，从而出现病证性质和症候表现不一致的复杂病理现象。

2.3.1 阴盛格阳

阴盛格阳，是指体内阴寒过盛，将阳气格拒于外，出现真寒假热的一种病理变化。其病证性质虽然是寒，而被格拒于外的阳气却表现出热的假象。如阳虚而生内寒，疾病发展至危重阶段，阴寒盛极，浮阳外越，就形成阴盛格阳的病理变化，其表现除有阴寒过盛之四肢厥逆、下利清谷、脉微欲绝等症外，又见身体反温（但欲盖衣被）、面颊泛红等假热之象。

false heat, as feverish sensation in body (but with preference for covering with quilt), red complexion, etc. as well.

2.3.2 Preponderance of yang refusing yin

The preponderance of yang refusing yin implies that the yang heat inside the body is excessive to refuse the yin entering, leading to a kind of pathological change of the true heat and false cold. Since the pathogenic heat is deeply hidden and fails to go out, the false cold can be seen on the body surface, but the property of the disease is the heat pattern. For example, in the warm-heat disease, the pathogenic heat is accumulated inside. The severe preponderance of heat causes the disharmony of yin and yang, the yin qi is refused, leading to the manifestations of yang excess, as vexation and feverish sensation in heart and chest, dry mouth, burning sensation at tongue, red tongue body, etc., and also the manifestations of false cold, as chills in four limbs, hidden pulse, etc. as well.

2.4 Mutual transformation of yin and yang

The mutual transformation of yin and yang implies that during the process of disease, the yang-heat pattern may reversely transform into the yin-cold pattern, while the yin-cold pattern may reversely transform into the yang-heat pattern.

2.4.1 Yang pattern transforming into yin

The property of the disease pertains to the yang heat originally, but the yang heat becomes hyperactive to a certain degree to transform into the yin cold. For example, in the early stage of some febrile diseases, there are the manifestations of heat, as high fever, thirst, red tongue body with yellow coating, rapid pulse, etc., pertaining to the yang-

2.3.2 阳盛格阴

阳盛格阴,是指阳热盛极,格阴于外,反似寒证的一种病理变化。由于热邪深伏,不能外达,故外见假寒,其本质仍属热证。如温热病热盛于内,由于热势盛极,阴阳不相调和,阴气即受阻格,其表现除有心胸烦热、口干舌焦、舌红等症外,又有阳极似阴的四肢厥冷、脉伏不起等症。

2.4 阴阳转化

阴阳转化,是指在疾病发展过程中,阳热证可逆转为阴寒证,阴寒证也可逆转为阳热证。

2.4.1 阳证转阴

疾病的性质本属阳热,但阳热亢盛至一定程度时,可向阴寒方向转化。如某些热病初期可见高热、口渴、舌红、苔黄、脉数等一派热象,显然属于阳热之证。由于治疗不当或邪毒太盛等原因,

heat pattern. Due to some factors as improper treatment or excessive pathogenic toxin may cause the critical manifestations of the yin cold, as sudden decrease of body temperature, chills in four limbs, wetness with cold sweat, extremely weak pulse, etc. This is the fundamental transformation of the property of the disease, essentially different from the condition of the true heat and false cold due to preponderance of yang refusing yin.

2.4.2   Yin pattern transforming into yang

The property of the disease pertains to the yin cold originally, but the yin cold becomes hyperactive to a certain degree to transform into the yang heat. For example, in the early stage of the diseases due to attack of the exogenous pathogenic cold, there are the manifestations of wind-cold attacking the exterior, as aversion to cold with light fever, headache, aching of whole body, thing-white tongue coating, superficial and taut pulse, etc. Later, the diseases may transform into the yang-heat pattern, with the manifestations of high fever, sweating, thirst, red tongue body with yellow tongue coating, rapid pulse, etc. This is the yin pattern transforming into yang. As the fundamental transformation of the property of the disease, it is completely different from the condition of the true cold and false heat due to preponderance of yin refusing yang.

2.5   Collapse of yin and yang

The collapse of yin and yang, including the collapse of yin and collapse of yang, implies a kind of pathological change in which the yin fluid or yang qi of the body is severely lost suddenly, so as to lead to the critical condition. The collapse of yin and col-

可突然出现体温下降、四肢厥逆、冷汗淋漓、脉微欲绝等阴寒危象。这是疾病性质的根本转变，与阳盛格阴的真热假寒证有本质区别。

2.4.2   阴证转阳

疾病的性质本属阴寒，但阴寒盛极至一定程度时，可向阳热方向转化。如外感寒邪，初期可见恶寒重发热轻、头身疼痛、苔薄白、脉浮紧等风寒束表之象，其后可发展为高热、汗出、口渴、舌红、苔黄、脉数等阳热之证。这就属于阴证转阳，寒证化热，与阴盛格阳的真寒假热证完全不同。

2.5   阴阳亡失

阴阳亡失，包括亡阴和亡阳两个方面，是指机体的阴液或阳气突然大量地亡失，导致生命垂危的一种病理变化。亡阴和亡阳也属于

lapse of yang, pertaining to the scope of the weakness of yin and weakness of yang, are featured by abrupt onset of disease, critical condition, etc.

2.5.1 Collapse of yang

The collapse of yang is caused by the factors of preponderance of the Xie (Pathogenic) Qi which cannot be dispelled by the Zheng (Anti-Pathogenic) Qi, body constitution of yang deficiency accompanied by over-fatigue, mistreatment with sweat-making method causing profuse sweating, so as to cause the sudden loss of the yang qi in the body, with the manifestations of profuse sweating, chills in skin, hands and feet, sleepiness, fatigue, extremely weak pulse, etc.

2.5.2 Collapse of yin

The collapse of yin is caused by the factors preponderance of the pathogenic heat, severe vomiting, profuse sweating, serious diarrhea, etc., so as to cause sudden and severe loss of yin fluid in the body, causing dry and shriveled body, folded skin, enophthalmus, scanty and sticky sweat, vexation, restlessness, thready-weak pulse, etc.

The collapse of yin and collapse of yang may occur alone. Due to the mutual rooted and mutual functioning relation between yin and yang, the loss of any one may lead to the rapid loss of the other. Therefore, in the collapse of yin, yang has no residence to stay. In the collapse of yang, yin has no residence to stay. In the end, the collapse of both yin and yang occurs. When the collapse of yin or collapse of yang occurs, if the rescuing methods are not prompt, there can be the critical condition of "separation of yin and yang leading to the Jing (Essence) Qi vanishing", to cause death.

阴阳偏衰的范畴,但其有发病急骤、病情危重的特点。

2.5.1 亡阳

亡阳常见于邪盛而正不胜邪、素体阳虚而疲劳过度、误用汗法而汗出过多等原因,导致机体阳气突然脱失,症见大汗淋漓、肌肤手足厥冷、蜷卧神疲、脉微欲绝等。

2.5.2 亡阴

亡阴常见于热邪炽盛、大吐、大汗、大泄等原因,导致机体阴液大量丢失,症见身体干瘪、皮肤皱褶、眼球凹陷、汗出少而黏、烦躁不安、脉细弱无力等。

亡阴和亡阳虽可单独出现,但由于阴阳互根互用的,任何一方亡失都会导致另一方的迅速消亡,所以亡阴之后阳气将无所依附,亡阳之后阴液不能独存,最终导致阴阳俱亡。因此,出现亡阴或亡阳时,如不及时抢救,必然出现"阴阳离决,精气乃绝"的严重局面,导致死亡。

3   Abnormalities of qi, blood and body fluid

The abnormalities of qi, blood and body fluid include the abnormality of qi, abnormality of blood and abnormality of body fluid. Each of abnormality includes two types of insufficiency and disturbance. The insufficiency causes the deficiency pattern, as the qi deficiency, blood deficiency, body fluid deficiency, etc., while the disturbance leads to the circulatory abnormality of qi, blood and body fluid.

3.1   Abnormality of qi

3.1.1   Qi insufficiency

The qi insufficiency causes the qi deficiency pattern, with the manifestations of sallow-yellow facial complexion, low spirit, lassitude, fatigue, light voice in speaking, susceptibility to catching cold, etc. Qi deficiency further causes the function decrease of the zang-fu organs, leading to the patterns of the heart qi deficiency, spleen qi deficiency, lung qi deficiency, kidney qi deficiency, etc.

3.1.2   Qi activity disturbance

The qi activity disturbance includes the pathological changes of qi stagnation, qi reverse-flow, qi sinking, qi blockage, qi escape, etc.

Qi stagnation: It refers to the pathological state of the unsmooth qi activity. If the qi circulation is obstructed, qi is accumulated at the local area, leading to the symptoms of distension, fullness, pain, etc. For example, the liver qi stagnation leads to distension and fullness in chest and hypochondria, or lower abdominal distension and pain. The qi stagnation in intestines and stomach causes epigastria distension and fullness, or abdominal disten-

3   气血津液失常

气血津液失常,分为气失常、血失常和津液失常三个方面,每一方面又有不足和失调两类表现。其不足则形成虚证,如气虚、血虚、津液亏虚等;失调则主要表现为气血津液运行失常。

3.1   气失常

3.1.1   气不足

气不足则形成气虚证,主要表现为面色萎黄、精神不振、倦怠乏力、语声低弱,以及容易感冒等症。气虚而导致脏腑功能减退,可出现心气虚、脾气虚、肺气虚、肾气虚等证。

3.1.2   气机失调

气机失调的病机变化有气滞、气逆、气陷、气闭、气脱等。

气滞,指气机不畅的病机状态。气机运行受阻,郁滞于局部,引起胀满、疼痛等症。如肝气郁滞,则胸胁胀满,或少腹胀痛;肠胃气滞,则胃脘胀满,或腹胀腹痛。

sion and abdominal pain.

Qi reverse-flow, qi sinking, qi blockage and qi collapse are the pathological changes due to the abnormality of the up-flow, down-flow, outflow and inflow of qi.

If qi up-flows excessively, it causes the qi reverse-flow. If qi is inadequate in up-flow, it causes the qi sinking. If qi fails to disperse and outflow, it causes the qi blockage. If qi loses its checking function and fails to inflow, it causes the qi escape.

Qi reverse-flow and qi blockage are mostly the excess patterns. The up-reverse flow of the liver qi may cause dizziness, blurring of vision, distension in head, or coma. The up-reverse flow of the stomach qi may lead to nausea and vomiting. The up-reverse flow of the lung qi may cause stuffy chest, unsmooth respiration, nasal obstruction and absence of sweating.

Qi sinking and qi escape are mostly the deficiency patterns. The down-sinking of the Zhong (Central) Qi leads to dizziness, blurring of vision, diarrhea, prolapse of internal organs and prolapse of rectum. The checking function loss of the lung qi causes spontaneous sweating. The checking functions loss of the kidney qi leads to incontinence of urination. The Yuan (Primary) Qi escape causes agape of mouth and four limbs, incontinence of urination and defecation, and wetness due to profuse sweating.

3.2 Abnormality of blood
3.2.1 Blood insufficiency

The blood insufficiency causes the blood deficiency pattern, with the symptoms of pale and lusterless complexion, dizziness, blurring of vision,

气逆、气陷、气闭、气脱，都是由于气的升降出入失常所导致的病机变化。

气升太过，则为气逆；气升不及，则为气陷；气失宣泄，不得外出，可形成气闭；气失固摄，不能内守，可导致气脱。

气逆、气闭多为实证，如肝气上逆则眩晕、头胀或昏厥；胃气上逆则恶心、呕吐；肺气郁闭则胸闷、呼吸不畅、鼻塞、无汗。

气陷、气脱多为虚证。如中气下陷则头昏目眩、大便下利、内脏下垂、脱肛；肺气不固则自汗不止；肾气不固则小便失禁；元气外脱则张口撒手、二便失禁、大汗淋漓。

3.2 血失常
3.2.1 血不足

血不足则形成血虚证，主要表现为面色淡白无华、头晕眼花、心悸少寐、口唇爪

palpitation, poor sleep, pale lips and nails, scanty and light-colored blood in menstruation, etc. If the blood is deficient, it fails to nourish the zang-fu organs, leading to the patterns of the heart blood deficiency and liver blood deficiency.

3.2.2 Blood circulation disturbance

The blood circulation disturbance includes two types of blood stasis and bleeding. The blood stasis refers to the pathological changes of the unsmooth flow of blood and obstruction of meridians, leading to pain, distension, swelling, masses, etc. Bleeding is caused by the injury of the vessels which makes the blood to flow away from the meridians, or by the spleen failing to control the blood, or by the liver failing to store the blood. As a result, various bleeding patterns occur, as spitting blood, hemoptysis, nasal bleeding, bloody feces, bloody urine, etc.

3.3 Abnormality of body fluid

3.3.1 Body fluid insufficiency

The body fluid insufficiency causes lack of moisture, leading to the dryness pattern. If the exogenous pathogenic dryness or heat attacks to body, there can be the exogenous dryness pattern. The five emotional factors transforming into the fire, or the factors of fever, profuse sweating, sever vomiting or diarrhea, bleeding, etc., consume the body fluid, leading to the endogenous dryness pattern. If the body fluid is insufficient, it fails to moisturize the skin, orifices and apertures, zang-fu organs, etc., leading to the symptoms of dry skin, dry mouth, dry throat, dry eyes, scanty urine, constipation, etc.

3.3.2 Body fluid disturbance

The body fluid disturbance implies the

甲色淡、妇女月经量少色淡等。血虚而脏腑失养，主要表现为心血虚和肝血虚证。

3.2.2　血行失调

血行失调主要表现为血瘀和出血。血瘀是血行不畅，经脉瘀阻，可导致疼痛、肿胀、癥积等病理变化。出血是因血脉损伤，血液离经；或脾不统血，或肝不藏血，导致各种出血证，如吐血、咯血、衄血、便血、尿血等。

3.3　津液失常

3.3.1　津液不足

津液不足，失于滋润，形成燥证。若感受燥热之邪气，则形成外燥证；若由五志化火，或发热、多汗、吐下过度、失血等原因使津液耗伤，则形成内燥证。津液不足，皮肤、孔窍、脏腑皆失其滋润，从而出现皮肤干燥、口干咽燥、两目干涩、小便短少、大便干结等症。

3.3.2　津液失调

津液失调即津液的运行

disturbance of body fluid circulation and metabolism, to cause internal retention of water-damp, leading to the diseases of phlegm-rheum, edema, etc. Its causative factor is actually the dysfunction of the spleen, lung and kidney. The failure of spleen in transporting and transforming the water-damp, or the failure of lung in dredging and regulating the water passage, or the failure of kidney in dominating the water metabolism, may disturb the transforming and transpiring function, leading to the retention and accumulation of water-damp.

The abnormality of qi, abnormality of blood and abnormality of body fluid are mutually influenced. For example, the qi deficiency leads to blood deficiency, while the blood deficiency causes qi deficiency. The qi stagnation leads to blood stasis, while the blood stasis causes qi stagnation. The blood insufficiency causes the body fluid insufficiency. In terms of the pathological mutations due to the disturbance of the relations among qi, blood and body fluid, please refer to "Section 4 Relationships among Qi, Blood and Body Fluid, Chapter 2 Qi, Blood and Body Fluid".

代谢障碍,水湿内停,从而导致痰饮、水肿等病证。其形成原因,主要在于脾、肺、肾三脏功能失调,使脾不能运化水湿,或肺不能通调水道,或肾不能主宰水液代谢,都可使气化失司,水湿停聚。

气失常、血失常、津液失常三方面的病机也可相互影响。如气虚可导致血虚,血虚也可导致气虚;气滞可导致血瘀,血瘀也可导致气滞;气滞则津液代谢障碍;血不足也可导致津液不足等。此类由气血津液关系失常所导致的病机变化,可参阅本书第二章第 4 节"气血津液之间的关系"。

Chapter 7 Prevention and Therapeutic Principles

第7章 预防与治则

The prevention and therapeutic principles in TCM are established upon the guide of the theories of yin-yang, five elements, qi, blood and body fluid, zang-fu organs, meridians and collaterals, etiology, pathogenesis, etc. As early as in Huang Di Nei Jing, it is advanced the theory of "treatment of the unformed disease", i. e. the important thought of preventive medicine. The theory of "search for the primary cause of disease in treatment" is the important therapeutic principle for diseases.

中医预防和治则,都是在阴阳五行、气血津液、脏腑经络、病因病机等理论指导下确立的。早在《黄帝内经》就提出"治未病"的理论,即是重要的预防医学思想。其提出"治病求本"的理论,即是重要的疾病治疗原则。

Section 1 Prevention

第1节 预防

The prevention implies that it is necessary to apply some measures for the purpose to prevent the occurrence and development of the diseases. The prevention in TCM is called "treatment of the unformed disease", including the thoughts of prevention and the methods of prevention.

预防,就是采取一定的措施,防止疾病的发生和发展。中医的预防原则,传统称为"治未病",包括预防思想和预防方法两方面内容。

1 Thoughts of prevention

The guiding thoughts of the preventive principles in TCM are as follows:

1 预防思想

中医预防原则的指导思想主要有以下三点。

1.1 Stress on the conception of entirety

The human body and the external environment form up a closely linked entirety, while the human body itself is also an organic entirety. Therefore, in the process of preventing the diseases, it is stressed on

1.1 强调整体观念

人体与外界环境是一个息息相关的整体,人体自身也是一个有机的整体,所以在预防疾病过程中既要重视

the coordinative relation between the human body and the environment, and also on the mutual relations among the zang-fu organs, meridians and collaterals, and body constituents, etc. inside the human body.

1.2　Stress on the Zheng (Anti-Pathogenic) Qi

The Zheng (Anti-Pathogenic) Qi concentrically reflects the anti-disease and recovery abilities of human body. In various types of preventive measures, it is the most basic and positive measure to protect and cultivate the Zheng (Anti-Pathogenic) Qi. Even when the Zheng (Anti-Pathogenic) Qi is sufficient and vigorous, can the human body not be attacked by the exogenous pathogens, and can the human body be easier to dispel the pathogens if it is sick. Therefore, it should be paid great attention to the life preservation in the preventive principles of TCM.

1.3　Stress on the integrity of body and mind

The health refers to not only the body health, but also the psychic health as well. The human's psychic and mental factors possess the important functions which cannot be underestimated in the occurrence of diseases. Therefore, the mental regulation and cultivation are placed as the top in various preventive measures according to the preventive principles in TCM.

2　Methods of prevention

2.1　Prevent the condition before disease occurrence

To prevent the condition before the disease occurrence implies that it is necessary to apply the preventive measures so as to avoid the occurrence of disease before the disease occurrence. Since the oc-

人体与环境的协调关系,又要重视人体脏腑经络形体之间的相互联系。

1.2　强调首重正气

正气集中体现于人体的抗病康复机能。在各种预防措施中,保护和培养正气是最根本、也是最积极的措施,只有正气强盛,人体才不易遭受外邪侵袭,一旦患病也容易祛邪外出。所以在中医预防原则中应特别重视养生。

1.3　强调身心合一

健康不仅是身体的健康,也包括心理的健康。人的心理精神因素在疾病发生中具有不可低估的重要作用,因此中医预防原则把精神调养放在各种预防措施的首位。

2　预防方法

2.1　未病先防

未病先防,就是在未病之前,先行预防,不使疾病发生。由于疾病的发生关系到正气不足和邪气侵袭两个方

currence of disease is related to two factors of the Zheng (Anti-Pathogenic) Qi insufficiency and the Xie (Pathogenic) Qi attack, it is necessary to start with these two aspects, i. e. to make the Zheng (Anti-Pathogenic) Qi not be deficient and to make the Xie (Pathogenic) not attack, so as to realize the purpose of prevention. In terms of the protection and cultivation of the Zheng (Anti-Pathogenic) Qi, it is advisable to apply the methods of the mind adaptability, the diet adaptability, life adaptability, exercise adaptability, etc. Besides, it is necessary to pay attention to the prevention of the Xie (Pathogenic) Qi attack.

2.1.1 Mind adaptability

To stress on the mind adaptability is possible to avoid the seven emotional factors from damaging the internal organs and disturbing qi and blood, to prevent the attack of the Xie (Pathogenic) Qi when the Zheng (Anti-Pathogenic) Qi deficiency which caused by the internal damage due to the emotional factors, and to protect and nourish the Zheng (Anti-Pathogenic) Qi for the purpose to strengthen the body constitution.

There are many methods of the mind adaptability, with the principles of purifying the heart and restrict passions, and being quiet in mind and indifferent to worldly gain. In the state of the spiritual quietness, qi and blood inside the human body are normally and orderly circulating, and qi of the heavenly and earthly yin and yang can connect and response to the human body. Not only the Xie (Pathogenic) Qi has no way to attack, but also the body constitution will be stronger and stronger.

面的因素,所以只要从这两方面着手,使正气不虚,或不让邪气侵入,就可达到预防的目的。从保护和培养正气方面来说,可以采取精神调养、饮食调养、起居调养及运动调养等方法。此外,还要注意避免病邪的侵袭。

2.1.1 精神调养

注重精神调养,可以避免七情损伤内脏及扰乱气血,可以防止因情志内伤而导致正虚邪入,可以护养正气而进一步增强体质。

精神调养的方法很多,其总的原则是要求人们清心寡欲、恬惔虚无。人体在精神宁静的状态下,气血不乱,运行有序,天地阴阳之气能与人体相通相应,不但邪气不得侵入,而且体质也会越来越强。

2.1.2　Diet adaptability

The diet adaptability acts to avoid the factors of over hunger, over fullness, unclean food intake, overindulgence in particular foods, etc. from damage and destroy the balance and coordination of zang-fu organs, qi and blood of human body, and also acts to make the human body gain the necessary nutrient substances from the food intake as well. Furthermore, the diet adaptability functions to reinforce and benefit the essence and qi, regulate yin and yang and improve the body constitution, so as to strengthen the anti-disease ability. There are many methods of the diet adaptability, which should be applied according to the different body constitutions. The general principles are to take the proper volume of food timely, to take the food with proper cold or warm property, to take both the coarse food and fine-prepared food, to pay attention to hygiene, to keep away from the bad diet habit and indulgence, etc.

2.1.3　Life adaptability

The life adaptability includes several aspects of the regular life habit, the moderate sexual activity, being properly dressed to adapt the climatic changes, the integration of strain and idleness, etc. The life adaptability, by complying with the changes of yin and yang in the nature, acts to protect the essence, qi, blood and body fluid of human body from being over consumed, thus the Xie (Pathogenic) Qi has no way to attack.

2.1.4　Exercise adaptability

The exercise adaptability functions to promote the circulation of qi and blood and enhance the functions of zang-fu organs of human body, and to

2.1.2　饮食调养

饮食调养的作用,主要是避免过饥过饱、饮食不洁、饮食偏嗜等因素损害和破坏人体脏腑、气血的平衡与协调,同时可从饮食获得人体所必需的营养物质。通过饮食调养,还可补益精气,调整阴阳,改善体质,进一步增强抗病能力。饮食调养的方法很多,应根据人的体质状况合理进行。其一般原则是,饮食应适时适量,寒温适宜,精粗搭配,讲究卫生,无不良饮食习惯及嗜好等。

2.1.3　起居调养

起居调养包括多方面内容,如作息应有规律,房事要有节制,衣着应适应时令气候变化,劳逸应当结合等。通过起居调养,可以顺应自然界阴阳变化,保护人体脏腑精气血津液而不使过分耗散,这样邪气就无侵入之机。

2.1.4　运动调养

运动调养,可以促进人体气血流通,增进脏腑功能,防止邪气留着而致病。古今

prevent the Xie (Pathogenic) Qi from retaining to cause the disease. There are many exercise methods in regime, as Five Animal Exercise, Eight Section Brocade Exercise, Tendon Changing Classic Exercise, Tai Chi Chuan Boxing, etc. These exercises are featured by the smooth and moderate movements and the association of activity and inertia, so as to function to guide the circulation of qi and blood and to regulate and adjust yin and yang, without damaging the tendons and bones and consuming qi and blood.

运动养生方法很多,如传统的五禽戏、八段锦、易筋经、太极拳等。其优点在于动作舒缓,动静结合,具有独到的导引气血、双调阴阳的功效,而无伤损筋骨、耗散气血的不良作用。

2.1.5　Prevention of the Xie (Pathogenic) Qi attack

Since the Xie (Pathogenic) Qi is the important condition to cause the disease, it is necessary to pay attention to the avoidance of the Xie (Pathogenic) Qi attack at the same time when the Zheng (Anti-Pathogenic) Qi is cultivated and nourished. But some pathogens are very poisonous, so the Zheng (Anti-Pathogenic) Qi is difficult to resist the attack even it is strong and sufficient. Only when the Xie (Pathogenic) Qi cannot attack, can the disease not occur.

2.1.5　避免邪侵

由于邪气是致病的重要条件,所以在培养正气的同时,也要注意避免被邪气所伤。有些病邪毒性很强,即使正气强盛,一般也难以抵御,只有不让邪气侵入,才能防止疾病的发生。

2.2　Prevent the development after disease occurrence

To prevent the development after the disease occurrence implies that it is necessary to apply the positive measures to block the transferring and mutating ways during the process of disease, so as to assist the improvement of disease. To prevent the development after the disease occurrence pertains to the principles of prevention in TCM, including two aspects of the diagnosis and treatment in early stage and the control of transference and mutation.

2.2　既病防变

既病防变,是指采取积极措施,阻断疾病过程中的传变途径,有助于疾病向愈。既病防变也属于中医预防原则的范畴,它包括早期治疗和控制传变两方面。

2. 2. 1 Diagnosis and treatment in early stage

In the early stage of the disease, the condition is mild and the Zheng (Anti-Pathogenic) Qi is not deficient, so it is easy to treat. If the treatment is improper, the Xie (Pathogenic) Qi enters from the exterior to the interior, and the condition is more severe. The Zheng (Anti-Pathogenic) Qi becomes consumed, so the treatment is more difficult. If the Zheng (Anti-Pathogenic) Qi is damaged seriously and the Xie (Pathogenic) Qi is becoming hyperactive gradually, the Xie (Pathogenic) Qi wins and the Zheng (Anti-Pathogenic) Qi declines, the treatment becomes troublesome, and the disease develops to the critical stage. Therefore, the diagnosis and treatment in early stage are an important therapeutic principle in TCM.

2. 2. 2 Control of transference and mutation

The transference and mutation implies that the disease may transfer and change in the different areas and layers of the exterior and the interior, the upper and the lower, the zang-fu organs, the meridians and collaterals, the Wei (Defense) Phase, Qi (Energy) Phase, Ying (Nutrient) Phase and Xue (Blood) Phase, etc. The certain regulation and way of transference and mutation can be found in various diseases. It is advisable to apply the apporpriately preventive measures according to the different regulation and way of transference and mutation, to prevent the transference and mutation of disease. It is another important part in the aspect to prevent the development after disease occurrence.

There are many different methods in the control of transference and mutation. It is necessary "to comfort the area which is not attacked", to en-

2. 2. 1 早期诊治

疾病初期,病情轻浅,正气未衰,比较易治。若治疗失时,病邪会由表入里,病情由轻变重,正气因此受到耗损,治疗也就由易变难。若正气耗损严重,邪气日益亢盛,以致邪胜正衰,不但治疗棘手,而且病情有向恶的危险。所以,早期诊治是中医学的一个重要原则。

2. 2. 2 控制传变

传变,是指疾病在表里、上下、脏腑、经络、卫气营血等不同部位或层次之间的传移变化。各种疾病的传变均有一定的规律和途径可循,根据其不同的传变规律和途径,采取相应的预防措施,不使疾病发生传变,是既病防变的又一重要内容。

控制传变的方法多种多样,如"先安未受邪之地",使可能被传变的脏腑正气转强

hance the Zheng (Anti-Pathogenic) Qi of the zang-fu organs which are possibly attacked, so as to prevent the attack of the Xie (Pathogenic) Qi. It is said in Jin Kui Yao Lüe that "if the liver is sick, it is known that the liver disease may transfers to the spleen, so it is necessary to strengthen the spleen first". It implies that it is to supplement the spleen qi to make the spleen qi sufficient and vigorous, so as to block the pathological progress in which the liver disease transfers to the spleen, for the purpose to control the transference and mutation of disease. In the febrile diseases, the pathogenic heat damages yin, first the stomach yin is injured, and later the kidney yin may be injured as well. In this condition, it is necessary to add the salty-cold herbs which nourish the kidney yin on the basic prescription of sweet-cold herbs which nourish the stomach yin, so as to prevent the pathogenic heat from attacking the kidney.

而不受邪。《金匮要略》就有"见肝之病，知肝传脾，当先实脾"之论，指出先充实脾气，令脾气得补而转旺，就可以切断其肝病传脾的病理进程，达到控制疾病传变的目的。又如温热病热邪伤阴，胃阴受损，进一步可耗伤肾阴，此时可在甘寒养胃之方中加入咸寒养肾阴的药物，防止热邪伤肾。

Section 2　Therapeutic Principles

第 2 节
治则

The therapeutic principles are established guided by the conception of holism and the treatment based upon pattern identification, possessing the general guiding significance to the establishment of therapeutic methods, prescription and application of herbs in the clinic.

The therapeutic principle is different from the therapeutic method, i. e. the former is the general principle to guide the therapeutic method, while the latter is the concrete application of the thera-

治则是在整体观念和辨证论治精神指导下制定的，对临床治疗立法、处方、用药，具有普遍指导意义。

治则与治法不同，治则是用以指导治疗方法的总则，治疗方法是治则的具体化。因此，任何治疗方法都

peutic principle. Therefore, any type of therapeutic method should pertain to a certain therapeutic principle.

The therapeutic principles introduced in this book include: ① search for the root of disease in treatment; ② strengthen Zheng (Anti-Pathogenic) Qi and eliminate Xie (Pathogenic) Qi; ③ regulate yin and yang; ④ treat disease according to climatic and seasonal conditions, geographical locations and individual conditions.

1　Search for the root of disease in treatment

The branch and root of the disease are the relevant concepts, including many implications and applied to illustrate the primary and secondary relation of various contradictions in the process of disease. In terms of the Xie (Pathogenic) Qi and Zheng (Anti-Pathogenic) Qi, the Zheng (Anti-Pathogenic) Qi is regarded as the root, while the Xie (Pathogenic) Qi as the branch. In terms of the etiology-pathogenesis and patterns-manifestations, the etiology and pathogenesis are regarded as the root, while the patterns and manifestations as the branch. In terms of the priority of the disease occurrence, the primary disease is regarded as the root, while the secondary disease as the branch. In terms of the acute disease and chronic disease, the chronic disease is regarded as the root, while the acute disease as the branch.

In the treatment of general diseases, it is not necessary to consider the priority of treatment of the branch or the root. It is always take the treatment of the root as the predominant way, even the treatment focuses on the etiology and pathogenesis

应从属于一定的治疗原则。

本书所要介绍的治疗原则,包括治病求本、扶正祛邪、调整阴阳、因人因地因时制宜等。

1　治病求本

疾病的标与本,是一个相对的概念,有多种含义,可用于说明病变过程中各种矛盾的主次关系。如从邪正而言,则正气为本,邪气为标;从病因病机与证候表现而言,则病因病机为本,证候表现为标;从疾病先后而言,原发病为本,继发病为标;从新病与旧病而言,旧病为本,新病为标。

在一般病证中,并不一定均存在着标本先后的问题,治病总是以治本为主,即针对疾病的病因病机进行治疗。但是,在复杂多变的病

of the disease. But in the treatment of some complicated and variable diseases or some critical stages of
the diseases, it is necessary to consider the treatment of the branch or the root in priority.

In the clinic application to "search for the root
of disease in treatment", it is necessary to master
two ways of "the routine treatment and contrary
routine treatment" and "the treatment of branch
and root".

1.1 Routine treatment and contrary routine treatment

The routine treatment and contrary routine
treatment are the concrete application of the therapeutic principle to "search for the root of disease in
treatment".

1.1.1 Routine treatment

The routine treatment is a kind of commonly-
used therapeutic principle to treat the disease
adverse to its property, so called "the adverse treatment". In this treatment, it is to apply the formulas
and herbs with the property opposite to that of the
disease, suitable for the treatment of the disease in
which the essence and appearance are compatible.
In most diseases, their essence and appearance are
compatible, truly reflecting the essence of the disease from the clinical manifestations, i.e. the manifestations of cold occurring in the cold pattern, the
manifestations of heat occurring in the heat pattern,
the manifestations of deficiency occurring in the deficiency pattern, and the manifestations of excess occurring in the excess pattern. Therefore, the routine
treatment is the mostly commonly-used in clinic.

(1) Heating method for cold: The cold implies
that the property of the disease is of cold, such as

证中,或在疾病的危重阶段,
就必须考虑治标治本的缓急
先后。

在临床运用治病求本这
一治疗法则时,必须正确掌
握"正治与反治""治标与治
本"两种情况。

1.1 正治与反治

正治与反治都是治病求
本这一治则的运用。

1.1.1 正治

正,有通常、常规之意。
正治,是逆其证候性质而治
的一种常用治疗法则,故又
称"逆治"。这一治则采用与
疾病证候性质相反的方药进
行治疗,适用于疾病的本质
与现象相一致的病证。临床
上绝大多数病证的本质与现
象是相一致的,临床表现真
实地反映出疾病本质,如寒
性病证出现寒象、热性病证
出现热象、虚证出现虚象、实
证出现实象。所以,正治在
临床上最为常用。

(1)寒者热之:寒,指证
候性质偏寒,如寒实、虚寒

the cold pattern of excess, the cold pattern of deficiency, etc. The heating method implies that the property of the therapeutic methods, formulas and herbs is of heat, such as the pungent-dispersing, the warming-reinforcing, etc. The heating method for cold implies that it is advisable to apply the warm-heat property formulas and herbs to treat the cold patterns.

(2) Cooling method for heat: The heat implies that the property of the disease is of heat, such as the heat pattern of excess, the heat pattern of deficiency, etc. The cooling method implies that the property of the therapeutic methods, formulas and herbs is of cold, such as the heat-reducing, yin-nourishing, etc. The cooling method for heat implies that it is advisable to apply the cold-cool property formulas and herbs to treat the heat patterns.

(3) Reinforcing method for deficiency: The deficiency implies that the property of the disease is of deficiency, such as the qi deficiency pattern, the blood deficiency pattern, etc. The reinforcing method implies that the property of the therapeutic methods, formulas and herbs is of reinforcing, such as the qi-reinforcing, the blood-reinforcing, etc. The reinforcing method for deficiency implies that it is advisable to apply the reinforcing action formulas and herbs to treat the deficiency patterns.

(4) Reducing method for excess: The excess implies that the property of the disease is of excess, such as the heat accumulation pattern, the blood stasis pattern, etc. The reducing method implies that the property of the therapeutic methods, formulas and herbs is of reducing, such as the heat-dispersing, the stasis-dissolving, etc. The reducing

等；热，指治法和方药性质偏热，如辛散、温补等。所谓寒者热之，即是用温热性质的方药来治疗寒性病证。

（2）热者寒之：热，指证候性质偏热，如实热、虚热等；寒，指治法和方药性质偏寒，如清热、滋阴等。所谓热者寒之，即是用寒凉性质的方药来治疗热性病证。

（3）虚则补之：虚，指证候性质偏虚，如气虚、血虚等；补，指治法和方药性质具有补虚作用，如补气、补血等。所谓虚者补之，即是用具有补益功用的方药来治疗虚证。

（4）实则泻之：实，指证候性质偏实，如热结、瘀血等；泻，指治法与方药性质具有祛邪作用，如泄热、化瘀等。所谓实则泻之，即是用具有祛邪功用的方药来治疗实证。

method for excess implies that it is advisable to apply the reducing action formulas and herbs to treat the excess patterns.

1.1.2 Contrary routine treatment

The contrary routine treatment is a kind of commonly-used therapeutic principle to treat the disease favorable to the false phenomena of the disease, so called "the favorable treatment". In this treatment, it is to apply the formulas and herbs with the property same as that of the false phenomena of the disease. Therefore, the contrary routine treatment is only suitable for the diseases in which the phenomena (clinical manifestations) do not comply with the essence (etiology and pathogenesis), as the patterns of the true cold with the false heat, the true heat with false cold, the true deficiency with false excess, the true excess with the false deficiency, etc.

(1) Heating method for heat: It is the method to apply the heat-property formulas and herbs to treat the diseases with the symptoms of false heat, as the disease in which the yin-cold is excessive internally and refuses yang from entering, leading to the diseases with the symptoms of false heat. The heating method for heat is only the representative concept, but actually it is the method to apply the warm-heat property herbs to treat the cold patterns. When the true cold is eliminated, the false heat disappears itself. For example, in the critical pattern of the deficiency-type yang floating outside, there are the manifestations of the false heat, as red complexion, superficial and big pulse, etc. It is necessary to apply the warm-heat property herbs to eliminate the true cold, and then the manifestations of

1.1.2 反治

反,与"正"相对,有反常、变异之意。反治,是顺从疾病假象而治的一种常用治疗法则,故又称"从治"。从,是言其所用方药的性质顺从疾病的假象。所以,反治只适用于疾病的征象(临床表现)与疾病的本质(如病因病机)不相一致的病证,如真寒假热、真热假寒、真虚假实、真实假虚等证。

(1) 热因热用:是用热性方药治疗具有假热症状的病证,适用于阴寒内盛,格阳于外,反见热象的一类疾病。可见,以热治热,仅是表面之象,而实际上还是用温热药物治疗寒性病症。真寒得除,假热自消。如虚阳外越的危重之证,可出现面色浮红、脉象浮大等假热症,必须用温热药物除其真寒,假热之象方能消除。从这一意义上看,"热因热用"的反治法,本质上还是属于"寒者热之"。

the false heat can be removed. From this sense, the contrary routine treatment of heating method for heat in essence pertains to "heating method for cold".

(2) Cooling method for cold: It is the method to apply the cold-property formulas and herbs to treat the disease with the symptoms of false cold, as the disease in which the pathogenic yang-heat is excessive internally and refuses yin from entering, leading to the diseases with the symptoms of false cold. The cooling method for cold is only the representative concept, but actually it is the method to apply the cold-cool property herbs to treat the heat patterns. When the true heat is eliminated, the false cold disappears itself. For example, in the extreme heat pattern, yang is excessive internally and refuses yin from entering, leading to the manifestations of the false cold, as chills in four limbs, alternately deep and superficial pulse, etc. It is necessary to apply the cold-cool property herbs to eliminate the true heat, and then the manifestations of the false cold can be removed. From this sense, the contrary routine treatment of cooling method for cold in essence pertains to "cooling method for heat".

(3) Blocking method for blocking: It is the method to apply the reinforcing formulas and herbs to treat the blocking diseases of deficiency type, i. e. the true deficiency pattern with false excess, such as stuffiness and fullness in chest and abdomen, retention of urine, constipation, scanty volume of blood in menstruation, amenorrhea, etc. caused by the deficiency of the Zheng (Anti-Pathogenic) Qi. In general conditions, the symptoms of blockage are

（2）寒因寒用：是用寒性方药治疗具有假寒症状的病证，适用于邪热极盛，阳盛格阴，热深厥深，反见假寒的一类疾病。可见，以寒治寒，仅是表面之象，而实际上还是用寒凉药物治疗热性病症。真热一清，假寒亦除。如热厥之证，阳盛于内，格阴于外，出现四肢厥冷，脉象沉浮，很似寒证，必须用寒凉药物清其真热，假寒之象方能消除。从这种意义上说，"寒因寒用"的反治法，本质上还是属于"热者寒之"。

（3）塞因塞用：是用补益方药治疗虚性闭塞不通的病证，适用于因正虚而致胸腹闷满、二便不通，或妇女经少，甚则闭经等闭阻不通的真虚假实证。在一般情况下，闭阻不通的证候常见于实证，多用通利之法治疗，但因虚致闭者亦不在少数，如

often seen in the excess patterns, so it is common to apply the dredging method to treat. But some blockage diseases are caused by the deficiency, as constipation caused by the yin-fluid insufficiency, amenorrhea caused by essence and blood deficiency, etc., and they are should be treated with "the reinforcing method for the purpose of dredging".

(4) Dredging method for dredging: It is the method to apply the dredging formulas and herbs to treat the over-discharge diseases of excess type, i. e. the true excess pattern with false deficiency, such as frequency of urination, frequency of defecation, abnormal uterine bleeding, etc. caused by the deficiency of the Zheng (Anti-Pathogenic) Qi. In general conditions, the symptoms of over-discharge are often seen in the deficiency patterns, so it is common to apply the reinforcing method to treat. But some over-discharge diseases are caused by the excess, as frequency and urgency of urination due to downward infusion of damp-heat in bladder, diarrhea and tenesmus due to damp-heat accumulation in large intestine, heavy blood flow in menstruation due to stagnant blood blocking uterus, etc., and they are should be treated with "the dredging method for dredging".

1.2   Treatment of branch and root

In the complicated and variable diseases, since there are the primary and secondary differences between the branch and root, there are the differences of the early and the later and of the moderate and the emergent. In general conditions, it is advisable to "search for the root of disease in treatment" in the clinical application of the treatment of branch and root. But in some conditions when the branch

阴液不足的便闭、精亏血少的闭经等，就应用"以补开塞"之法治疗。

（4）通因通用：是用通利方药治疗实性通泄不止的病证，适用于因邪实所致的二便频数、妇女崩漏等有下泄见症的真实假虚证。在通常情况下，通泄之症多见于虚证，故多用补益之法治疗。但临床上因实致通泄者也时有可见，其时就用"以通治通"之法治疗。如湿热下注膀胱，可见尿频尿急；湿热蕴结大肠，可见下利后重；瘀血阻滞胞宫，可见月经量多淋漓。凡见此等病证，多可以"通因通用"治之。

1.2   治标与治本

在复杂多变的病症中，常有标本主次的不同，因而在治疗上就应有先后缓急的区别。标本治法的临床应用，一般是"治病必求于本"。但在某些情况下，标病甚急，如不及时解决，可危及患者生命及影响疾病的治疗，则

disease is very emergent and critical, and will damage the patient's life and influence the treatment of disease, it is necessary to apply the principles of "the treatment of branch for emergent condition and the treatment of root for moderate condition", to treat the branch disease first, and the root disease later. If the branch and root diseases are same serious, it is advisable to consider both the branch and root, and to treat both the branch and root simultaneously.

1.2.1　Treatment of branch for emergent condition

　　In the clinic, the symptoms of severe bleeding, panting, loss of consciousness, mania, high fever, unceasing vomiting and diarrhea, severe pain, etc. pertain to the pattern of emergent branch, and they are critical to damage the patient's life, so it is advisable to apply "the treatment of branch for emergent condition", so as to relieve the critical symptoms first, and then to treat the root. For the mild and the severe and the moderate and emergent between the chronic disease and acute disease and between the primary disease and secondary disease, it is advisable to establish the therapeutic program according the principles of "the treatment of branch for emergent condition and the treatment of root for moderate condition". For example, in the patient with the chronic lung disease catches cold, it is advisable to apply the heat-reducing, lung-dispersing and phlegm-dissolving methods to treat the recently attacked disease, and then to treat the original disease after the exterior heat is relieved.

1.2.2　Treatment of root for moderate condition

　　The principle of "the treatment of root for

应采取"急则治其标,缓则治其本"的法则,先治其标病,后治本病。若标本并重,则应标本兼顾,标本同治。

1.2.1　急则治其标

　　临床上如出现大量出血、呼吸喘促、神昏狂乱、高热不退、吐泻不止、剧烈疼痛等均属标急之证,足以危及生命,均可采用"急则治其标"的方法,以缓解其危重的症状,然后再治其本。旧病与新病、原发病与继发病之间的轻重缓急,也可按"急则治其标,缓则治其本"的原则来确定治疗方案。如慢性肺部疾患患者复感外邪时,一般多先治以清热宣肺化痰等法以除新感,待表解热退之后,再治其宿疾。

1.2.2　缓则治其本

　　缓则治其本的治则,对

moderate condition" possesses the guiding significance in the treatment of the chronic diseases or the recovery stage of the acute diseases. For example, in pulmonary tuberculosis, the yin deficiency of lung and kidney or the deficiency of qi and yin is regarded as the root, while cough with bloody sputum, nocturnal sweats, etc. are as the branch. In the treatment, it is not advisable to apply the cough-stopping and sweat-stopping herbs, but advisable to apply the herbs to nourish and reinforce yin of lung and kidney, or to reinforce both qi and yin to treat the root. After the yin deficiency of lung and kidney or the deficiency of qi and yin is cured, the symptoms of cough with bloody sputum, nocturnal sweats, etc. will be relieved. For another example, in chronic edema, the pathogenesis is deficiency of spleen and kidney which fail to transport and transform the water. Edema is the symptom, the branch of the disease, so it is advisable to strengthen the spleen and warm the kidney so as to assist the transforming function, never possible to apply the attacking method to discharge the water.

1. 2. 3 Treatment of both branch and root

The treatment of both branch and root is a kind of therapeutic principle in the treatment when the branch disease and root disease are same serious and complicated, i. e. it is necessary to consider and treat both the branch disease and root disease simultaneously, without particular stress on any of them, for the purpose of gaining the better therapeutic effects. For example, in the person with weak body constitution catches cold, his qi-deficiency or blood-deficiency body constitution is regarded as the root, while catching cold as the branch. The attack of the

于慢性疾病或急性疾病的恢复期有着重要的指导意义。如肺痨咳嗽，一般多以肺肾阴虚、气阴两亏为其本，咳嗽、痰中带血、盗汗等为其标，故治疗多不主张选用强烈的止咳、敛汗之剂，而多采用滋补肺肾之阴，或气阴双补之法来治其本。肺肾之虚、气阴之亏恢复，则其咳嗽、痰血、盗汗等亦可随之缓解。他如慢性水肿，其病机多为脾肾两虚，气化失司。水肿是症状，是病之标，治疗宜以健脾温肾以助气化为主，而不可只图一时之快而滥用攻水消伐之品。

1. 2. 3 标本兼治

标本兼治是在标病与本病错杂并重时采取的一种治则。就是说，当单治本病不顾其标病，或单治标病不顾其本病，必须标本兼顾同治。这样，才能取得较好的治疗效果。例如虚人感冒，患者素体气虚或血虚为本，有反复外感为标，其外感病虽不重，但因其正虚无力抗邪，故外邪不易祛除。因此，必须

exogenous pathogens is not very severe, but the Zheng (Anti-Pathogenic) Qi is too deficient to resist against the pathogens to eliminate them. Therefore, it is necessary to apply the therapeutic methods to benefit qi and relieve the exterior, or to nourish the blood and relieve the exterior. Herein, the qi-benefiting method or the blood-nourishing method is to strengthen the Zheng (Anti-Pathogenic) Qi and to treat the root, while the exterior-relieving method is to eliminate the Xie (Pathogenic) Qi and to treat the branch. Such a treatment of both branch and root functions to strengthen the Zheng (Anti-Pathogenic) Qi and eliminate the Xie (Pathogenic) Qi so as to cure the disease.

2　Strengthen Zheng (Anit-Pathogenic) Qi and eliminate Xie (Pathogenic) Qi

The conflict between the Xie (Pathogenic) Qi and Zheng (Anti-Pathogenic) Qi runs through the whole process of disease. The wining or losing result of the conflict between the Xie (Pathogenic) Qi and Zheng (Anti-Pathogenic) Qi determines the development, transference and mutation of the disease. If the Zheng (Anti-Pathogenic) Qi wins and the Xie (Pathogenic) Qi is eliminated, the disease improves and becomes cured gradually. If the Xie (Pathogenic) Qi wins and the Zheng (Anti-Pathogenic) Qi is declined, the disease is worsened and even the death occur. In order to make the disease improved and cured, it is necessary to strengthen the Zheng (Anti-Pathogenic) Qi and eliminate the Xie (Pathogenic) Qi, so as to make the Zheng (Anti-Pathogenic) Qi to defeat the Xie (Pathogenic) Qi. Therefore, to strengthen the Zheng (Anti-Pathogenic) Qi and

采用益气解表、养血解表治法，益气、养血是扶正治本，解表是祛邪治标。这样标本同治，才能使正盛邪退而病愈。

2　扶正祛邪

疾病的过程始终贯穿着邪正相争，邪正相争的盛衰与胜负，决定着疾病的发展演变与转归。若正胜邪退，则疾病好转并逐渐痊愈；若邪胜正衰，则疾病恶化或归于死亡。为使疾病向好转、痊愈方向转化，就必须扶助正气，祛除邪气，促使正气战胜邪气。因此，扶正祛邪是指导临床治疗的一个重要原则。

eliminate the Xie (Pathogenic) Qi are the important principle to guide the clinc treatment.

2.1 Concept of strengthening the Zheng (Anti-Pathogenic) Qi and eliminating the Xie (Pathogenic) Qi

Strengthening the Zheng (Anti-Pathogenic) Qi refers to the method to support and assist the Zheng (Anti-Pathogenic) Qi, i. e. "the reinforcing method". In the reinforcing method, there are many measures, as herbal medicine, acupuncture and moxibustion, tuina-massage, diet regulation, qigong exercise, etc., all of which possess the reinforcing function. The reinforcing method is applied to treat the deficiency patterns, so it is said "the reinforcing method for the deficiency". All types of deficiency patterns, as qi deficiency, blood deficiency, yin deficiency, yang deficiency, body fluid insufficiency, kidney essence depletion, etc., can be treated by the reinforcing method. The therapeutic method of strengthening the Zheng (Anti-Pathogenic) Qi is able to correct the deficient condition, enhance the Zheng (Anti-Pathogenic) Qi, and increase the anti-disease ability, so as to assist the body to eliminate the Xie (Pathogenic) Qi. But it is not advisable to apply the reinforcing method in the treatment of the excess patterns due to the preponderance of the Xie (Pathogenic) Qi, because the reinforcing method makes the Xie (Pathogenic) Qi retaining inside the body, so that the Xie (Pathogenic) Qi cannot be eliminated.

Eliminating the Xie (Pathogenic) Qi refers to the method to remove the Xie (Pathogenic) Qi, i. e. "the reducing method" or "the attacking method". The reducing method is able to treat the excess

2.1 扶正祛邪的概念

所谓扶正，就是扶助正气，通常称为"补法"。补法有多种手段，如药物、针灸、推拿、饮食调理、气功锻炼等，都具有补益的功效。补法适用于虚证，故有"虚则补之"的理论。凡气虚、血虚、阴虚、阳虚、津液不足、肾精亏少等，都可用补法。通过扶正治法，可以纠正虚损，增强正气，提高抗病能力，从而有助于祛除邪气。但邪气亢盛的实证不宜用补法，因为补法易使邪气留恋于体内，不利于祛邪。

所谓祛邪，就是祛除邪气，通常称为"泻法"，也称"攻法"。泻法适用于实证，故有"实则泻之"的理论。凡

patterns, so it is said "the reducing method for the excess". All types of excess patterns, as attack of the exogenous pathogens, food retention, internal accumulation of phlegm-damp, internal retention of water, qi stagnation, excessive heat or hyperactive fire, accumulation of pathogenic cold, etc., can be treated by the reducing method. The therapeutic method to eliminating the Xie (Pathogenic) Qi is able to remove the Xie (Pathogenic) Qi, and stop the further damage of the Zheng (Anti-Pathogenic) Qi of human body by the Xie (Pathogenic) Qi, so as to assist the Zheng (Anti-Pathogenic) Qi to recover. But it is not advisable to apply the reducing method in the treatment of the deficiency patterns due to the weakness of the Zheng (Anti-Pathogenic) Qi, because the reducing method injures the Zheng (Anti-Pathogenic) Qi, so that the Zheng (Anti-Pathogenic) Qi cannot be recovered.

2.2 Application of strengthening the Zheng (Anti-Pathogenic) Qi and eliminating the Xie (Pathogenic) Qi

In the application of the principle of strengthening the Zheng (Anti-Pathogenic) Qi and eliminating the Xie (Pathogenic) Qi, it is necessary to carefully analyze the conditions of both the Xie (Pathogenic) Qi and Zheng (Anti-Pathogenic) Qi, identify the deficiency property from the excess property of the patterns and manifestations, and make a clear distinction between the primary and secondary relations of the Xie (Pathogenic) Qi excess and the Zheng (Anti-Pathogenic) Qi deficiency, so as to apply the different therapeutic methods accordingly. In the general conditions, the reinforcing method is applied for the pure deficiency pat-

有外邪侵袭、食积停滞、痰湿内蕴、水气内停、瘀血内阻、气机郁滞、热盛火旺、寒邪结滞等，都可用泻法。通过祛邪治法，可以祛除邪气，中止邪气对人体正气进一步的损害，从而有利于正气的恢复。但正气不足的虚证不能用泻法，因为泻法易损伤正气，不利于扶正。

2.2　扶正祛邪的运用

运用扶正祛邪的原则时，要仔细地分析邪正双方的情况，辨别证候的虚实性质，分清邪盛与正衰的主次关系，分别采用不同的治法。一般情况下，单纯虚证可以用扶正法，单纯实证可以用祛邪法，若属于正虚邪实相兼的虚实错杂证，则应扶正与祛邪并用。根据正虚与邪实的主次和缓急的不同，扶正与祛邪并用有三种不同的用法，即先攻后补、先补后攻

terns, while the reducing method for the pure excess patterns. As for the complicated patterns with both the Zheng (Anti-Pathogenic) Qi deficiency and the Xie (Pathogenic) Qi excess, it is advisable to apply both the methods of strengthening the Zheng (Anti-Pathogenic) Qi and eliminating the Xie (Pathogenic) Qi. According to the different conditions of the primary and the secondary, and the moderate and the emergent of the Zheng (Anti-Pathogenic) Qi deficiency and the Xie (Pathogenic) Qi excess, there are three methods of strengthening the Zheng (Anti-Pathogenic) Qi and eliminating the Xie (Pathogenic) Qi, i. e. attacking first and reinforcing later, reinforcing first and attacking later and simultaneous application of attacking and reinforcing.

2.2.1　Attacking first and reinforcing later

It is the method to eliminate the Xie (Pathogenic) Qi first and to strengthen the Zheng (Anti-Pathogenic) Qi later. In the complicated pattern of the Zheng (Anti-Pathogenic) Qi deficiency and the Xie (Pathogenic) Qi excess, if the Xie (Pathogenic) Qi is preponderant but the Zheng (Anti-Pathogenic) Qi is not so weak and tolerable to the attacking method, the method of attacking first and reinforcing later is applied. If strengthening the Zheng (Anti-Pathogenic) Qi is paid more attention, it is possible to assist the Xie (Pathogenic). Therefore, it is advisable to attack the Xie (Pathogenic) Qi first, and then to apply the reinforcing method after the Xie (Pathogenic) Qi is basically removed. For example, in metrorrhageia and metrostaxis due to stagnant blood, if the stagnant blood is not removed, bleeding cannot be stopped. It is necessary

和攻补兼施。

2.2.1　先攻后补

即先祛邪后扶正。在正虚邪实的虚实错杂证中,若邪气盛,急待祛邪,而正气虽虚,尚可耐攻;若兼顾扶正反会助邪,此时应先攻邪,待邪气大势已去,然后再用补法。如瘀血所致崩漏证,因瘀血不去,出血不止,虽然失血当补,但恐补血滋腻之药不利于祛瘀,出血不止则血虚难复,此时可先用活血化瘀,瘀血去而血能循经而行,血可自止,然后再用调经补血之法缓治其本。

to reinforce the blood for the blood loss as a rule,
but those reinforcing herbs are too sticky to dissolve
the stagnant blood. If bleeding cannot be stopped,
the blood deficiency condition will never be cured.
In such a condition, it is advisable to apply the
method to activate the blood and dissolve the stasis
first, and the method to regulate menstruation and
reinforcing blood later as the treatment of the root,
after the stagnant blood is dissolved to stop bleeding
and the blood can flow normally inside the meridians.

2.2.2 Reinforcing first and attacking later

It is the method to strengthen the Zheng (Anti-
Pathogenic) Qi first and eliminate the Xie (Pathogenic) Qi later. In the complicated pattern of the
Zheng (Anti-Pathogenic) Qi deficiency and the Xie
(Pathogenic) Qi excess, if the Xie (Pathogenic) Qi
is not too preponderant to be removed immediately,
but the Zheng (Anti-Pathogenic) Qi is too weak to
be tolerable to the attacking method, the method of
strengthening the Zheng (Anti-Pathogenic) Qi and
eliminating the Xie (Pathogenic) Qi is applied. If
the method of eliminating the Xie (Pathogenic) Qi
is applied too early, it is possible to damage the
Zheng (Anti-Pathogenic) Qi. Therefore, it is advisable to strengthen the Zheng (Anti-Pathogenic) Qi
first, and then to apply the attacking method after
the Zheng (Anti-Pathogenic) Qi is recovered and able
to to lerate the attacking method. For example, the
ascites due to pathogenic water retaining in the
abdomen, if the Zheng (Anti-Pathogenic) Qi is deficient and is not tolerable to the attacking herbs, it
is advisable to apply the method to strengthen the
Zheng (Anti-Pathogenic) Qi first, and the attacking

2.2.2 先补后攻

即先扶正后祛邪。适用
于正虚邪实的虚实错杂证,
此时虽有邪气当祛,但正气
虚衰较甚,不耐攻伐,若过早
地用攻法治疗,会更伤正气,
恐有正气不支之虞,所以应
先用补法扶正,使正气恢复
到能承受攻伐时再攻其邪。
如鼓胀病水邪盘踞腹中,而
正气虚衰日久,正气不耐峻
药攻逐,应先扶正,待正气稍
复后再用攻邪逐水之法,方
为稳妥。

method to dispel the retained water later after the Zheng (Anti-Pathogenic) Qi is somewhat recovered.

2.2.3 Simultaneous application of attacking and reinforcing

It is the method to strengthen the Zheng (Anti-Pathogenic) Qi and eliminate the Xie (Pathogenic) Qi simultaneously. In the complicated pattern of the Zheng (Anti-Pathogenic) Qi deficiency and the Xie (Pathogenic) Qi excess, if the single method to strengthen the Zheng (Anti-Pathogenic) Qi may cause the retention of the Xie (Pathogenic) Qi, or if the single method to eliminate the Xie (Pathogenic) Qi may damage the Zheng (Anti-Pathogenic) Qi, it is advisable to apply the simultaneous application of attacking and reinforcing. For example, in the treatment of common cold due to qi deficiency, it is advisable to apply the methods to reinforce qi and to relieve the exterior simultaneously.

3　Regulate yin and yang

It is believed in TCM that the basic cause of the disease is the disharmony of yin and yang. Therefore, the key to the treatment of disease is to regulate yin and yang, so as to bring back the equilibrium and harmony between yin and yang. The disharmony between yin and yang reflects the preponderance of yin or yang and the weakness of yin or yang, so the significance to regulate yin and yang is to decrease it for the surplus and to supplement it for the insufficiency, so as to correct the pathological state of preponderance or weakness, to realize the purpose to bring back the equilibrium and harmony between yin and yang.

2.2.3　攻补兼施

即扶正与祛邪兼用。适用于正虚邪实的虚实错杂证,若单用补则有恋邪之忧,单用攻又恐伤正,兼用则有相得益彰之利,此时应当攻补兼施。如气虚感冒,可用补气兼解表法治疗。

3　调整阴阳

中医学认为,疾病的根本原因是阴阳失调。因此,治疗疾病的关键在于调整阴阳,使之恢复阴阳平和状态。由于阴阳失调主要表现为阴阳偏盛和阴阳偏衰,所以调整阴阳的意义就在于,通过损其有余和补其不足,纠正偏盛和偏衰的病理状态,达到恢复阴阳平和的目的。

3.1　Decrease it for the surplus

To decrease it for the surplus is to decrease the preponderant state, to make the preponderant yin or yang to be back to the normal state. The preponderance of yin or yang causes the excess pattern, and the therapeutic method to treat the excess pattern is to "reduce", so the principle to "decrease it for the surplus" is also called "the reducing method for excess" in the therapeutics of TCM.

The preponderance is divided into the preponderance of yin and preponderance of yang, so the preponderance of yin causes the cold pattern of excess, while the preponderance of yang causes the heat pattern of excess. The therapeutic method for the cold pattern of excess is "the heating method for the cold", i. e. to apply the warm-heat property herbs to warm and dispel the yin-cold. The therapeutic method for the heat pattern of excess is "the cooling method for the heat", i. e. to apply the cold-cool property herbs to cool and reduce the yang-heat.

Since yin and yang are opposite, the preponderance of yin damages yang, while the preponderance of yang injures yin. Therefore, in the treatment of the patterns of yin or yang preponderance, it is necessary to pay attention to the injured party and properly to consider the treatment for the insufficiency, i. e. it is advisable to assist yang at the same time when warming and dispelling the yin-cold, and to nourish yin at the same time when cooling and reducing the yang-heat.

3.2　Supplement it for the insufficiency

To supplement it for the insufficiency is to supplement the weak state, to make the weak yin or

3.1　损其有余

损其有余,就是削弱其偏盛,使过于亢盛的阴或阳恢复到正常状态。由于阴阳偏盛所导致的证候性质为实证,治疗实证的大法为"泻",所以"损其有余"的原则在治疗学上也称"实则泻之"。

阴阳偏盛分为阴偏盛和阳偏盛,阴偏盛则形成实寒证,阳偏盛则形成实热证。针对实寒证,相应的治法是"寒者热之",即用温热药等以温散其阴寒;针对实热证,相应的治法是"热者寒之",即用寒凉药等以清泻其阳热。

由于阴阳是对立的,阴盛可以伤阳,阳盛可以伤阴,所以在治疗阴阳偏盛的病证时,应注意其相对一方受损伤的情况,必要时应当兼顾其不足,即在温散阴寒时兼顾扶阳,清泻阳热时兼顾滋阴。

3.2　补其不足

补其不足,就是补益其偏衰,使过于衰弱的阴或阳

yang to be back to the normal state. The weakness of yin or yang causes the deficiency pattern, and the therapeutic method to the deficiency pattern is to "reinforce", so the principle of "supplement it for the insufficiency" is also called "the reinforcing method for the deficiency" in the therapeutics of TCM.

The weakness is divided into the weakness of yin and weakness of yang, so the weakness of yin causes the heat pattern of deficiency, while the weakness of yang causes the cold pattern of deficiency. The therapeutic method for the heat pattern of deficiency is to nourish yin, i. e. to apply the nourishing-reinforcing herbs to nourish yin and reinforce blood. The therapeutic method for the cold pattern of deficiency is to reinforce yang, i. e. to apply the warming-reinforcing herbs to enhance yang and reinforce qi. Besides, one more thing should be paid attention to. In terms of the cold pattern of deficiency caused by the weakness of yang, it can be the water-rheum retention inside the human body due to deficiency of yang qi which fails to transform the water, it is not advisable to apply the attacking and reducing method to dissolve the water-rheum, but necessary to warm and reinforce the yang qi as the root. When the yang qi is inspired, its transforming function is normal, so the water-rheum can be dissolved, as it is said by the ancients that "the method to benefit the source of fire can dissolve the yin accumulation". In terms of the heat pattern of deficiency caused by the weakness of yin, it can be the internal production of the fire-heat due to deficiency of yin which fails to restrain yang. It is not advisable to apply the cooling

恢复到正常状态。由于阴阳偏衰所导致的证候性质为虚证,治疗虚证的大法为"补",所以"补其不足"的原则在治疗学上也称"虚则补之"。

阴阳偏衰分为阴偏衰和阳偏衰,阴偏衰则形成虚热证,阳偏衰则形成虚寒证。针对虚热证,相应的治法是补阴,即用滋补药等以滋阴补血;针对虚寒证,相应的治法是补阳,即用温补药等以壮阳补气。特别需要注意的是,阳偏衰的虚寒证,可因阳虚气化无力而导致水饮等在体内滞留,此时不可妄用攻泻法以图祛除水饮,而应从根本上温补阳气,阳气一旦振兴,气化流通,其水饮自然消散,所以古人有"益火之源,以消阴翳"的说法;阴偏衰的虚热证,可因阴虚不能制阳而出现火热内生,此时不可妄用清泻法以图祛除火热,而应从根本上填补阴精,阴精一旦充满,阴阳调和,阳得以潜藏,其火热自然平息,所以古人有"壮水之主,以制阳光"的理论。

and reducing method to dispel the fire-heat, but necessary to supplement and reinforce the yin essence as the root. When the yin essence is full and sufficient, yin and yang becomes harmonious, so yang can be restrained by yin and the fire-heat can be diminished. As it is said by the ancients that "the method to strengthen the dominator of water can restrain the yang brightness".

Furthermore, yin and yang are mutually rooted, so the weakness of yin may involve yang to cause yang deficiency, while the weakness of yang may involve yin to cause yin deficiency. As a result, both yin and yang become deficient, so it is advisable to reinforce both yin and yang for such a condition. In the treatment of the pure yin deficiency pattern, it is advisable to add some yang-reinforcing herbs in the yin-nourishing prescription, so that the transforming function of yang may assist the yin essence to be transformed and produced. This is called "to search for yin from yang". In the treatment of the pure yang deficiency, it is advisable to add some yin-nourishing herbs in the yang-reinforcing prescription, so that the moisturizing and nourishing function of the yin essence may assist yang to be transformed and produced. This is called "to search for yang from yin".

Since there are the yin-yang attributions and mutual relations in the meridians and collaterals, between qi and blood, between zang and fu organs, between up-flow and down-flow movements of qi, between outflow and inflow movements of qi, etc., the therapeutic principle to "regulate yin and yang" can be specified into the appropriately therapeutic methods, such as to recuperate meridians and collat-

此外,由于阴阳是互根的,阴偏衰可以累及阳而导致阳衰,阳偏衰也可累及阴而导致阴衰,最终使阴阳俱衰,治疗时应阴阳并补。对于单纯的阴虚证,在滋阴方中可适当佐以补阳药,借阳的气化功能以帮助阴精的化生,这叫做"阳中求阴";对于单纯的阳虚证,在补阳方中可适当佐以滋阴药,借阴精的涵养功能以帮助阳的化生,这叫做"阴中求阳"。

由于经络、气血、脏腑、升降出入等都具有各自的阴阳属性及其相互关系,所以"调整阴阳"的治疗原则也可以用来概括其他相关的治疗方法。如调理经络失常、调理气血失常、调理脏腑失常、调理升降出入失常等等,都

erals from abnormality, to recuperate qi and blood from abnormality, to recuperate zang-fu organs from abnormality, to recuperate up-flow, down-flow, out-flow and inflow from abnormality, etc., all of which pertain to the scope to "regulate yin and yang".

4　Treat disease according to individual conditions, geographical locations and climatic and seasonal conditions

The occurrence, development, transference and improvement of the disease are influenced by many different factors, such as the individual differences, geographical and environment conditions, seasonal and climatic conditions, etc., all of which are the important factors influencing the property, seriousness and reaction to the treatment of the disease. Therefore, it is necessary to treat the disease according to the individual conditions, geographical locations and climatic and seasonal conditions.

4.1　Treat disease according to individual conditions

It is necessary to consider the principle of prescribing herbs according to the patient's age, gender, body constitution and life habit in the treatment of disease.

4.1.1　Age

The physiological functions of human body and the volume of qi and blood vary along with the change of the age, so the herbal prescriptions are different. As to a child, whose body is vigorous, but whose qi and blood are not full and sufficient, whose zang-fu organs are tender and delicate, he is easily attacked by pathogenic cold or heat, so his condition is often of deficiency or excess, with rapid

可归属于"调整阴阳"的范畴。

4　因人、因地、因时制宜

疾病的发生、发展与转归,受多方面因素的影响,如个体差异、地域环境、时令气候等,都是影响疾病性质、程度及对治疗的反应性的重要因素。因此在治疗时,还应根据不同情况,因人、因地、因时制宜。

4.1　因人制宜

因人制宜,是根据病人的年龄、性别、体质和生活习惯的不同特点,来考虑治疗用药的原则。

4.1.1　年龄

人体的生理功能和气血的盛衰,随着年龄的变化而有不同,治疗用药也应有区别。一般地说,小儿生机旺盛,但气血未充,脏腑娇嫩,易寒易热,易虚易实,病情变化较快,故治小儿病,忌用峻攻,少用补益,用药量宜轻,

changes. Therefore, in the treatment of the child's disease, it is not advisable to apply the attacking method and to apply the moderately reinforcing method, with the prescription and herbs of low dose. As to an old person, whose body is declining, whose qi and blood are getting deficient, he is easily diseased by the deficiency pattern or the excess pattern in which the weak body constitution should be considered, so it should be highly careful to apply the pathogen-attacking method. Due to the deficiency of qi and blood in the old people, his response to the herbs decreases, therefore, it is advisable to apply the herbs of higher dose by applying the reinforcing method to treat the old person's deficiency pattern for a longer period of time.

4.1.2 Gender

　　Man and women are different in physiology. Women have the different conditions of menstruation, leucorrhea, pregnancy, delivery, etc. from men, it should be considered in the treatment. For example, during menstruation, it is not advisable to apply the cold-cool property herbs and astringing herbs which will block the menstrual flow. In the period just after menstruation, the blood and vessels are deficient, so it is advisable to apply more reinforcing methods than reducing methods. During pregnancy, it is necessary to protect the fetus, and not advisable to apply the purging herbs, the blood-breaking herbs, the lubricating herbs, the fleeing herbs, or the poisonous herbs, which may damage the fetus. In the period just after delivery, qi and blood are deficient, so it is advisable to apply more reinforcing methods than reducing methods. Simultaneously, it is necessary to consider the lochia dis-

剂型及服药方法也应考虑小儿的特点；老年人生机减退，气血渐衰，患病多虚，即使是实证也应考虑其体质偏虚的一面，用攻邪法要慎重，但老年人气血虚衰后对药物的反应性也降低，因此老年虚证用补益法往往需要更大的剂量和较长的疗程。

4.1.2 性别

　　男女性别不同，各有其生理特点。如女子有经、带、胎、产等情况，有别于男子，治疗时应加以考虑。如在月经期，用药不应有碍经血运行，一般忌过用寒凉收涩药；经期后血去脉虚，宜多补少泻。妊娠期需注意护胎，凡峻下、破血、滑利、走窜伤胎或有毒药物，当禁用或慎用。产后大多气血亏虚，应多补少泻，但同时应兼顾恶露的排出情形，若恶露未净，一般宜用温补疏通之剂，不宜用凉补敛涩之剂，以免留瘀不去。由于女子以肝为先天，肝气易郁，故治疗妇科病常需疏理肝气。

charge, advisable to apply the warming-reinforcing herbs and dredging herbs rather than the cooling-reinforcing herbs and astringing herbs if the lochia is not discharge smoothly, so as to avoid the lochia retention. Furthermore, since the liver is regarded as the congenital basis in women, the liver qi is easily stagnated, so it is advisable to soothe the liver and promote qi flow for the treatment of women's diseases.

4.1.3 Body constitution

There are different types of body constitution, so the treatment and herbs are different accordingly. Generally speaking, as to the person with strong body constitution which is tolerable to attacking method but intolerable to reinforcing method, it is advisable to apply the attacking herbs with higher dose and the reinforcing herbs with lower dose. As to the person with weak body constitution which is tolerable to reinforcing method but intolerable to attacking herbs, it is advisable to apply the attacking herbs with lower dose and the reinforcing herbs with higher dose. As to the person with the body constitution of yang excess or yin deficiency, it should be highly cautious in applying the warm-heat property herbs, because the over-dose of such herbs may assist the fire or consume yin. As to the person with the body constitution of yang deficiency or yin excess, it should be highly cautious in applying the cold-cool property herbs, because the over-dose of such herbs may damage yang qi or assist the damp to produce phlegm.

4.1.4 Life habit

The different life habits will cause different influences on the body constitution, it should be con-

4.1.3 体质

人的体质有不同的类型,对于不同类型的体质,治疗用药应有不同。一般来说,体质强者耐攻伐而不耐补益,故用攻邪法药量可大,而用补益法不宜过量;体质弱者耐补益而不耐攻伐,故用攻邪法药量宜小,而用补益法药量可大。素体阳盛或阴虚之人,慎用温热之剂,若过量则有助火或伤阴之虞;素体阳虚或阴盛之人,慎用寒凉之剂,以防损伤阳气或助湿生痰。

4.1.4 生活习惯

生活习惯不同,对体质的影响也不同,治疗时必须

sidered in the treatment. For example, alcohol drinking for long period of time may cause liver yin insufficiency or phlegm-damp blocking spleen, overindulgence of particular foods for long period of time may cause qi and blood deficiency or yin and yang disharmony, lack of physical exercises may cause functional decrease of zang-fu organs or slow circulation of qi and blood, etc. The people from different regions, different countries and different races have their different life habits. The differences in the life habits may deduce their body constitutions, as the important reference in the diagnosis and treatment.

4.2 Treat disease according to geographical locations

It is necessary to consider the principles to prescribe herbs according to the different features of the different geographical locations.

In different areas, due to the differences in height above sea level, in the climatic conditions and in the life habits, the human body will be relevantly differences physiologically and pathologically, so the treatment and herbs should be different according to the local geographical locations and life habits. For example, in the plateau of northwest China, it is cold and dry with a little amount of rain. People there live in the mountain area and prefer intake of dairy products and meats, and the body is strong and the skin is fine and close, so the exogenous pathogens are not easy to attack. If attacked by the exogenous pathogens, it is advisable to apply the dispersing method with the exterior-relieving herbs of heavy dose. In the coastal area of southeast China, the land is low-lying, and it is

加以注意。如一贯嗜酒，往往肝阴不足与痰湿困脾；长期偏食，易致气血偏衰或阴阳不和；运动不足，往往脏腑功能减退，气血运行迟缓等。不同地区、不同国家、不同民族的人，其生活习惯上的差异更大，从这些生活习惯的差异可以推断其体质的倾向，作为治疗时的重要参考。

4.2 因地制宜

因地制宜，是根据不同地区的地理特点，来考虑治疗用药的原则。

不同地区，由于地势的高低，以及气候条件与生活习惯的不尽相同，人体生理功能特点和病变特点也有相应的差异，所以治疗用药应根据当地环境和生活习惯而有所变化。如中国西北高原地区，气候寒冷，干燥少雨，人们依山陵而居，多食乳酪及肉类，故体质壮实，腠理致密，外邪不易侵犯，若感受外邪需用发散法治疗，当用解表重剂；东南沿海地区，地势低洼，温热多雨，人们傍水而居，多食鱼米，故体质较弱，腠理疏松，易受外邪侵袭，若

warm and humid with large volume of rain. People there live beside the water and prefer intake of sea foods and rice, and the body is weak and the skin is loose, so the exogenous pathogens are easy to attack them. If attacked by the exogenous pathogens, it is advisable to apply the dispersing method with the exterior-relieving herbs of light dose.

4.3 Treat disease according to climatic and seasonal conditions

It is necessary to consider the principle to prescribe herbs according to the different features in the different climatic and seasonal conditions.

The climatic changes in the four seasons may influence the physiological functions and pathological changes of the human body, so it is necessary to consider the application of herbs according to these features of the climatic changes. Generally speaking, in spring and summer, yang qi ascends and increases, the skin of human body is loose and open, so the exogenous pathogenic wind and cold are easy to attack the body. In the treatment, it is not advisable to apply the over-dose pungent-warm herbs and dispersing herbs, so as to avoid over opening and dispersing to damage and consume qi and yin. In autumn and winter, it is cool and changes to cold with yin excess and yang deficiency, the skin of human body is fine and close, so the yang qi is stored and kept inside. In the treatment, it is not advisable to apply the cold-cool property herbs so as to avoid the damage of yang, except for the severe heat pattern. It is said in Huang Di Nei Jing that "herbs heat-property are applied avoiding warm seasons" and "herbs cold-property are applied avoiding cold seasons", to illustrate the therapeutic principles of

感受外邪需用发散法治疗,当用解表轻剂。

4.3 因时制宜

因时制宜,是根据时令气候的不同特点,来考虑治疗用药的原则。

四时气候的变化,对人体的生理功能、病理变化均能产生一定的影响,因此在治疗上应根据这种气候变化的特点来考虑用药。一般来说,春夏季节,气候由温渐热,阳气升发,人体腠理疏松开泄,即使患外感风寒,也不宜过用辛温发散药物,以免开泄太过,耗伤气阴;而秋冬季节,气候由凉变寒,阴盛阳衰,人体腠理致密,阳气内敛,此时若非大热之证,当慎用寒凉药物,以防伤阳。《黄帝内经》把这种夏季慎用热药、冬季慎用寒药的治疗法则归纳为"用热远热""用寒远寒"。

careful application of herbs heat-property in summer and herbs cold-property in winter.

12 Earthly Branch (EB) 十二地支

Zi	子	The First Earthly Branch (EB 1)
Chou	丑	The Second Earthly Branch (EB 2)
Yin	寅	The Third Earthly Branch (EB 3)
Mao	卯	The Fourth Earthly Branch (EB 4)
Chen	辰	The Fifth Earthly Branch (EB 5)
Si	巳	The Sixth Earthly Branch (EB 6)
Wu	午	The Seventh Earthly Branch (EB 7)
Wei	未	The Eighth Earthly Branch (EB 8)
Shen	申	The Ninth Earthly Branch (EB 9)
You	酉	The Tenth Earthly Branch (EB 10)
Xu	戌	The Elventh Earthly Branch (EB 11)
Hai	亥	The Twelfth Earthly Branch (EB 12)

Shanghai Pujiang Education Press(Shanghai University of Traditional Chinese Medicine Press)

1550 Haigang Haigang Ave, Shanghai, P. R. China 201306

All righrs reserved. No part of this book may be reproduced, stored in a retrieval system, or transmitted in any form or by means, electronic, mechanical, photocopying, recording or otherwise, without the prior permission in writing of the Publisher.

图书在版编目(CIP)数据

中医基础理论/李其忠主编. —上海：上海浦江教育出版社
有限公司,2017.8
((英汉对照)精编实用中医文库/陈凯先,李其忠,何星海主编)
ISBN 978-7-81121-512-0

Ⅰ.①中… Ⅱ.①李… Ⅲ.①中医医学基础—英、汉 Ⅳ.①R22

中国版本图书馆 CIP 数据核字(2017)第174502号

上海浦江教育出版社出版

社址：上海海港大道 1550 号上海海事大学校内　　邮政编码：201306
分社：上海蔡伦路 1200 号上海中医药大学内　　邮政编码：201203
电话：(021)38284910(12)(发行)　38284923(总编室)　38284916(传真)
E-mail: cbs@shmtu. edu. cn　　URL: http://www. pujiangpress. cn
上海盛通时代印刷有限公司印装　上海浦江教育出版社发行
幅面尺寸：170 mm×240 mm　印张：19.5　字数：371 千字
2017 年 8 月第 1 版　2017 年 8 月第 1 次印刷
责任编辑：黄　健　封面设计：赵宏义
定价：88.00 元